# Cardiology
## A Practical Handbook

**David Laflamme**

# Cardiology
## A Practical
## Handbook

Foreword by Dr Paul Dorian

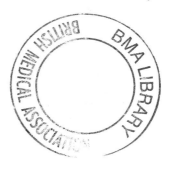

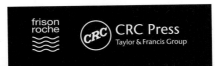

frison roche

**CRC Press**
Taylor & Francis Group

## From the same publisher

Prescription guidelines in cardiology, R. Haïat, G. Leroy, 5<sup>th</sup> edition, 2015
**www.cardio-log.com**

## Cover illustrations

*HeartWare HVAD,* ventricular assist device, HeartWare International,
Framingham, MA, USA (with permission)

*EnSite NavX Navigation & Visualization Technology,* St. Jude Medical,
St. Paul, MN, USA (with permission)

*Edwards SAPIEN XT* transcatheter heart valve, Edwards Lifesciences LLC,
Irvine, CA, USA (with permission)

## Artistic direction and graphic design

Julie Laflamme

© Copyright

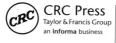 frison-roche    19 rue des Lyanes, 75020 Paris, 2016
**infos@editions-frison-roche.com / www.editions-frison-roche.com**

ISBN 978-2-87671-585-1

**CRC Press**
Taylor & Francis Group
an **informa** business

6000 Broken Sound Parkway, NW
Suite 300, Boca Raton, FL 33487
711 Third Avenue
New York, NY 10017
2 Park Square, Milton Park
Abingdon, Oxon OX14 4RN, UK

ISBN 978-1-4987-7981-4

There has been a near exponential increase in the amount of information available on the pathophysiology and management of heart diseases over the past decades. Meanwhile, our understanding of the underlying pathology and physiology has deepened and broadened with new methodologies to monitor cardiac structure and function. These developments have led to an overwhelming amount of information available to students, trainees, and physicians on all aspects of cardiac disease. What is in short supply is a comprehensive yet concise and clear description of the important cardiac conditions and disorders, an approach to their management, and an easily consulted and well indexed summary to be used at the bedside or in the clinic.

The Cardiology Handbook fills an extremely important, not well occupied niche in providing junior and senior practitioners alike with a brief yet detailed summary of "what you need to know" about virtually all important cardiovascular conditions.

This handbook does not aim to be a comprehensive review of all of the evidence pertaining to pathophysiology, investigation, and treatment of cardiovascular disorders. It does however wonderfully clearly get "straight to the point" and I think will be a frequently used and extremely effective resource for a brief "look up" in the clinic, in the emergency room, and on the wards.

I anticipate this handbook will be a treasured resource for senior medical students, trainees in internal medicine, emergency medicine, anesthesia, and other specialties where cardiovascular disorders are commonly seen. The effective use of figures and tables makes this appealing both visually and cognitively, and for those unfamiliar with the complex and varied terrain of cardiovascular medicine, will prove an outstanding trail map to allow successful navigation of unfamiliar terrain. In an era where there is often "too much information", this handbook provides just the right amount.

Sincerely,

*Paul Dorian*

**Paul Dorian**, MD, FRCPC, FHRS
Dexter H.C. Man Chair in Cardiology
Director Division of Cardiology, University of Toronto
Past President, Canadian Heart Rhythm Society

# Table of contents

## 01 | CARDIAC DIAGNOSTIC ASSESSMENT

**1.1/** Cardiac physical examination ............2
**1.2/** Electrocardiogram (ECG) ................8
**1.3/** Stress test ..................................22
**1.4/** Transthoracic echocardiography (TTE)..27
**1.5/** Transesophageal echocardiography (TEE) ................................................39
**1.6/** Stress echocardiography ..................43
**1.7/** Chest x-ray (CXR) ........................45
**1.8/** Coronary angiography......................48
**1.9/** Hemodynamic assessment ..............53
**1.10/** Cardiac nuclear medicine ..............60
**1.11/** Cardiac magnetic resonance imaging (cardiac MRI) ..............................63
**1.12/** Cardiac CT scan ..........................65
**1.13/** Cardiopulmonary exercise testing ......66
**1.14/** Exposure to radiation during cardiac examinations ................................67

## 02 | CORONARY ARTERY DISEASE (CAD) & MYOCARDIAL INFARCTION

**2.1/** Stable angina ..............................72
**2.2/** Biomarkers..................................80
**2.3/** Myocardial infarction: Definition..........81
**2.4/** Unstable angina & NSTEMI ..............83
**2.5/** STEMI ........................................88
**2.6/** Acute coronary syndrome: Adjuvant treatments................................95
**2.7/** Complications of myocardial infarction ................................98
**2.8/** Revascularization – PCI ................103
**2.9/** Revascularization – Coronary artery bypass graft ..........................106
**2.10/** Prinzmetal angina (vasospastic angina) ..................................108
**2.11/** Cardiac syndrome X........................108

## 03 | HEART FAILURE

**3.1/** Heart failure: assessment ..............112
**3.2/** Systolic heart failure: management ...115
**3.3/** Diastolic heart failure (preserved LVEF) ..................................123
**3.4/** Decompensated heart failure............125
**3.5/** Heart transplantation ..................130
**3.6/** Long-term ventricular assist device ..................................133
**3.7/** Right heart failure ........................136
**3.8/** Palliative care ............................136

## 04 | VALVULAR HEART DISEASE

**4.1/** Aortic stenosis............................140
**4.2/** Chronic aortic regurgitation ............145
**4.3/** Acute aortic regurgitation ............148
**4.4/** Mitral stenosis............................148
**4.5/** Chronic mitral regurgitation ............151
**4.6/** Acute mitral regurgitation ............155
**4.7/** Tricuspid stenosis ........................156
**4.8/** Tricuspid regurgitation ..................156
**4.9/** Pulmonary stenosis ......................157
**4.10/** Pulmonary regurgitation ..............157
**4.11/** Multivalvular heart disease ............158
**4.12/** Valvular prostheses......................158
**4.13/** Infective endocarditis....................160
**4.14/** Cardiovascular implantable electronic device infection ..........167
**4.15/** Rheumatic fever ..........................168

## 05 | DISEASES OF THE PERICARDIUM & MYOCARDIUM

**5.1/** Diseases of the pericardium: etiologies..................................172
**5.2/** Acute pericarditis ........................173
**5.3/** Incessant and recurrent pericarditis..174
**5.4/** Cardiac tamponade........................174
**5.5/** Constrictive pericarditis ................177
**5.6/** Congenital anomalies of the pericardium ..............................179
**5.7/** Cardiomyopathies - Classification .....179
**5.8/** Hypertrophic cardiomyopathy ..........181
**5.9/** Dilated cardiomyopathy ................184
**5.10/** Restrictive cardiomyopathy..............184
**5.11/** Cardiac amyloidosis ....................187
**5.12/** Arrhythmogenic right ventricular dysplasia (ARVD) ..................188
**5.13/** Isolated left ventricular noncompaction ........................190
**5.14/** Takotsubo (stress) cardiomyopathy ...191
**5.15/** Myocarditis................................191
**5.16/** Indications for endomyocardial biopsy..................................193
**5.17/** Cardiac tumors............................194
**5.18/** Cardiac complications of cancer .......196

# Table of contents

## 06 ARRHYTHMIAS

**6.1/** Physiology .................................200
**6.2/** Bradyarrhythmias ......................201
**6.3/** Supraventricular tachyarrhythmias ...204
**6.4/** Atrial fibrillation .......................210
**6.5/** Ventricular tachyarrhythmias ...........219
**6.6/** Channelopathies ......................224
**6.7/** Syncope .................................227
**6.8/** Antiarrhythmic drugs (AAD) .........229
**6.9/** Amiodarone ............................232
**6.10/** Permanent pacemaker (PPM)...........233
**6.11/** Cardiac resynchronization therapy (CRT) .................................239
**6.12/** Implantable cardioverter-defibrillator (ICD) .................................241

## 07 ADULT CONGENITAL HEART DISEASE & HEART DISEASE IN PREGNANT WOMEN

**7.1/** Segmental assessment & fetal circulation .........................248
**7.2/** Atrial septal defect (ASD) .................248
**7.3/** Patent foramen ovale (PFO).............250
**7.4/** Ventricular septal defect (VSD).........250
**7.5/** Atrioventricular canal defect .........251
**7.6/** Patent ductus arteriosus .................252
**7.7/** Left ventricular outflow tract obstruction .........................253
**7.8/** Coarctation of the aorta (CoA) .........254
**7.9/** Right ventricular outflow tract obstruction .........................256
**7.10/** Tetralogy of Fallot (TOF) .................257
**7.11/** Transposition of the great arteries (D-TGV)...............................259
**7.12/** Congenitally corrected Transposition of the great arteries (L-TGV)...............261
**7.13/** Ebstein's anomaly.........................262
**7.14/** Marfan syndrome .........................263
**7.15/** Fontan procedure .........................265
**7.16/** Eisenmenger syndrome .................266
**7.17/** Cyanotic heart disease.....................267
**7.18/** Anomalous pulmonary venous connection.........................268
**7.19/** Congenital coronary artery anomalies .........................268
**7.20/** Vascular annulus .........................269
**7.21/** Cor triatriatum .........................270
**7.22/** Heart disease in pregnant women.....270

## 08 PERIPHERAL VASCULAR DISEASE

**8.1/** Aneurysm of the thoracic aorta.........276
**8.2/** Acute aortic syndrome .....................279
**8.3/** Abdominal aortic aneurysm (AAA).....282
**8.4/** Other aortic diseases .....................283
**8.5/** Peripheral artery disease (PAD).........285
**8.6/** Atherosclerotic renovascular disease.................................289
**8.7/** Cerebrovascular disease.................290
**8.8/** Pulmonary embolism .....................295
**8.9/** Heparin-induced thrombocytopenia (HIT)...................300
**8.10/** Pulmonary hypertension .................301

## 09 MISCELLANEOUS

**9.1/** Preoperative assessment (non cardiac surgery).......................310
**9.2/** Primary & secondary prevention of cardiovascular disease .................314
**9.3/** Smoking cessation .........................315
**9.4/** Dyslipidemia.............................316
**9.5/** Hypertension .............................323
**9.6/** Diabetes .................................329
**9.7/** Physical activity .........................333
**9.8/** Weight & Diet .........................336
**9.9/** Obstructive sleep apnea syndrome ...338
**9.10/** Driving & Air travel.........................339
**9.11/** Cardiovascular complications of systemic diseases .......................341
**9.12/** Cardiovascular complications of trauma .............................343
**9.13/** Poisoning.................................344
**9.14/** Swan-Ganz catheter placement........346
**9.15/** Cardiopulmonary resuscitation.........347

## ABBREVIATIONS                353

## ★ CLINICAL TRIALS CITED       359

## INDEX                          363

*To my parents, Diane and Marcel,*
*for their constant support,*
*and to Anne-Sophie, for*
*her extraordinary patience.*

Cardiology is a fascinating medical specialty. This vast discipline combines various fields of expertise, including research, prevention, clinical evaluation, diagnostic examinations, therapeutic management, invasive interventions and rehabilitation.

As a result of the spectacular progress over the last two decades, cardiology now comprises sophisticated and advanced diagnostic and therapeutic tools (validated by evidence-based medicine) allowing cardiologists to more effectively manage their patients, who have greatly benefited in terms of survival and/or quality of life.

In relation to such an effervescent and increasingly complex discipline, physicians who have the privilege to practice cardiology must have access to resources that enable them to acquire, update, refine and organize their knowledge.

The purpose of this book is to provide a concise overview of modern cardiology. More than 10,000 pages of references have been condensed and organized into less than 350 pages. This pocket book provides practising clinicians with specific and accurate information on a particular subject. It is also designed to allow students, interns and all other personnel working in the field of cardiology to acquire and organize their valuable knowledge.

The design of this cardiology handbook was a captivating but colossal task. The information presented in this book is derived from numerous valid and up-to-date sources and has been verified by various reviewers, experts in their respective fields. The various recommendations are also derived from American, European or Canadian learned society evidence-based guidelines.

I sincerely hope that this book will inspire or maintain your passion for cardiology and I wish you an enjoyable read.

**David Laflamme**, MD, FRCPC, Cardiologist
Hôpital Charles-LeMoyne, Longueuil, Canada
laflamme@cardiomedik.com

February 2016

The author has no conflicts of interest to declare concerning this book.

# Scientific revision

- **Dr Andrew M. Freeman**, MD, FACP, FACC, Director, Clinical Cardiology and Operations, Assistant Professor of Medicine, National Jewish Health, Denver, CO
  *Chapter 1 - Cardiac diagnostic assessment*

- **Dr Tiziano M. Scarabelli**, MD, PhD, FACP, FAHA, Associate Professor of Internal Medicine and Pharmacology; Director, Center for Heart and Vessel Preclinical Studies, St John Hospital & Medical Center, Wayne State University, Detroit, MI
  *Chapter 1 - Cardiac diagnostic assessment*

- **Dr Edward Koifman**, Levied Heart Center, Chaim Sheba Medical Center, Tel Hashomer, Israel
  *Chapter 2 - Coronary artery disease & Myocardial infarction*

- **Dr Émilie Belley-Côté**, MD, FRCPC, Cardiologist - Intensivist, Research fellow, Population Health Research Institute, McMaster University, Hamilton, Ontario
  *Chapter 3 - Heart failure*

- **Dr Shikhar Agarwal**, MD, MPH, Section of Interventional Cardiology, Heart and Vascular Institute, Cleveland Clinic, Cleveland, OH
  *Chapter 4 - Valvular heart disease*

- **Dr Ankur Kalra**, MD, FACP, Interventional Cardiology Fellow, Beth Israel Deaconess Medical Center, Harvard Medical School, Boston, MA
  *Chapter 5 - Diseases of the pericardium & myocardium*

- **Dr Charles Dussault**, MD, FRCPC, Clinical Cardiac Electrophysiology fellow Harvard Medical School, Boston, MA
  *Chapter 6 - Arrhythmias*

- **Dr Tabitha G. Moe**, MD, Adult Congenital Cardiology, Arizona Pediatric Cardiology, Phoenix Children's Heart Center, Phoenix, AZ
  *Chapter 7 - Adult congenital heart disease & Heart disease in pregnant women*

- **Dr Ryan Maybrook**, MD, Cardiology fellow, Division of Cardiovascular Diseases, University of Kansas Medical Center, Kansas City, KS
  *Chapter 8 - Peripheral vascular disease*

- **Dr Jaya Mallidi**, MD, MHS, Cardiology Fellow, Division of Cardiology, Baystate Medical Center, Tufts University, Springfield, MA
  *Chapter 9 - Miscellaneous*

Every physician is responsible for his or her acts. Although the recommendations and management presented in this book are based on valid, reliable and up-to-date references at the time of writing, the author and publisher decline all responsibility and remind the reader that every physician must practice medicine according to current medical and scientific guidelines, taking into account his or her own capacities and limitations, and, if necessary, seeking advice from more experienced specialists.

# Cardiac diagnostic assessment 01

| 1.1/ | Cardiac physical examination | 2 |
| 1.2/ | Electrocardiogram (ECG) | 8 |
| 1.3/ | Stress test | 22 |
| 1.4/ | Transthoracic echocardiography (TTE) | 27 |
| 1.5/ | Transesophageal echocardiography (TEE) | 39 |
| 1.6/ | Stress echocardiography | 43 |
| 1.7/ | Chest x-ray (CXR) | 45 |
| 1.8/ | Coronary angiography | 48 |
| 1.9/ | Hemodynamic assessment | 53 |
| 1.10/ | Cardiac nuclear medicine | 60 |
| 1.11/ | Cardiac magnetic resonance imaging (cardiac MRI) | 63 |
| 1.12/ | Cardiac CT scan | 65 |
| 1.13/ | Cardiopulmonary test | 66 |
| 1.14/ | Exposure to radiation during cardiac examinations | 67 |

# 1.1/ CARDIAC PHYSICAL EXAMINATION

## EXAMINATION OF THE PATIENT

**GENERAL INSPECTION:** Diaphoresis; Signs of hypoperfusion; Cachexia; Mitral facies; Cheyne-Stokes breathing

**CUTANEOUS INSPECTION:** Cyanosis (central vs peripheral); Pallor; Telangiectasias (Osler-Weber-Rendu; scleroderma); Tanned skin (hemochromatosis); Jaundice (liver disease); Ecchymoses (coagulopathy); Petechiae (thrombocytopenia); Purpura (vasculitis; endocarditis); characteristic axillary skin fold (pseudoxanthoma elasticum); Lentiginosis (LEOPARD; Carney); Lupus pernio - erythema nodosum (sarcoidosis); blue sclera (osteogenesis imperfecta); nicotine stains (smoking)

> **Familial hypercholesterolemia:** Arcus senilis; pathognomonic tendinous xanthomas (extensor tendons; MCP; Achilles tendon); Xanthelasma
> **Familial hypertriglyceridemia (LPL deficiency):** Eruptive xanthomas; Lipemia retinalis
> **Dysbetalipoproteinemia:** Tuberous xanthomas (elbows; knees); Palmar xanthomas

**SIGNS OF ENDOCARDITIS:** Roth's spots; Janeway lesions; Osler's nodes; splinter hemorrhages; mucosal petechiae

**FUNDOSCOPY:** hypertensive retinopathy (arteriovenous nicking; exudates; hemorrhages; cotton-wool spots; papilledema); diabetic retinopathy; endocarditis (Roth's spot); Hollenhorst plaque (cholesterol embolism); Lipemia retinalis

## VITAL SIGNS

**BLOOD PRESSURE:** in both arms (± legs)

> **Large pulse pressure (> 50% of SBP):** Age - HTN; AR; Patent ductus arteriosus; Ruptured aneurysm of the sinus of Valsalva; Fever; Anemia; Hyperthyroidism; Pregnancy; AV fistula; Paget's disease
> **Narrow pulse pressure (< 25% of SBP):** Cardiac tamponade; Heart failure; Cardiogenic shock; Aortic stenosis
> **BP difference between the two arms > 10 mmHg:** Normal variant; PAD; Inflammatory vascular disease (Takayasu; giant cell arteritis); Supravalvular aortic stenosis; CoA; Aortic dissection
> **BP difference between the arms and legs > 20 mmHg:** Hill's sign (significant AR); CoA; severe PAD
> **Pulsus paradoxus:** ↘ SBP > 10 mmHg on inspiration
> **Orthostatic hypotension:** ↘ SBP > 20 mmHg or ↘ DBP > 10 mmHg during the first 3 minutes after standing up
> **Valsalva response**

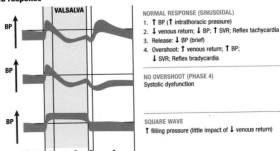

NORMAL RESPONSE (SINUSOIDAL)
1. ↑ BP (↑ intrathoracic pressure)
2. ↓ venous return; ↓ BP; ↑ SVR; Reflex tachycardia
3. Release: ↓ BP (brief)
4. Overshoot: ↑ venous return; ↑ BP; ↓ SVR; Reflex bradycardia

NO OVERSHOOT (PHASE 4)
Systolic dysfunction

SQUARE WAVE
↑ filling pressure (little impact of ↓ venous return)

**OTHER VITAL SIGNS**: Pulse; heart rate regularity; Respiratory rate; Oxygen saturation; Temperature; Weight; Height; Waist

> **Body surface area (m²)** = **0.007184 x weight (kg) x height (cm)**                           +

---

## NECK

### CAROTID PULSE

> **Shape**: ▶▶| Hemodynamic assessment (arterial recording)
> **Carotid sinus massage:** abnormal response if **asystole > 3 seconds (sinus arrest or AV block) and/or significant and symptomatic fall in SBP**                    +

### JUGULAR VEINS

> **Jugular vein vs carotid artery**: Biphasic; Height modified by inspiration and position and hepatojugular reflux (HJR); Impalpable; Compressible                        +
> **Height**: distance between the sternal angle and the summit of venous pulsation; **normal < 3 cmH₂O**

$$\text{normal} < 3\ cmH_2O$$

> • **CVP (cmH₂0):** height above the sternal angle + 5 cmH₂0                                +
> • **Normal CVP: < 8 cmH₂0 (< 6 mmHg)**                                                     +
> • **Conversion: 1.36 cmH₂0 = 1 mmHg**                                                      +
> **Waves**: ▶▶| Hemodynamic assessment (atrial recording)

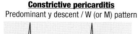

**Normal pattern**
a wave > v wave

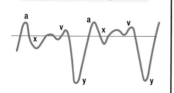

**Tricuspid stenosis (or RVH)**
Predominant a wave

**Constrictive pericarditis**
Predominant y descent / W (or M) pattern

**Tricuspid regurgitation**
Predominant v wave

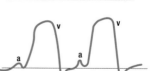

> **Kussmaul's sign**: inspiratory increase (or absence of decrease) of CVP (constriction; RCM; RV infarction; pulmonary embolism; TS; RA tumor; right heart failure)
> **Hepatojugular reflux (HJR)**: Right upper quadrant (RUQ) compression (25 mmHg) x 15 seconds
> • **Abnormal response: sustained ↗ of CVP > 3 cm throughout compression** (patient breathing normally); **reflects right heart failure and/or wedge pressure > 15 mmHg**     +

# PRECORDIUM

**INSPECTION OF THE RIB CAGE:** pectus excavatum; pectus carinatum; kyphoscoliosis; barrel chest; surgical scars; breathing; PPM / ICD

**INSPECTION OF THE PRECORDIUM:** position and dimensions of the apical impulse

**PALPATION:** patient in 30° supine position

> **Apical impulse:** with the fingertips; left lateral supine position as required; **medial to the midclavicular line; 4th or 5th intercostal space; diameter < 2 cm**          +
>   - **Apical pulsation:** corresponds to isovolumic contraction of the LV
>   - **Hyperdynamic apex:** increased amplitude of apical impulse but of normal duration; AR; patent ductus arteriosus; MR; VSD; hyperthyroidism; anemia; pregnancy
>   - **Sustained apical impulse: the impulse persists during or after the carotid upstroke; associated with pressure overload** (AS; HCM; HTN)          +
>   - **Enlarged apical impulse:** dilatation > 2 cm and/or shift downwards and to the left; associated with **LV volume overload**          +
>   - **Palpable S3:** LV volume overload
>   - **Palpable S4:** noncompliant LV / ↗ end-diastolic pressure
>   - **Triple apical impulse:** HCM (early-systole; end-systole due to dynamic LVOT obstruction; S4)
> **Ectopic pulsation:** LV aneurysm (mid-precordial or anterior axillary)
> **Left parasternal heave:** associated with RVH
> **Thrill:** palpate the 4 areas (palm of the hand at the level of the MCP joints)
> **Pulsation in the 2nd right intercostal space:** ascending aortic aneurysm
> **Pulsation in the 2nd left intercostal space:** PA dilatation

# AUSCULTATION - SYSTOLIC HEART SOUNDS

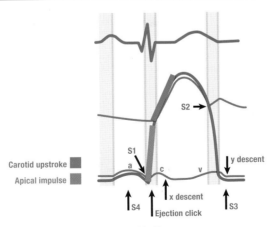

**LOOK FOR:** S1; Ejection click; Mid-systolic click; S2

**S1:** $M_1$-$T_1$ (interval: 20-30 ms); maximum at the apex; T1 mainly in the 5th left intercostal space; **precedes the carotid upstroke**

> ⬈ **Intensity of S1 (S1 ≥ S2 in the 2ⁿᵈ left intercostal space)**: Rheumatic MS (early stage); Hyperdynamic state (⬈ dP/dt); PR < 120 ms; ⬈ flow through mitral valve (VSD; patent ductus arteriosus)
> ⬊ **Intensity of S1**: Calcified MS (⬊ mobility); Systolic dysfunction; PR > 200 ms; acute AR
> **Variable intensity of S1:** AF; AV dissociation; Tamponade
> **Split S1 (split sound in the 5ᵗʰ left intercostal space)**: RBBB; ASD (delayed T1); ST (delayed T1); Ebstein's anomaly

**S2**: A2-P2; maximum in the 2ⁿᵈ left intercostal space

> **Normal physiological splitting**: on inspiration; 2ⁿᵈ left intercostal space; interval: 20-60 ms

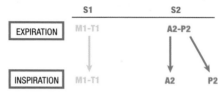

> **Normal but narrow inspiratory splitting**: PHT (associated with ⬈ P2)
> **Increased splitting**: RBBB; severe MR (early A2); VSD (early A2); RVOT obstruction (late P2)
> **Fixed splitting (A2-P2 variation < 20 msec)**: ASD; right heart failure (absence of variation of ejection volume according to RV preload)
> **Paradoxical splitting**: LBBB; RV PPM; AS; HCM; LV systolic dysfunction; AR (prolonged ejection)

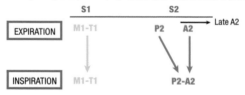

> ⬈ **intensity of A2**: HTN; CoA; Ascending aortic aneurysm; Transposition of the great arteries; supravalvular AS
> ⬊ **intensity of A2**: Valvular AS; AR
> ⬈ **intensity of P2: P2 > A2 in the 2ⁿᵈ left intercostal space or P2 heard at the apex or palpable P2**: PHT; Supravalvular RVOT obstruction
> ⬊ **intensity of P2**: Valvular PS; pulmonary regurgitation (except if secondary to PHT); Transposition of the great arteries
> **Single S2**: ⬊ A2 (AS) or ⬊ P2 (PS); Transposition of the great arteries

**VALVULAR EJECTION CLICK: coincides with carotid upstroke** (120-140 ms after QRS); high-pitched sound; diffuse radiation; best heard in lower left parasternal region; associated with bicuspid aortic valve (valve still pliable) or **congenital PS (⬊ click on inspiration; valve still pliable)**    +

> **Vascular ejection click**: Aortic root dilatation; PA dilatation (idiopathic; post-stenotic; PHT)

**MID-SYSTOLIC CLICK OF MVP: non-ejection click** (after the carotid pulsation); high-pitched sound; earlier if the patient stands up; ± MR murmur

## AUSCULTATION - DIASTOLIC HEART SOUNDS

**LOOK FOR**: S2; Opening snap; Pericardial knock; S3; Tumor plop; S4; Friction rub

**MITRAL OPENING SNAP**: High-pitched sound; stethoscope diaphragm at the apex; **A2-opening snap interval inversely proportional to the severity of MS** (40-120 ms after S2); interval decreases with tachycardia; ↘ intensity of opening snap when the valve is calcified

**PERICARDIAL KNOCK**: Constrictive pericarditis; early diastolic sound (at the end of the y descent); 100-120 ms after S2

**S3**: left lateral supine position; stethoscope bell at the apex; 140-160 ms after S2; during rapid ventricular filling (at the end of the y descent); associated with <u>ventricular volume overload</u> ┼

> **Etiologies:** Dilated cardiomyopathy; heart failure; MR; AR; VSD; patent ductus arteriosus; diastolic dysfunction; young subjects in good health; normal pregnancy
> **Right S3:** lower left parasternal region; ↗ on inspiration; TR; right heart failure; PHT

**S4**: left lateral supine position; stethoscope bell at the apex; occurs during atrial kick (after the P wave); associated with a <u>poorly compliant ventricle</u> and <u>↗ filling pressure</u> ┼

> **Etiologies:** HTN; AS; HCM; LVH; Ischemia; Acute AR; Acute MR; Age
> **Right S4:** lower left parasternal region; ↗ on inspiration; RVOT obstruction; PHT

**SUMMATION GALLOP:** fusion of S3 and S4 during tachycardia

**TUMOR PLOP:** prolapse of the tumor through the AV valve; sound varies with position

**PERICARDIAL FRICTION RUB: 1 or 2 or 3 components** (rapid ventricular filling; atrial kick; ventricular systole); forced expiration while leaning forward; stethoscope diaphragm in left parasternal region

## AUSCULTATION - MURMURS

**IDENTIFY:** Moment of the cycle; Configuration (crescendo; decrescendo; crescendo-decrescendo; plateau); Site; Radiation; Tone; Intensity; Modifiers (breathing; special maneuvers)

> **1/6**: Very faint murmur (barely perceptible)
> **2/6**: Faint murmur but heard immediately
> **3/6**: Moderate murmur
> **4/6**: Palpable thrill
> **5/6**: Very loud; heard even when only part of the stethoscope is in contact with the chest
> **6/6**: Heard even when the stethoscope is not in contact with the chest

**BENIGN MURMUR:** 1-2/6 in left parasternal region; Ejection murmur; S2 of normal intensity with normal physiological splitting; No other heart sounds or murmurs; No LVH (on examination or ECG); Murmur not increased by Valsalva maneuver or standing

**INDICATIONS FOR TTE:** Diastolic or continuous or holosystolic or end-systolic or early systolic murmur or associated with ejection click or ≥ 3/6 with mid-systolic peak or radiating to the neck or back or signs or suspicion of MR, MVP, HCM or VSD on dynamic auscultation

| SYSTOLIC MURMUR | |
|---|---|
| **Mid-systolic (often diamond-shaped)** S1     S2 | • Benign<br>• Ejection murmur: High output state (pregnancy; hyperthyroidism; anemia; AV fistula; AR; PR; ASD)<br>• Aortic stenosis (supravalvular; valvular; subvalvular)<br>• Aortic sclerosis<br>• HCM<br>• PS (supravalvular; valvular; subvalvular)<br>• CoA<br>• Functional / ischemic MR |

| **Holosystolic** 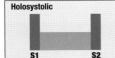 <br> S1 S2 | • MR <br> • TR <br> • VSD (restrictive) |
|---|---|
| **Early systolic**  <br> S1 S2 | • Acute MR <br> • Primary TR (without PHT) <br> • VSD: small muscular VSD or large VSD with significant PHT |
| **End-systolic**  <br> S1 S2 | • MVP <br> • Functional / ischemic MR (↗ on exercise) <br> • Tricuspid valve prolapse |

## DIASTOLIC MURMUR (ALWAYS INVESTIGATE)

| **Early diastolic** 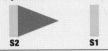 <br> S2 S1 | • AR <br> • Graham-Steell: PR secondary to PHT (decrescendo; high-pitched; signs of associated PHT) <br> • PR without PHT (faint murmur) |
|---|---|
| **Mid-diastolic** 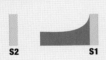 <br> S2 S1 | • MS <br> • TS <br> • Austin-Flint (absence of opening snap) <br> • Myxoma <br> • ↗ diastolic flow through AV valve (MR; TR; VSD; patent ductus arteriosus; ASD; abnormal pulmonary venous return) <br> • Carey Coombs murmur (mitral valvulitis during acute rheumatic fever) |
| **End-diastolic**  <br> S2 S1 | • MS (presystolic accentuation) <br> • TS <br> • Austin-Flint <br> • Myxoma <br> • Rytand's murmur: diastolic mitral regurgitation in a context of complete AV block |

## CONTINUOUS MURMUR (OFTEN PATHOLOGICAL)

| **Starts at systole and continues uninterrupted during diastole** 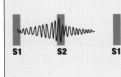 <br> S1 S2 S1 | • Patent ductus arteriosus (Gibson's murmur; machinery murmur) <br> • Aortopulmonary window <br> • Coronary arteriovenous fistula <br> • Ruptured aneurysm of the sinus of Valsalva <br> • Neck venous hum <br> • Mammary murmur of pregnancy <br> • Stenosis of peripheral branch of pulmonary artery <br> • Lutembacher's syndrome: MS + ASD <br> • CoA / Intercostal collateral vessels <br> • Pulmonary or systemic AV fistula <br> • Bronchial collateral vessels |
|---|---|

# DYNAMIC AUSCULTATION

| MANEUVERS | AS | HCM | MVP | MR | OTHER |
|-----------|-----|-----|-----|-----|-------|
| **Valsalva** (↘ preload) | ↘ | ↗ | ↗ duration of murmur | ↘ | ↘ AR |
| **Standing up** (↘ preload) | ↘ | ↗ | ↗ duration of murmur | ↘ | |
| **Squatting or leg raising** (↗ preload) | unchanged or ↗ | ↘ | ↘ duration of murmur | ↗ | ↗ AR - ↗ VSD |
| **Hand grip** (↗ afterload) | unchanged or ↘ | ↘ | ↘ duration of murmur | ↗ | ↗ AR - ↗ VSD ↗ MS (↗ HR) |
| **Amyl nitrate** (↘ afterload) | ↗ | ↗ | ↗ duration of murmur | ↘ | ↗ MS (↗ HR) ↘ AR - ↘ VSD ↘ Austin Flint |
| **Post-PVC** (↗ contractility) | ↗ | ↗ | ↘ duration of murmur (↗ LV volume) | unchanged | |

**INSPIRATION:** louder right heart sounds/murmurs (except for pulmonary valve ejection click); ↗ splitting of S2

# PHYSICAL EXAMINATION - OTHER EXAMINATIONS

**LUNGS:** crackles; effusion; wheezing; pleural friction rub

**ABDOMEN:** Liver (pulsation); Ascites; Splenomegaly; Aorta; Murmurs

**LOOK FOR PRESACRAL EDEMA**

**UPPER LIMBS:** clubbing; arachnodactyly; signs of endocarditis; nicotine stains; sclerodactyly; pulse in both arms

**LOWER LIMBS:** murmurs; lower limb edema; pulse in both legs; capillary refill; discoloration; ulcer; coldness; atrophic changes; hair loss
> **Radiofemoral delay:** CoA
> **Pulse:** 0 = absent; 1 = decreased; 2 = normal; 3 = bounding

**BRIEF NEUROLOGICAL EXAMINATION**

# 1.2/ ELECTROCARDIOGRAM (ECG)

## SYSTEMATIC APPROACH

a) **HEART RATE:** 1500 / number of small squares between 2 QRS or 300-150-100-75-60-50-43-38
b) **RHYTHM** (►►I Chapter 6 - Arrhythmias)
c) **P WAVE:** morphology
d) **AV CONDUCTION**
e) **QRS:** frontal axis; intraventricular conduction; precordial QRS transition; voltage / chamber hypertrophy
f) **REPOLARIZATION:** ST segment - T wave - QT interval - U wave
g) **MYOCARDIAL INFARCTION / Q WAVE**

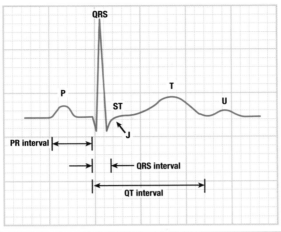

| NORMAL VALUES | |
|---|---|
| **Calibration** | • **Vertical: 10 mm = 1 mV**<br>• **Horizontal: 1 mm = 40 msec** |
| **P wave duration and amplitude** | < 120 ms and < 2.5 mm in amplitude |
| **P wave axis** | 60° (positive I-II-aVL-aVF; negative aVR)<br>Normal axis: 0-90° |
| **PR interval** | 120-200 ms |
| **QRS duration** | ≤ 110 ms |
| **QRS axis** | -30° to +90° |
| **Precordial QRS transition** | R = S in V3 or V4 |
| **QRS amplitude** | • **Limbs:** > 5 mm      • **Precordial:** > 10 mm |
| **J Point / ST segment** | **Elevation**<br>• **V2-V3:** < 2 mm (men > 40 years); < 2.5 mm (men < 40 years); < 1.5 mm (women)<br>• **Other leads:** < 1 mm<br>**Depression:** < 0.5 mm |
| **T wave** | • **Positive:** I-II-V3-V4-V5-V6<br>  **> V5-V6:** T wave inversion < 1 mm in 2%<br>• **Negative:** aVR<br>• **Variable:** aVL-III-V1-V2<br>• **Maximum amplitude V2:** < 14 mm (men) and 10 mm (women) |
| **QTc** | • **Men:** < 450 ms      • **Women:** < 460 ms |

## TECHNICAL CONSIDERATIONS

**ARM LEAD REVERSAL:** P and QRS and T wave inverted in I and aVL but not in V6

**PRECORDIAL LEAD MALPOSITION:** abnormal precordial QRS transition

**RIGHT HEART OR POSTERIOR LEADS:** V3R-V4R or V7-V8-V9

**ARTIFACTS:** tremor; Parkinson's disease (pseudo-flutter)

## SINUS RHYTHM

▶▶│ Chapter 6 - Arrhythmias

**SINUS RHYTHM (SR):** origin of sinoatrial node; HR 60 -100 bpm

> **Sinus tachycardia**: HR > 100 bpm
> **Sinus bradycardia**: HR < 60 bpm
> **Normal atrial activation**: RA to AV node and to LA; P axis 0° to +90° (positive P wave I-II-aVL-aVF); biphasic P wave in V1-V2; duration < 120 ms
> **Retrograde atrial activation**: retrograde AV conduction or ectopic atrial pacemaker close to AV node; negative P wave in II and aVF

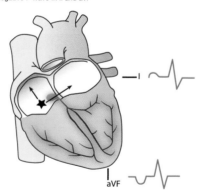

**SINUS ARRHYTHMIA:** phasic respiratory variation of the duration of the PP interval; variation ≥ 120 ms or PPmax - PPmin / PPmin > 10%

## SUPRAVENTRICULAR ARRHYTHMIAS

▶▶│ Chapter 6 - Arrhythmias

## VENTRICULAR ARRHYTHMIAS

▶▶│ Chapter 6 - Arrhythmias

| | NORMAL | RA ABNORMALITY | LA ABNORMALITY |
|---|---|---|---|
| **II** | RA    LA | RA  Peaked P wave  LA  > 2.5 mm | RA  > 40 ms  LA  > 120 ms |
| **V1** | RA  LA | RA  > 1.5 mm  > 60 ms  LA | RA  > 40 ms  > 1 mm  LA |
| | • Axis 60° <br> • Duration < 120 ms | • Axis > 75° | • Axis terminal portion -30° to -90° (negative in III) |

**INTRA-ATRIAL CONDUCTION BLOCK:** Duration of P wave > 120 ms; biphasic P wave in inferior leads; does not satisfy the criteria for RA or LA anomaly

> **Abnormal activation:** RA activation → Bachmann's bundle block → LA activation from coronary sinus (from inferior to superior)

## AV CONDUCTION

▶▶| Chapter 6 - Arrhythmias

**NORMAL PR INTERVAL:** 120-200 ms

**LONG PR INTERVAL:** PR > 200 ms; 1st degree AV block

**SHORT PR INTERVAL:** PR < 120 ms in sinus rhythm; rule out accessory pathway

> **Lown-Ganong-Levine syndrome**: atrio-His accessory pathway (James fibers) short-circuiting the AV node; narrow QRS

**X:Y AV CONDUCTION:** failure of AV node to conduct certain atrial impulses to the ventricle; **the refractory period of the AV node is longer when it is stimulated more rapidly (decremental conduction)**

> **AV block with variable conduction**: 2:1 3:1...; frequent in atrial flutter

**AV DISSOCIATION:** independent atrial and ventricular rhythms; 3 situations:

1) 3rd degree AV block; RR interval > PP interval
2) Accelerated junctional rhythm or junctional tachycardia or VT (without retrograde VA conduction); RR < PP; ± fusion or capture beats
3) Sinus bradycardia with junctional or ventricular escape (without retrograde VA conduction); RR < PP; ± isorhythmic dissociation

## FRONTAL QRS AXIS

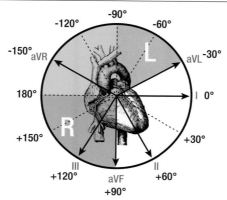

| Normal axis | -30° to + 90° | | I +<br>aVF + (if aVF - → II +) |
|---|---|---|---|
| Right axis deviation | +90° to +180° | I -<br>aVF + | **DDx:** RVH; LPHB; dextrocardia; lateral infarction; secundum ASD; vertical heart (COPD); pulmonary embolism |
| Left axis deviation | -30° to -90° | I +<br>aVF -<br>and II - | **DDx:** LVH; LAHB; primum ASD; complete AV canal defect; Tricuspid atresia (under-developed RV); pregnancy; ascites; inferior infarction |
| Extreme "North-West" axis deviation | - 90° to 180° | | I -<br>aVF - |

**INDETERMINATE AXIS:** Equiphasic QRS in all frontal leads (with no dominant QRS); axis perpendicular to the frontal plane

## QRS: INTRAVENTRICULAR CONDUCTION

**ABERRANT CONDUCTION OF SUPRAVENTRICULAR BEATS:** arrival of a supraventricular beat during the relative refractory period of intraventricular conduction tissue; conduction with wide QRS (RBBB > LBBB morphology)

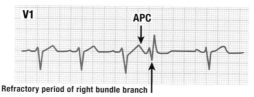

**ASHMAN PHENOMENON: Long RR then short RR → wide QRS** (frequent RBBB morphology); **long RR associated with ↗ refractory period of His-Purkinje tissue**

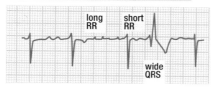

### LAHB (LEFT ANTERIOR HEMIBLOCK)

1) Left axis deviation -45° to -90°
2) qR in I and aVL
3) rS in III and aVF
4) QRS duration < 120 ms
5) R wave peak time in aVL > 45 ms
   > Late precordial QRS transition
   > **Rule out differential diagnoses**: LVH; COPD; inferior infarction

### LPHB (LEFT POSTERIOR HEMIBLOCK)

1) Right axis deviation +90° to +180°
2) rS in I and aVL
3) qR in III and aVF
4) QRS duration < 120 ms
   > **Rule out differential diagnoses**: RVH; COPD; lateral infarction; dextrocardia; arm lead reversal

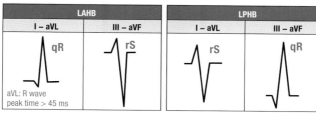

| LAHB | | LPHB | |
|---|---|---|---|
| I – aVL | III – aVF | I – aVL | III – aVF |
| qR / aVL: R wave peak time > 45 ms | rS | rS | qR |

### LBBB (LEFT BUNDLE BRANCH BLOCK)

1) QRS ≥ 120 ms
2) Wide monophasic R wave in I-aVL-V5-V6
3) Absence of septal q wave in I-V5-V6
4) R wave peak time > 60 ms in V5-V6
5) ST and T in opposite direction to QRS (appropriate discordance)

| Acute myocardial infarction with a LBBB (Sgarbossa criteria) | 1) **ST elevation ≥ 1 mm in leads with positive QRS (inappropriate concordance)** <br> 2) ST depression ≥ 1 mm V1-V2-V3 (inappropriate concordance) <br> 3) ST elevation ≥ 5 mm in leads with negative QRS (extreme discordance) |
|---|---|
| Old myocardial infarction in LBBB | 1) **Cabrera's sign:** Notch of the upslope of the S wave in V2-V3-V4 <br> 2) **Chapman's sign:** Notch of the upslope of the R wave in V5-V6-I-aVL |

### INCOMPLETE LEFT BUNDLE BRANCH BLOCK

**1)** QRS 110-119 ms
**2)** LVH pattern
**3)** R wave peak time > 60 ms in V5-V6
**4)** Absence of septal q wave in I-V5-V6

### RBBB (RIGHT BUNDLE BRANCH BLOCK)

**1)** QRS ≥ 120 ms
**3)** rsr', rsR', or rSR' in V1 or V2 (width of R' or r' > width of r)
**4)** S > 40 ms in I and V6 (S larger than R in V6)
> In a minority of patients, wide monophasic R wave in V1 and/or V2 (with R wave peak time > 50 ms in V1)
> **If axis deviation:** consider bifascicular block (RBBB with LAHB or RBBB with LPHB)
> **If bifascicular block with ↗ PR:** consider lesion of 3 branches with prolonged HV interval

### INCOMPLETE RIGHT BUNDLE BRANCH BLOCK

**1)** QRS 110-119 ms
**2)** Other criteria similar to RBBB

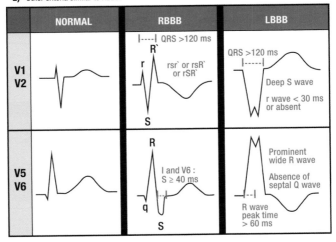

### NONSPECIFIC INTRAVENTRICULAR CONDUCTION DISORDER

**1)** QRS > 110 ms
**2)** Absence of criteria of RBBB or LBBB

### VENTRICULAR PRE-EXCITATION

**1)** PR interval < 120 ms (in sinus rhythm)
**2)** **Delta Wave:** slow rise of the initial portion of the QRS
**3)** QRS ≥ 120 ms
**4)** Secondary ST and T anomalies
> Possible pseudo-infarction (Q waves)
> **Concertina effect:** the degree of pre-excitation can vary according to conduction and the refractory period of the accessory pathway and AV node

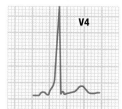

| SITE OF ACCESSORY PATHWAY | V1 | aVF | aVL |
|---|---|---|---|
| **Left lateral** | + | + | - |
| **Posterior or left septal** | + | - | + |
| **Posterior or right septal** | - | - | + |
| **Anterior or right lateral** | - | + | + |

## QRS: PRECORDIAL R WAVE TRANSITION

**NORMAL VENTRICULAR ACTIVATION: 1)** Left-to-right septal activation (septal q wave in I-aVL-V5-V6; septal r wave in aVR and V1; **2)** Anterior LV then lateral LV activation; **3)** Posterobasal LV activation

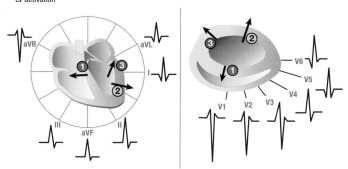

**NORMAL PRECORDIAL TRANSITION:** rS V1 → qR V6; R = S in V3 or V4

> **DDx of abnormal precordial transition**: lead malposition; dextrocardia; anterior or anteroseptal or posterior myocardial infarction; LVH; RVH; LAHB; LBBB; RBBB; dilated or infiltrative cardiomyopathy; pre-excitation (right or anteroseptal accessory pathway); COPD; pneumothorax; chest wall anomaly...

**LOW VOLTAGES:** QRS amplitude **< 5 mm on frontal leads and < 10 mm on precordial leads**

> **DDx**: COPD; obesity; cardiomyopathy; infiltrative disease - amyloidosis - tumor; myocarditis; extensive MI; pericardial effusion; constrictive pericarditis; pleural effusion; myxedema; anasarca; calibration; left pneumothorax

**ELECTRICAL ALTERNANS**: QRS amplitude varies between beats

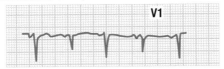

> **DDx**: pericardial effusion; severe cardiomyopathy; severe AR; supraventricular tachycardia
> **P wave alternans**: pathognomonic of pericardial effusion
> **T wave alternans**: long QT syndrome

## QRS: CHAMBER HYPERTROPHY

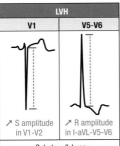
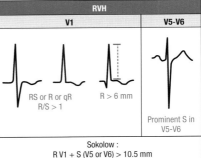

| LVH | |
|---|---|
| **V1** | **V5-V6** |
| ↗ S amplitude in V1-V2 | ↗ R amplitude in I-aVL-V5-V6 |
| Sokolow & Lyon : S V1 + R (V5 or V6) > 35 mm | |

| RVH | | |
|---|---|---|
| **V1** | | **V5-V6** |
| RS or R or qR R/S > 1 | R > 6 mm | Prominent S in V5-V6 |
| Sokolow : R V1 + S (V5 or V6) > 10.5 mm | | |

**LEFT VENTRICULAR HYPERTROPHY (LVH)**: multiple criteria

> **Sokolow & Lyon:** S V1 + R (V5 or V6) ≥ 35 mm
> **Cornell voltage:** S V3 + R aVL ≥ 28 mm (men) and ≥ 20 mm (women)
> **R aVL:** > 11 mm (> 18 mm if left axis deviation)

| ROMHILT-ESTES SCORE | | |
|---|---|---|
| Frontal leads: R or S max ≥ 20 mm **or** SV1 or SV2 ≥ 30 mm **or** RV5 or RV6 ≥ 30 mm | 3 points | ≥ 5 points: definite LVH |
| ST-T abnormality (without Digoxin) ST-T abnormality (with Digoxin) | 3 points 1 point | |
| LA abnormality | 3 points | 4 points: probable LVH |
| Left axis deviation (-30° to -90°) | 2 points | |
| QRS duration ≥ 90 ms | 1 point | |
| R wave peak time V5 or V6 ≥ 50 ms | 1 point | |

> **Other**: secondary repolarization abnormalities; left axis deviation; LA abnormality; Prolonged R wave peak time in V5-V6

- **LVH associated with LBBB**: consider concomitant LVH if: **A)** LA abnormality; **B)** QRS > 155 ms; **C)** Precordial voltage criteria
- **LVH associated with RBBB**: consider concomitant LVH if: **A)** LA abnormality; **B)** Left axis deviation; **C)** S V1 > 2 mm; **D)** R V5 or V6 > 15 mm; **E)** Left axis deviation and precordial SR max > 29 mm; **F)** R in I > 1 mm

## RIGHT VENTRICULAR HYPERTROPHY (RVH): multiple criteria

- **Sokolow**: R V1 + S (V5 or V6) > 10.5 mm
- **R/S V1**: > 1
  - **DDx of prominent R wave in V1-V2**: Lead malposition; Dextrocardia; posterior myocardial infarction; Duchenne muscular dystrophy; RVH (right axis deviation); septal HCM; RBBB; Preexcitation (left posterior or lateral pathway); pediatric ECG
- **R V1**: > 6 mm
- **R wave peak time V1**: > 35 ms
- **R/S V5 or V6**: < 0.75 (V5) or < 0.4 (V6)
- **S V5 or V6**: > 10 mm (V5) or > 3 mm (V6)
- **Other**: Right axis deviation; T wave inversion V1-V2-V3; RA abnormality; S1S2S3; S1Q3
- **RVH associated with RBBB**: consider concomitant RVH if **R in V1 > 15 mm** and right axis deviation

## BIVENTRICULAR HYPERTROPHY: look for criteria of both RVH and LVH

- **LVH**: consider concomitant RVH if → prominent S in V5 or V6; right axis deviation; unusual biphasic R/S complexes on several precordial leads (late precordial transition); RA hypertrophy
- **RVH**: consider concomitant LVH if → combined R/S amplitude in V2 to V4 > 60 mm; LA hypertrophy; prominent R wave in right and left precordial leads

---

## REPOLARIZATION: ST - T - QT - U

| ST ELEVATION (AT J POINT IN ≥ 2 CONTIGUOUS LEADS | |
|---|---|
| V2 – V3 | • Men ≥ 40 years: ≥ 2 mm<br>• Men < 40 years: ≥ 2.5 mm<br>• Women: ≥ 1.5 mm |
| All other leads | ≥ 1 mm |
| V3R – V4R – V7 – V8 – V9 | ≥ 0.5 mm |

**DDX OF ST ELEVATION:** Myocardial ischemia / STEMI; normal variant (early repolarization); LV aneurysm; pericarditis; myocarditis; cardiomyopathy; Prinzmetal angina / Vasospasm; Takotsubo; LVH; LBBB; pre-excitation; PPM; Brugada syndrome; pulmonary embolism; hyperkalemia; intracranial haemorrhage / SAH; hypothermia (Osborn); post-ECV; lead malposition; hypercalcemia; Rx (class IC AAD)…

- **Early repolarization:** 2-5% of the population; concave ST segment elevation (V2-V3-V4-V5) from J point; notch at J point; prominent T wave

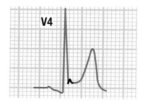

**01**

Cardiac diagnostic assessment

| ST DEPRESSION (AT J POINT ON ≥ 2 CONTIGUOUS LEADS) |
| --- |
| ≥ 0.5 mm (horizontal or descending) |

**DDX OF ST DEPRESSION:** ischemia; LVH; RVH; LBBB; RBBB; pre-excitation; myocarditis; pericarditis; cardiomyopathy; amyloidosis; hypokalemia; Digoxin; pulmonary embolism; intracranial hemorrhage; stroke; acute systemic disease; sepsis; fever; acidosis; anemia; postoperative period after cardiac surgery; hyperventilation...

| T WAVE INVERSION (ON ≥ 2 CONTIGUOUS LEADS) |
| --- |
| ≥ 1 mm; leads with R/S > 1 |

**DDX OF T WAVE INVERSION:** persistent juvenile pattern; RBBB; LBBB; pre-excitation; LVH; RVH; apical HCM; ARVD; Brugada; acute CNS lesion; PVC; ventricular pacing ("*memory T wave*")

> **Persistent juvenile pattern:** T wave inversion in V1-V2-V3 persisting since childhood

**GIANT T WAVE INVERSION (>10 MM):** Apical HCM; ischemia; Wellens' syndrome; post-STEMI; CNS lesion

> **Wellens' syndrome:** deep T wave inversion in V2-V3-V4 with ↗ QT interval associated with proximal LAD lesion

| SYMMETRICALLY PEAKED T WAVES |
| --- |
| ≥ 5 mm (frontal leads); ≥ 10 mm (precordial leads) |

**DDX OF SYMMETRICALLY PEAKED T WAVES:** hyperkalemia; acute ischemia (early STEMI); CNS lesion; LVH or LBBB (asymmetrical T waves)

| PROLONGED QT INTERVAL |
| --- |
| QTc ≥ 450 ms (men) or ≥ 460 ms (women) |

**DDX OF PROLONGED QT INTERVAL:** medication - **www.qtdrugs.org** (interrupt agent when **QTc > 500 ms or increases by > 60 ms**); long QT syndrome; hypocalcemia; hypokalemia; ﹢ hypomagnesemia; hypothermia; CNS lesion; ischemia; severe bradycardia...

> **Normal QT:** < 1/2 RR interval
> - **Bazett's equation:** $QTc = QT (msec) / \sqrt{R\text{-}R (s)}$ (HR < 100 bpm) ﹢
> - **Linear model:** $QTc = QT + 1.75 \times (HR - 60)$
> - **Significant change on medication:** > 60 ms
> **Measurement of QT:** longest interval (often V2-V3); draw a tangent from the most pronounced descent of the T wave to intersect the TP segment
> **QT associated with prolonged QRS:** JTc interval (QT duration - QRS duration) (normal < 370 ms)

**SHORT QT INTERVAL: QTc ≤ 390 msec** (HR < 100 bpm) ﹢

> **Etiologies:** hypercalcemia; hyperkalemia; Digoxin; congenital short QT syndrome

**PROMINENT U WAVE (> 2 MM):** hypokalemia; hypercalcemia; Digoxin; class IA and IC AAD; thyrotoxicosis; intracranial hemorrhage; congenital long QT syndrome

> **U wave inversion:** leads on which the T wave is positive; sign of ischemia

SUBENDOCARDIAL ISCHEMIA

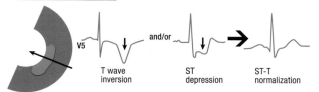

T wave inversion    and/or    ST depression    ST-T normalization

TRANSMURAL ISCHEMIA

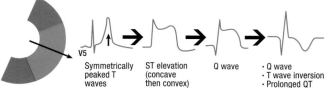

Symmetrically peaked T waves    ST elevation (concave then convex)    Q wave    • Q wave
• T wave inversion
• Prolonged QT

| ST ELEVATION OR SYMMETRICALLY PEAKED T WAVES ||
|---|---|
| **V1-V2** | Anteroseptal infarction |
| **V3-V4** | Anteroapical infarction |
| **V5-V6 (± aVL - I)** | Anterolateral infarction |
| **V1-V2-V3-V4-V5-V6** | Extensive anterior infarction |
| **aVL-I** | Lateral infarction |
| **II-III-aVF** | Inferior infarction |
| **V3R-V4R (± V1) (+ II-III-aVF)** | RV infarction |
| **V7–V8–V9 (mirror changes in V1–V2)** | Posterior infarction |

| ABNORMAL Q WAVE (IN ≥ 2 CONTIGUOUS LEADS) ||
|---|---|
| **V2-V3** | QS or Q duration ≥ 20 ms |
| **I-II-aVL-aVF**<br>**V4-V5-V6**<br>**V7-V8-V9** | QS or<br>Q ≥ 30 ms and > 1 mm |
| **V1-V2** | Consider old posterior infarction if R > 40 ms with R/S ≥ 1 in absence of conduction disorder |

**DDX OF Q WAVES (PSEUDO-INFARCTION):** septal Q waves (V4-V5-V6; I; aVL; aVF); normal variant in V1 or III; LVH; RVH; LBBB; LAHB; pre-excitation; myocarditis; RCM - Infiltration (amyloidosis; sarcoidosis; tumor); HCM; DCM; dextrocardia; hyperkalemia; chest deformity; pneumothorax; COPD; pulmonary embolism...

---

## CLINICAL ENTITIES

**ACUTE PERICARDITIS: 4 phases**
1) Diffuse ST elevation (concave); PR segment depression; mirror image in aVR
2) Normalisation of ST segment with depression of J point
3) T wave inversion
4) Normalisation of T waves

**PERICARDIAL EFFUSION:** low voltage; electrical alternans

**PULMONARY EMBOLISM:** sinus tachycardia; QR or qR in III-aVF / V1-V2-V3 (pseudo-infarction); S1Q3T3 (12% of patients); ST depression (sometimes elevation) and T wave inversion in V1-V2-V3; complete or incomplete RBBB; delayed precordial QRS transition; right axis deviation

**HYPERTROPHIC CARDIOMYOPATHY (HCM):** LVH; LAH; left axis deviation; pseudo-infarction (Q waves - inferior - lateral - precordial leads); giant T wave inversion in precordial leads (apical HCM)

**PRIMUM ASD:** RBBB; left axis deviation; RAH

**SECUNDUM ASD:** Incomplete RBBB; right axis deviation; RAH; notch in the upslope of the R wave in inferior leads

**MITRAL STENOSIS:** RVH; right axis deviation; LAH ± RAH

**LEFT VENTRICULAR ANEURYSM:** persistent convex ST elevation (3 weeks post-MI) in the presence of a Q wave

**DEXTROCARDIA:** inverted P and QRS and T waves in I and aVL; positive QRS in aVR; inverted precordial QRS transition

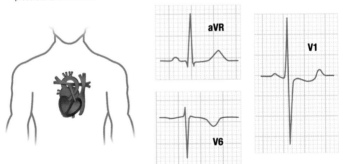

**COPD:** RVH; RAH; right axis deviation; ↘ QRS amplitude on frontal leads (electrical isolation due to hyperinflation); delayed precordial transition (cardiac position modified by hyperinflation and lowering of the diaphragm); persistent S wave in all precordial leads; low amplitude R wave in V6; pseudoinfarction (Q waves); MAT - APCs - AF - Flutter

**ACUTE CNS LESION**: giant T wave inversions on precordial leads (sometimes positive and prominent); ↗ QT interval; U waves; transient ST elevation; ± Torsade de pointes

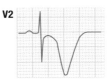
V2

**DIGOXIN IMPREGNATION: scooped ST**; flattened T wave; ↘ QT interval; ↗ PR interval; U wave

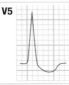
V5

**DIGOXIN TOXICITY**: sinus bradycardia; sinus arrest; ectopic atrial tachycardia; "regularized" AF (junctional escape rhythm); junctional tachycardia; AV block; PVCs; VT; bidirectional VT; VF

**HYPERCALCEMIA**: ↘ QT interval; sharp T wave upstroke; ↗ PR interval

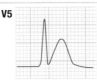
V5

**HYPOCALCEMIA**: ↗ QT interval (due to ↗ ST interval; T wave unchanged)

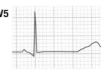
V5

**HYPERKALEMIA: symmetrically peaked T waves**; ↘ QT interval → ↗ **QRS duration** and ↗ QT interval; conduction disorders (RBBB; LBBB; bifascicular block; AV block) → **flattened P wave** (or even loss of P wave with sinoventricular rhythm; unexcitable atrial muscle); ST elevation → ventricular flutter / sinusoidal rhythm → asystole

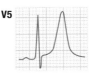
V5

**HYPOKALEMIA: prominent U wave**; ST depression; flat T wave; ↗ QT interval; blocks; atrial - ventricular - junctional tachyarrhythmias / Torsade de pointes

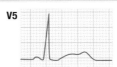
V5

**HYPOTHERMIA (< 34°C):** Osborn wave; bradycardia; ↗ QT interval; ↗ QRS duration; ↗ PR interval; artefacts secondary to rigors; junctional bradycardia; ventricular arrhythmia; asystole

> **Osborn wave:** notch and elevation of J point (maximal in V5-V6)

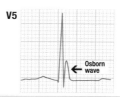

V5

← Osborn wave

**HYPOTHYROIDISM:** low voltage; sinus bradycardia; flat T wave; ↗ PR interval; conduction disorders; ↗ QT interval

## 1.3/ STRESS TEST

### INDICATION

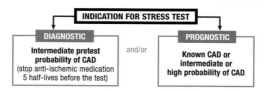

INDICATION FOR STRESS TEST

| DIAGNOSTIC | PROGNOSTIC |
|---|---|
| **Intermediate pretest probability of CAD** (stop anti-ischemic medication 5 half-lives before the test) | **Known CAD or intermediate or high probability of CAD** |

and/or

|  | SENSITIVITY | SPECIFICITY |
|---|---|---|
| **General population** | 68 % | 77 % |
| **LMCA or 3–vessel disease** | 86 % | 53 % |

### CONTRAINDICATIONS

| ABSOLUTE | RELATIVE |
|---|---|
| • Acute infarction ≤ 48 h<br>• High-risk unstable angina<br>• Decompensated heart failure<br>• Uncontrolled arrhythmia with symptoms or hemodynamic instability<br>• Myocarditis or acute pericarditis<br>• Severe symptomatic aortic stenosis<br>• Acute pulmonary embolism<br>• Acute aortic dissection | • Left main coronary artery stenosis<br>• Moderate stenotic valvular heart disease<br>• Electrolyte disorders<br>• Severe HTN: > 200/110 mmHg<br>• Tachyarrhythmia or bradyarrhythmia<br>• HCM<br>• Advanced AV block<br>• Mentally unable to perform the exercise<br>**ANOMALIES ON BASELINE ECG**<br>• Pre-excitation<br>• LBBB<br>• Ventricular pacing<br>• ST depression > 1 mm<br>• Digoxin and LVH with repolarization abnormalities (false-positive) |

**COMPLICATIONS:** 3.5 infarctions - 4.8 arrhythmias - 0.5 deaths per 10,000 examinations performed

# PROTOCOLS

| STAGE | % SLOPE | SPEED (mph) | TIME (min) | VO$_2$ (mL/kg/min) | METs |
|---|---|---|---|---|---|
| **BRUCE PROTOCOL** | | | | | |
| 0 | 0 | 1.7 | -6 to -3 | | |
| 0.5 | 5 | 1.7 | -3 to 0 | 11 | 3 |
| 1 | 10 | 1.7 | 3 | 17 | 4.5 |
| 2 | 12 | 2.5 | 6 | 25 | 7 |
| 3 | 14 | 3.4 | 9 | 35 | 10 |
| 4 | 16 | 4.2 | 12 | 47 | 13 |
| **CORNELL PROTOCOL** | | | | | |
| 1 | 0 | 1.7 | 2 | 7 | 2 |
| 2 | 5 | 1.7 | 4 | 11 | 3 |
| 3 | 10 | 1.7 | 6 | 17 | 4.5 |
| 4 | 11 | 2.1 | 8 | 19 | 5.5 |
| 5 | 12 | 2.5 | 10 | 25 | 7 |
| 6 | 13 | 3 | 12 | 30 | 8.5 |
| 7 | 14 | 3.4 | 14 | 35 | 10 |
| 8 | 15 | 3.8 | 16 | 40 | 11.5 |
| 9 | 16 | 4.2 | 18 | 47 | 13 |
| **NAUGHTON PROTOCOL** | | | | | |
| 1 | 0 | 2 | 2 | 7 | 2 |
| 2 | 3.5 | 2 | 4 | 10.5 | 3 |
| 3 | 7 | 2 | 6 | 14 | 4 |
| 4 | 10.5 | 2 | 8 | 17.5 | 5 |
| 5 | 14 | 2 | 10 | 21 | 6 |
| 6 | 17.5 | 2 | 12 | 24.5 | 7 |
| 7 | 12.5 | 3 | 14 | 28 | 8 |

**1 MET: = 3.5 mL O$_2$/kg/min** (O$_2$ consumption in a resting subject)

**ESTIMATED VO$_2$:** = [(2.68 x mph) x (0.1 + (% slope x 1.8))] + 3.5

**MONITORING: ECG - HR - BP - Rating of perceived exertion (Borg scale)** at the end of each stage; at the end of exercise; every 2-3 min during recovery (for 6-10 min or normalization of ECG)

**BRUCE PROTOCOL:** change of speed and slope at each 3-min stage; modified Bruce with the addition of 2 initial stages if necessary

**CORNELL PROTOCOL:** more gradual increase of exertion (each Bruce stage is subdivided into 2 substages)

**NAUGHTON PROTOCOL:** 2-min stages; increase of 1 MET per stage; used during evaluation of VO$_2$ max

Cardiac diagnostic assessment

**RAMP PROTOCOL**: the slope and speed increase progressively according to the patient's previously estimated functional class (according to an activity scale expressed in METs) to achieve exercise lasting about 8 to 12 minutes

**POST-INFARCTION: A)** Prescription of physical activity; **B)** Effects of treatment; **C)** Prognostic value (unknown coronary anatomy)

> **Submaximal stress test (3-4 days):** Modified Bruce or Naughton; stop if HR ≥ 120 bpm or ≥ 70% of predicted HRmax or 5 METs or Angina or Dyspnea or ↘ ST 2 mm or ↘ BP or ≥ 3 consecutive PVCs

> **Stress test limited by symptoms (3 weeks):** standard test

## ELECTROCARDIOGRAPHIC EVALUATION

**ST SEGMENT:** depression compared to PQ segment, **80 ms from point J (ST80)** or 60 ms from point J if HR > 130 bpm (ST60)

| | | |
|---|---|---|
| **Normal response: ascending ST depression** | • ST80 depression < 1.0 mm<br>• Ascending slope ≥ 1 mV/s (1 mV = 10 mm) |  J  ST80 |
| **Abnormal response: horizontal ST depression** | • J and ST80* depression ≥ 1 mm<br>• Horizontal slope (< 0.7 to 1 mV/s) |  3 BEATS |
| **Abnormal response: descending ST depression** | • J and ST80* depression ≥ 1 mm<br>• Descending slope (< -1 mV/s) |  3 BEATS |
| **Gray zone: ST depression with slow rise** | • ST80 depression ≥ 1.0 mm<br>• Ascending slope ≥ 1 mV/s<br>• Evaluate according to the patient's pretest probability of CAD |  ST80  Slope = 3 mV/s |
| **Transmural ischemia: ST elevation** | • J and ST60 elevation ≥ 1 mm<br>• Absence of Q wave<br>• Localize ischemia |  3 BEATS |

* ST60 if HR > 130 bpm

**MORE SPECIFIC LEADS: V4-V5-V6**; isolated ST abnormalities in II and aVF often associated with false-positive results

**ST DEPRESSION**: does not localize the ischemia

**ST ELEVATION IN AVR:** associated with left main coronary / ostial LAD stenosis

**U WAVE INVERSION:** associated with significant CAD

**BASELINE RBBB:** ignore leads V1-V2-V3-V4 during the stress test

**FALSE-POSITIVE:** baseline ST abnormality; anemia; cardiomyopathy; Digoxin; hyperventilation; hypokalemia; intraventricular conduction disorders; LVH; pre-excitation; severe AS; severe HTN; severe hypoxia; severe volume overload; supraventricular tachycardia; MVP

## INDICATIONS TO TERMINATE THE TEST

| ABSOLUTE | RELATIVE |
|---|---|
| • ↘ BP ≥ 10 mmHg with ischemia<br>• Severe and intolerable angina (CCS 3 to 4/4 on tolerance scale)<br>• Ataxia; Faintness<br>• Hypoperfusion (cyanosis; pallor)<br>• Technical difficulty<br>• Patient wants to stop<br>• Sustained VT<br>• ST elevation: ≥ 1 mm (in absence of Q wave and elsewhere than in aVR or V1) | • ↘ BP ≥ 10 mmHg<br>• ST depression: > 2 mm<br>• Marked change of QRS axis<br>• Arrhythmia: polymorphic PVCs; triplet PVCs; supraventricular tachycardia; block; bradyarrhythmia<br>• Fatigue - Dyspnea - Wheezing - Leg cramps - Claudication<br>• Intraventricular conduction disorder unable to be distinguished from VT<br>• Worsening retrosternal chest pain<br>• Exaggerated hypertensive response: BP > 250/115 |

## OTHER ELEMENTS TO BE EVALUATED

**NON-DIAGNOSTIC TEST: insufficient exercise (< 85% of predicted HRmax for age)**      +

**> Predicted HRmax for age: = 220 - age**

**MAXIMUM FUNCTIONAL CAPACITY:** # METs; powerful prognostic marker

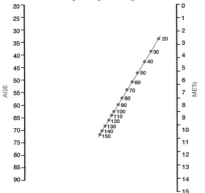

**Percentage of predicted exercise capacity for age**

**Source:** Morris CK, Myers J, Froelicher VF, et al. JACC 1993; 22; 175-182.

**DOUBLE PRODUCT**: HR x SBP / 1000 (normal: 20-35 mmHg x bpm x $10^{-3}$)

**ANGINA**: generally occurs after ST abnormalities

**SYSTOLIC BLOOD PRESSURE**: peak generally observed between 160 and 200 mmHg

> **Abnormal response**: failure to reach 120 mmHg or ↘ > 10 mmHg or ↘ below baseline SBP; associated with significant ischemia or cardiomyopathy or LVOT obstruction or antihypertensive medication or significant dehydration

> **Exaggerated hypertensive response**: SBP > 210 mmHg in men or > 190 mmHg in women; risk of developing HTN in the future in a currently normotensive patient; indicates an insufficient reduction of systemic vascular resistance by arteries and arterioles during exercise; ABPM may be indicated

**CHRONOTROPIC INCOMPETENCE**: failure to achieve > 80-85% of predicted HRmax for age (with significant exercise); associated with poor prognosis

> **Chronotropic index**: observed HR reserve (maximum HR on stress test - HR at rest) / (predicted HRmax for age - HR at rest); chronotropic incompetence if **< 80 %**

**DE NOVO LBBB ON EXERTION**: associated with ↗ risk of mortality and significant CAD

**RECOVERY OF HR AT 1 MIN**: = peak HR - HR after 1 minute of rest

> **Abnormal HR recovery**: < 12 bpm (standing) or 18 bpm (supine); associated with poor prognosis

**PVCS DURING RECOVERY**: associated with ↗ risk of mortality (compared to patients with PVCs on exertion only)

**DUKE TREADMILL SCORE (DTS)**

| **DTS = EXERCISE TIME (MIN) - (5 X MAXIMUM ST DEPRESSION IN MM) -4 X (ANGINA SCORE)** | |
|---|---|
| **ANGINA SCORE** | **ONE-YEAR MORTALITY** |
| • Angina requiring termination = 2 | • DTS -11 and less: 5.0% |
| • Angina not requiring termination = 1 | • DTS between +4 and -10: 1.25% |
| • No angina = 0 | • DTS ≥ +5: 0.25 % |

*Mark DB, Hlatky MA, Harrell FE Jr et al. Ann Intern Med. 1987; 106:793.*

## FACTORS OF POOR PROGNOSIS

**DUKE TREADMILL SCORE: -11 and less** +

**LOW FUNCTIONAL CAPACITY: < 5 METs** +

**LOW THRESHOLD ANGINA OR ISCHEMIA: < 70% predicted HRmax or HR < 120 bpm or ≤ 4 METs** +

**SEVERE ST DEPRESSION: ≥ 2 mm** +

**MULTIPLE LEADS: ischemia on ≥ 5 leads** +

**PERSISTENCE: ischemia ≥ 3 min during recovery** +

**ST ELEVATION: ≥ 1 mm** (except for aVR) +

**ABNORMAL BP RESPONSE**: failure to achieve 120 mmHg or ↘ > 10 mmHg or ↘ below baseline SBP

**SUSTAINED OR SYMPTOMATIC VT**

# 1.4/ TRANSTHORACIC ECHOCARDIOGRAPHY (TTE)

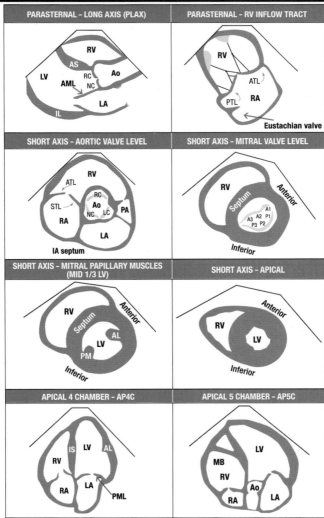

**PARASTERNAL – LONG AXIS (PLAX)**

RV
AS
LV
RC
AML
NC
Ao
LA
IL

**PARASTERNAL – RV INFLOW TRACT**

RV
ATL
PTL
RA
Eustachian valve

**SHORT AXIS – AORTIC VALVE LEVEL**

RV
ATL
RC
STL
Ao
NC
LC
PA
RA
LA
IA septum

**SHORT AXIS – MITRAL VALVE LEVEL**

RV
Septum
Anterior
A1
A3 A2 P1
P3 P2
Inferior

**SHORT AXIS – MITRAL PAPILLARY MUSCLES (MID 1/3 LV)**

RV
Septum
Anterior
LV
AL
PM
Inferior

**SHORT AXIS – APICAL**

Anterior
RV
LV
Inferior

**APICAL 4 CHAMBER – AP4C**

RV
IS
LV
AL
RA
LA
PML

**APICAL 5 CHAMBER – AP5C**

LV
MB
RV
Ao
RA
LA

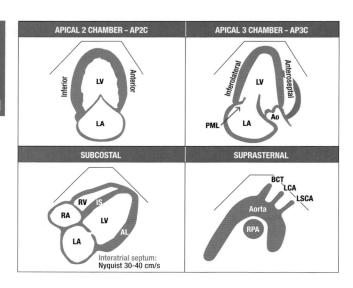

## LV - RV - LA - RA - PA EVALUATION

| | LEFT VENTRICLE | | | |
|---|---|---|---|---|
| | **NORMAL** | **SLIGHTLY ABNORMAL** | **MODERATELY ABNORMAL** | **SEVERELY ABNORMAL** |
| **LVDD: Diastolic diameter (mm)** | F: 38-52<br>M: 42-58 | F: 53-56<br>M: 59-63 | F: 57-61<br>M: 64-68 | F: ≥ 62<br>M: ≥ 69 |
| **LVSD: Systolic diameter (mm)** | F: 22-35<br>M: 25-24 | F: 36-38<br>M: 41-43 | F: 39-41<br>M: 44-45 | F: ≥ 42<br>M: ≥ 46 |
| **Indexed diastolic volume (mL/m²)** | F: 29-61<br>M: 34-74 | F: 62-70<br>M: 75-89 | F: 71-80<br>M: 90-100 | F: ≥ 81<br>M: ≥ 101 |
| **Index systolic volume (mL/m²)** | F: 8-24<br>M: 6-10 | F: 25-32<br>M: 32-38 | F: 33-40<br>M: 39-45 | F: ≥ 41<br>M: ≥ 46 |
| **Interventricular septum (mm)** | F: 6-9<br>M: 6-10 | F: 10-12<br>M: 11-13 | F: 13-15<br>M: 14-16 | F: ≥ 16<br>M: ≥ 17 |
| **Posterior wall (mm)** | F: 6-9<br>M: 6-10 | F: 10-12<br>M: 11-13 | F: 13-15<br>M: 14-16 | F: ≥ 16<br>M: ≥ 17 |
| **Indexed LV mass (g/m²) by linear method** | **LV mass = 0.6 g +**<br>**0.8 x (1.04 x [(LVDD + PW + Septum)³ - LVDD³])** | | | |
| | F: 43-95<br>M: 49-115 | F: 96-108<br>M: 116-131 | F: 109-121<br>M: 132-148 | F: ≥ 122<br>M: ≥ 149 |

| Relative wall thickness (RWT) | RWT = 2 x PW / LVDD | | | |
|---|---|---|---|---|
| | F: 0.22-0.42<br>M: 0.24-0.42 | F: 0.43-0.47<br>M: 0.43-0.46 | F: 0.48-0.52<br>M: 0.47-0.51 | F: ≥ 0.53<br>M: ≥ 0.52 |

| | **CONCENTRIC REMODELING**<br>Indexed mass: ≤ 95 g/m² (F) and ≤ 115 g/m² (M)<br><br>RWT > 0.42 | **CONCENTRIC LVH**<br>Indexed mass: > 95 g/m² (F) and > 115 g/m² (M)<br><br>RWT > 0.42 |
|---|---|---|
| | **NORMAL GEOMETRY**<br>Indexed mass: ≤ 95 g/m² (F) and ≤ 115 g/m² (M)<br><br>RWT ≤ 0.42 | **ECCENTRIC LVH**<br>Indexed mass: > 95 g/m² (F) and > 115 g/m² (M)<br><br>RWT ≤ 0.42 |

| LVEF (%) (Simpson biplane) | LVEF = ED volume - ES volume / ED volume | | | |
|---|---|---|---|---|
| | F: 54-74<br>M: 52-72 | F: 41-53<br>M: 41-51 | 30-40 | < 30 |

| LVEF (%) (Dumesnil) | **LVEF = stroke volume / ED volume**<br>• Stroke volume = 0.785 x LVOT diameter ² x LVOT VTI<br>• ED volume = 7 x LVDD³ / (2.4 + LVDD) | | | |
|---|---|---|---|---|

| Endocardial shortening fraction (%) | **% shortening = LVDD - LVSD / LVDD** | | | |
|---|---|---|---|---|
| | F: 27-45<br>M: 25-43 | F: 22-26<br>M: 20-24 | F: 17-21<br>M: 15-19 | F: ≤ 16<br>M: ≤ 14 |

| Cardiac output (L/min) | **• CO = HR x (0.785 x LVOT diameter ² x LVOT VTI)**<br>**• CO = HR x (ED volume - ES volume)** |
|---|---|
| | Normal cardiac output : 4 - 6 L/min |

| dP/dt (isovolumic contraction) | **dP/dt = 32 / time for velocity of MR jet to increase from 1 m/s to 3 m/s** |
|---|---|
| | Normal dP/dt: > 1200 mmHg/sec |

| LIMP (Left MPI) | **LIMP = IVCT + IVRT / ET ejection time** |
|---|---|
| | • Global myocardial performance index<br>• ▶▶⏐ RV MPI (right ventricle)<br>• Normal LV MPI : < 0.39 ± 0.05 |

| **RIGHT VENTRICLE** | | | | |
|---|---|---|---|---|

| RV dilatation (qualitative; AP4C) | Size of RV < size of LV; apex belongs to LV | Size of RV similar to size of LV; apex belongs to LV | Size of RV similar to size of LV; apex shared between the two | RV > LV; apex belongs to RV |
|---|---|---|---|---|

| | | |
|---|---|---|
| **Basal RV diameter AP4C (mm)** | Dilatation:<br>> 41 mm | RV-focused apical 4-chamber view; LV apex centered and not truncated, while displaying the largest basal RV diameter |
| **Mid–cavity RV diameter AP4C (mm)** | Dilatation:<br>> 35 mm | |
| **Longitudinal RV diameter AP4C (mm)** | Dilatation:<br>> 83 mm | |
| **RVOT diameter (mm)** | • Proximal: PLAX (dilatation if > 30 mm) or PSAX above the Ao valve (dilatation if > 35 mm)<br>• Distal: PSAX above the P valve (dilatation if > 27 mm) | |
| **RV wall thickness (mm)** | RVH: > 5 mm<br>Subcostal; end-diastole; at the extremity of T valve leaflets | |
| **Septal curvature** | <u>Pressure overload</u><br>D-shaped septum in systole and diastole | <u>Volume overload</u><br>D-shaped septum in diastole |

SYSTOLE     SYSTOLE

DIASTOLE     DIASTOLE

| | | |
|---|---|---|
| **FAC: RV fractional area change (%)** | RV systolic dysfunction:<br>< 35% | **FAC = (end-diastolic area - endsystolic area) / end-diastolic area x 100%**<br>AP4C; include the trabeculae in the cavity |
| **RV S' (Tissue Doppler)** | RV systolic dysfunction:<br>< 9.5 cm/s | AP4C; Velocity of longitudinal systolic excursion of basal segment of the free wall of the RV; angle dependant |
| **TAPSE (tricuspid annular plane systolic excursion)** | RV systolic dysfunction:<br>< 17 mm | AP4C; RV longitudinal function;<br>Tricuspid lateral annular longitudinal excursion by M-mode (mm) |

| RIMP (Right MPI): Global myocardial performance index | Tissue Doppler: RV dysfunction if > 0.54  Pulsed Doppler: RV dysfunction if > 0.43 | **RIMP = IVCT + IVRT / ET ejection time**<br>• **Tissue Doppler**: tricuspid annulus: ET = duration S`; IVCT + IVRT + ET = interval between the end of A` and the start of E`<br>• **Pulsed Doppler**:<br>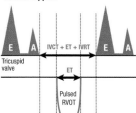 |
|---|---|---|

| LEFT AND RIGHT ATRIA | | | | |
|---|---|---|---|---|
| **LA diameter PLAX (mm)** | F: 27-38<br>M: 30-40 | F: 39-42<br>M: 41-46 | F: 43-46<br>M: 47-52 | F: ≥ 47<br>M: ≥ 52 |
| **Indexed LA volume (mL/m²)** | **LA volume = (0.85 x A1 x A2) / L**<br>Area and long axis on biplane views (AP4C and AP2C) | | | |
| | 16-34 | 35-41 | 42-48 | ≥ 48 |
| **Indexed RA volume (mL/m²)** | **RA volume = RA area ² / L** (AP4C, single-plane)<br>Normal:   F: 21 ± 6     M: 25 ± 7 | | | |
| **Indexed RA length AP4C (cm/m²)** | **Long axis** (parallel to the interatrial septum)<br>Normal:   F: 2.5 ± 0.3   M: 2.4 ± 0.3 | | | |
| **Indexed RA diameter AP4C (cm/m²)** | **Short axis** (lateral wall of RA to interatrial septum)<br>Normal:   1.9 ± 0.3 | | | |
| **RA pressure (CVP) estimated by subcostal view of inferior vena cava (mmHg)** | • IVC ≤ 21 mm and collapse > 50%:<br>  RA pressure = 3 mmHg (0-5 mmHg)<br>• IVC > 21 mm and collapse < 50%:<br>  RA pressure = 15 mmHg (10-20 mmHg)<br>• **Intermediate**: RA pressure = 8 mmHg (5-10 mmHg)<br>• **Ventilated patient**: IVC ≤ 12 mm associated with<br>  RA pressure < 10 mmHg | | | |

| PULMONARY ARTERY | | | | |
|---|---|---|---|---|
| **Systolic PAP (mmHg)** | **sPAP = 4 x TR pressure gradient ² + RA pressure**<br>In the absence of RVOT obstruction | | | |
| | < 35 | 35 - 50 | 50 - 80 | > 80 |
| **Diastolic PAP (mmHg)** | **dPAP = 4 x PR end–diastolic velocity ² + RA pressure** | | | |

| Mean PAP (mmHg) | • mPAP = 1/3 sPAP + 2/3 dPAP<br>• mPAP = 4 x early diastolic PR velocity² + RA pressure<br>• **Mahan:** mPAP = 79 − (0.45 x PA acceleration time)<br>  &gt; If PA acceleration time < 120 ms:<br>    mPAP = 90 − (0.62 x PA acceleration time)<br>  &gt; **PA acceleration time:** start of QRS to peak<br>    pulmonary flow velocity; pulsed Doppler | | | |
| Pulmonary artery diameter (mm) | 15-21 | 22-25 | 26-29 | ≥ 30 |

## DIASTOLIC FUNCTION

| | E' (cm/s)<br>E/E' | LA<br>(mL/m²) | E/A<br>DT (ms)<br>IVRT (ms) | PV FLOW<br>AR - A (ms) | VALSALVA |
|---|---|---|---|---|---|
| **DIASTOLIC FUNCTION - GRADING** | | | | | |
| **NORMAL PATTERN** | E'sep ≥ 8<br>E'lat ≥ 10<br>E/E' ≤ 8<br> | < 34 | E/A 0.8 - 1.5<br>DT 160-200<br> | PV S > D<br>Ar - A < 0<br> | Reduction of E/A ratio < 0.5<br> |
| **GRADE I: ABNORMAL RELAXATION PATTERN** | E'sep < 8<br>E'lat < 10<br>E/E' ≤ 8<br> | ≥ 34 | E/A < 0.8<br>DT > 200<br>IVRT ≥ 100<br> | PV S > D<br>Ar - A < 0<br> | Reduction of E/A ratio < 0.5<br> |
| Normal filling pressures (generally)<br><br>> 60 years: E/A < 1 and DT > 200 ms in the absence of LVH or heart disease → normal for age | | | | | |
| **GRADE II: PSEUDO-NORMAL PATTERN** | E'sep < 8<br>E'lat < 10<br>E/E' 9-12<br> | ≥ 34 | E/A 0.8 - 1.5<br>DT 160-200<br> | VP D > S<br>Ar - A ≥ 30<br> | Reduction of E/A ratio ≥ 0.5<br> |
| ↗ Filling pressures | | | | | |

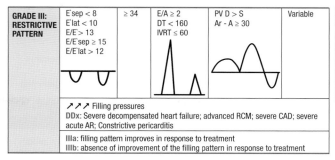

| **GRADE III: RESTRICTIVE PATTERN** | E'sep < 8<br>E'lat < 10<br>E/E' > 13<br>E/E'sep ≥ 15<br>E/E'lat > 12 | ≥ 34 | E/A ≥ 2<br>DT < 160<br>IVRT ≤ 60 | PV D > S<br>Ar - A ≥ 30 | Variable |
|---|---|---|---|---|---|
| | ↗ ↗ ↗ Filling pressures<br>**DDx:** Severe decompensated heart failure; advanced RCM; severe CAD; severe acute AR; Constrictive pericarditis | | | | |
| | IIIa: filling pattern improves in response to treatment<br>IIIb: absence of improvement of the filling pattern in response to treatment | | | | |

**IVRT**: Continuous Doppler LVOT; interval between end of Ao ejection and start of mitral filling (E wave)

**FUSION OF E AND A:** E wave > 20 cm/s at the beginning of the A wave

**FILLING PRESSURES**

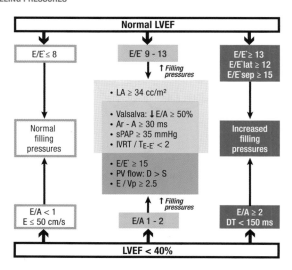

> **Increased filling pressures**: Wedge pressure > 12 mmHg or LVEDP > 16 mmHg
> **$T_{E-E'}$** = (interval between QRS and onset of E) - (interval between QRS and onset of E')
> **Vp**: velocity of propagation of diastolic flow on color M-mode
> **AF**: ↗ filling pressures if **IVRT ≤ 65 ms or DT of pulmonary vein diastolic flow ≤ 220 ms or septal E/E' ≥ 11**

+

# SEGMENTAL WALL MOTION

**LEFT VENTRICLE: divided into 16 segments** (+ apical cap)
> **Interventricular septum**: between the attachments of the RV to the LV

**LEFT VENTRICULAR CHAMBER: 3 levels → A)** Base - **B)** Mid 1/3 (papillary muscles) -
**C)** Apex

**SEGMENTAL WALL MOTION: evaluate endocardial excursion and segmental thickening**   +

| – 1 –<br>NORMAL (or<br>hyperdynamic) | – 2 –<br>HYPOKINESIA | – 3 –<br>AKINESIA | – 4 –<br>DYSKINESIA | – 5 –<br>ANEURYSM |
|---|---|---|---|---|
| Thickening > 40%<br>in systole | Thickening<br>10-40% | Thickening < 10%<br>(negligible) | Paradoxical<br>systolic movement | Diastolic<br>deformity |

| WMSI = Sum of each segment / Number of segments evaluated |
|---|
| Normal = 1; WMSI > 1.7 associated with perfusion defect > 20% (MIBI) |

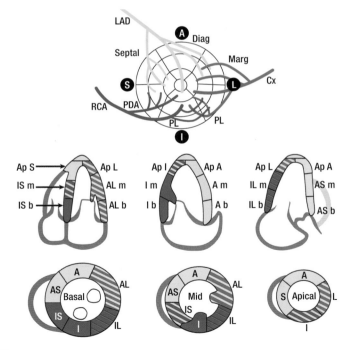

# VALVULAR HEART DISEASE

| | AORTIC STENOSIS | SEVERE |
|---|---|---|
| **Maximum jet velocity** | Look for parallel alignment between continuous Doppler and the jet | > 4 m/s |
| **Mean gradient** | Mean of instantaneous mean gradients during ejection | > 40 mmHg |
| **Valve area by continuity equation** | **Aortic valve area = 0.785 x LVOT diameter² x LVOT VTI / Aortic valve VTI** | < 1 cm² |
| | • LVOT VTI and LVOT diameter obtained at the same distance from the valve<br>• Proximal velocity (LVOT) > 1.5 m/s: use peak velocity and maximum gradient to grade severity<br>   > Maximum gradient = 4 (maximum v² – proximal v²) | |
| **LVOT VTI / Ao valve VTI ratio** | Independent of measurement of LVOT | < 0.25 |
| **Velocity > 4 m/s and Area > 1 cm²: high output; significant AR; tall patient**<br>**Velocity < 4 m/s and Area < 1cm²: low output; small patient; significant MR** | | |

| | MITRAL STENOSIS | SEVERE |
|---|---|---|
| **Mean gradient** | Mean of instantaneous mean gradients during filling | > 10 mmHg |
| **Valve area by planimetry** | • Method of choice in rheumatic MS<br>• At the extremity of the leaflets (PSAX) | < 1 cm² |
| **Valve area by pressure half-time** | **Mitral valve area = 220 / PHT** | < 1 cm² |
| | • Use the slope of the E wave at mid-diastole<br>• Method of choice in rheumatic MS<br>• Caveats: immediately after balloon valvuloplasty; severe AR (short PHT); abnormal LV relaxation (long PHT); ↗ LVEDP (short PHT); prosthetic valve (do not calculate prosthetic area but report PHT) | |
| **Valve area by continuity equation** | **Mitral valve area = 0.785 x LVOT diameter² x LVOT VTI / mitral valve VTI** | < 1 cm² |
| **Valve area by PISA** | **Mitral valve area = [6.28 x PISA radius x Aliasing velocity / Peak MS velocity] x alpha/180°** | < 1 cm² |

INDICATE HR AT THE TIME OF MEASUREMENTS; EVALUATE PAP

| BVR SCORE – BALLOON VALVULOPLASTY REGISTRY (WILKINS SCORE) | | | | |
|---|---|---|---|---|
| | – 1 –<br>**Mobility of leaflets** | – 2 –<br>**Thickening of leaflets** | – 3 –<br>**Calcification of leaflets** | – 4 –<br>**Thickening of subvalvular apparatus** |
| **1 point** | Very mobile valve; restriction of the extremity of the leaflets | Leaflets measure 4-5 mm | A single hyperechodense zone | Minimal thickening under the leaflets |

Cardiac diagnostic assessment

| 2 points | Normal mobility of the base and middle parts of the leaflets | Localized thickening (5-8 mm) | Several localized hyperechodense zones on the leaflets | Thickening of the chordae (1/3 of their length) |
|---|---|---|---|---|
| 3 points | Mobility of the base of the valve | Thickening of all of the leaflet (5-8 mm) | Hyperechodensities as far as the middle portion of the leaflets | Thickening of the chordae as far as their distal third |
| 4 points | Minimal or absent movement of the leaflets | Considerable thickening of the entire leaflet (8-10 mm) | Extensive hyperechodensities on the majority of the leaflets | Severe thickening as far as the papillary muscles |

**Score ≤ 8 associated with a favorable result of balloon valvuloplasty**

| MITRAL REGURGITATION | | SEVERE |
|---|---|---|
| **Vena contracta** | Narrowest portion of the jet distal to the regurgitating orifice; avoid AP2C; Nyquist 50-60 cm/s | ≥ 7 mm |
| **Regurgitant volume** | **VOLUMETRIC METHOD**<br>Regurgitant volume = (0.785 x Mitral annulus diameter $^2$ x anterograde mitral VTI)<br>- (0.785 x LVOT diameter $^2$ x LVOT VTI)<br>• Mitral annulus diameter: mean of PLAX and AP4C<br>• Significant AR: use pulmonic valve flow<br><br>**PISA**: Regurgitant volume = EROA x MR VTI | ≥ 60 cc |
| **EROA (Effective Regurgitation Orifice Area)** | **VOLUMETRIC METHOD**<br>EROA = Regurgitant volume / MR VTI<br>**PISA**<br>EROA = 6.28 x PISA radius $^2$ x "aliasing" velocity / peak MR velocity<br><br><br>• PISA corresponds to the time of peak MR velocity<br>• "Aliasing" velocity adjusted to the direction of regurgitation to obtain hemispheric convergence flow (Nyquist 20-40 cm/s) | ≥ 0.40 cm²<br><br>(≥ 0.20 cm² if functional MR) |
| **Regurgitant fraction** | Regurgitant fraction = Regurgitant volume / (0.785 x Mitral annulus diameter $^2$ x anterograde mitral VTI) | ≥ 50 % |
| **PISA radius** | Nyquist 40 cm/s | ≥ 9 mm |
| **MR jet** | • Nyquist 50-60 cm/s<br>• Severe MR: Large central jet > 10 cm² (or > 40% LA area) or eccentric jet adhering to the wall of the LA (Coanda effect) | |

| E wave | Dominant E wave | **> 1.2 m/s** |
|---|---|---|
| **Envelope of the jet on continuous Doppler** | • Severe MR: dense envelope; early peak and triangular shape<br>• MVP: mid- or end-systolic envelope | |
| **Pulmonary venous flow** | Severe MR: systolic reversal | |
| **LA dilatation and LV dilatation; Carpentier's mechanism** | | |

| | **AORTIC REGURGITATION** | **SEVERE** |
|---|---|---|
| **Vena contracta** | Narrowest portion of the jet distal to the regurgitating orifice; PLAX; Nyquist 50-60 cm/s | **≥ 6 mm** |
| **Regurgitant volume** | **VOLUMETRIC METHOD**<br>Regurgitant volume = (0.785 x LVOT diameter $^2$ x LVOT VTI)<br>- (0.785 x Mitral annulus diameter $^2$ x anterograde mitral VTI)<br>• Mitral annulus diameter: mean of PLAX and AP4C<br>• Significant MR: use pulmonic valve flow<br><br>**PISA**: Regurgitant volume = EROA x AR VTI | **≥ 60 cc** |
| **EROA (effective regurgitation orifice area)** | **VOLUMETRIC METHOD**<br>EROA = Regurgitant volume / AR VTI<br>**PISA**<br>EROA = 6.28 x PISA radius $^2$ x<br>"aliasing" velocity / peak AR velocity | **≥ 0.3 cm²** |
| **Regurgitant fraction** | **Regurgitant fraction =**<br>**Regurgitant volume / (0.785 x LVOT diameter $^2$ x LVOT VTI)** | **≥ 50 %** |
| **Jet width / LVOT diameter** | PLAX; 1 cm inside the Ao valve; Nyquist 50-60 cm/s | **≥ 65 %** |
| **Jet area / LVOT area** | PSAX | **≥ 60 %** |
| **Pressure half-time** | • Continuous Doppler<br>• End-diastolic speed > 4 m/s<br>• ↘ PHT: HTN; ↘ LV compliance; ↗ LVEDP | **< 200 ms** |
| **Envelope of the jet on continuous Doppler** | Severe AR: dense envelope (compare with density of the anterograde flow); rapid deceleration | |
| **Holodiastolic flow reversal in descending aorta** | • Pulsed Doppler (after the origin of the L subclavian)<br>• Also look for reversed flow in abdominal aorta<br>• **Reversal VTI ≈ anterograde flow VTI**<br> | |
| **LV dilatation; Ao dilatation; look for eversion or malcoaptation of leaflets; severe acute AR → restrictive mitral filling pattern** | | |

# PROSTHETIC VALVE

**LOOK FOR**: normal 60° opening of leaflets (normal movement of acoustic shadows); dehiscence / rocking movement; vegetation; thrombus; pannus; structural degeneration; abscess; intracardiac mass; pseudoaneurysm; fistula; periprosthetic regurgitation

> **Thrombus**: large mass; similar density to that of myocardium; recent symptoms; recent subtherapeutic INR; more frequent on mechanical mitral valve prosthesis
> **Pannus**: small, dense mass; not visualized in 30% of cases; more frequent in aortic valve prostheses

**PROSTHETIC VALVE HEMODYNAMIC MEASUREMENTS**: vary according to the model and dimensions of the prosthesis (compare with manufacturer's data); vary according to cardiac output

**RECOVERY PRESSURE PHENOMENON**: Ao transprosthetic gradient overestimated on TTE compared to catheterization (especially if proximal aortic diameter < 30 mm and small prosthesis)

**PROSTHETIC REGURGITATION**: distinguish physiological regurgitation specific to the prosthesis from pathological regurgitation; metallic mitral valve can hide MR due to shadowing

> **Central pathological regurgitation**: immobility of a mechanical leaflet; prolapse or perforation of a biological leaflet; mass - vegetation - thrombus
> **Periprosthetic pathological regurgitation**: dehiscence; rocking movement

**PATIENT-PROSTHESIS MISMATCH**: area of the effective prosthetic orifice too small for the patient's body surface area; **valve functions normally but with ↗ transvalvular gradients; normal prosthetic area (non-indexed) for the type of prosthesis**     +

> **Mild**: Indexed EOA > 0.85 cm²/m²
> **Moderate**: Indexed EOA: 0.65-0.85 cm²/m²
> **Severe**: Indexed EOA < 0.65 cm²/m²; associated with ↗ mortality (especially if LV dysfunction)
> **Mitral prosthesis**: aim for indexed EOA > 1.2 cm²/m²

| PROSTHETIC AORTIC VALVE DYSFUNCTION | | | |
|---|---|---|---|
| | **PEAK VELOCITY** | **VTI 1/2 RATIO** | **ACCELERATION TIME (AORTIC SYSTOLIC FLOW)** |
| **Obstruction (degeneration; thrombus; pannus)** | > 3 m/s | < 0.25 | > 100 ms Delayed and parabolic peak |
| **Regurgitation or ↗ cardiac output** | > 3 m/s | Normal (≥ 0.25) | AT < 80 ms Early triangular peak |
| **Patient-prosthesis mismatch** | **Indexed EOA < 0.85 cm²/m²** | | |
| | > 3 m/s | ≥ 0.25 | AT < 80 ms |

| PROSTHETIC MITRAL VALVE DYSFUNCTION | | | |
|---|---|---|---|
| | **PEAK VELOCITY** | **GRADIENT** | **PHT** | **PROSTHETIC MITRAL VALVE VTI / LVOT VTI RATIO** |
| **Obstruction (degeneration; thrombus; pannus)** | ≥ 1.9 m/s | > 5 mmHg | > 130 ms | > 2.2 |
| **Regurgitation** | ≥ 1.9 m/s | > 5 mmHg | < 130 ms | > 2.2 |
| **Hyperdynamic state / High output state** | ≥ 1.9 m/s | > 5 mmHg | < 130 ms | < 2.2 (normal) |

# ECHOCARDIOGRAPHIC MASS

**MASSES / STRUCTURES:** Eustachian valve / crista terminalis bridge / Chiari network (RA); vegetation; thrombus; degenerative valve disease; calcification; pacemaker lead; central catheter; lipomatous interatrial septum; pericardial cyst; hydatid cyst; hiatal hernia; tuberculoma; Lambl's excrescences / valvular strands (filiform structures; lenght 3-10 mm; atrial aspect of AV valves and ventricular aspect of semilunar valves; on the line of leaflet closure); benign or malignant cardiac tumor (or metastasis)

**THROMBUS:** absence of opacification with contrast; adherent to a hypokinetic or akinetic region

# CONTRAST ECHOCARDIOGRAPHY

**AGITATED SALINE:** 10 mL of saline solution; 0.25 mL of air emulsified with 2 syringes; right heart imaging

> **Intracardiac shunt:** opacification of L chambers within 3 beats (± Valsalva)     +
> **Intrapulmonary shunt (AVMs):** opacification of L chambers after 5 beats     +
> **Persistent left SVC:** injection into left arm → opacification of coronary sinus

**MICROBUBBLES:** lipid microspheres containing gas and able to cross the pulmonary circulation allowing visualization of left cardiac structures; useful for LVEF - segmental wall motion - stress echocardiography - L chamber mass / thrombus (no enhancement in the presence of thrombus) - aneurysm / pseudoaneurysm - HCM - LV noncompaction

> **Complications:** 0.01 %
> **Contraindications:** perflutren allergy; significant PHT; R → L shunt
> **Microbubbles mode:** reduction of mechanical index (0.4-0.5)

# TISSUE AND STRAIN DOPPLER

**TISSUE DOPPLER IMAGING (TDI):** evaluates the velocity of longitudinal movement of a cardiac structure (low velocities); angle dependant

**STRAIN (%):** longitudinal deformation evaluation; percentage change in length of the muscle during contraction (negative value by convention) or relaxation (positive value by convention)

**STRAIN RATE:** instantaneous measurement of the deformation (contraction or relaxation)

**TISSUE TRACKING:** distance covered (displacement) by a structure over a given time interval

| TISSUE DOPPLER (S WAVE) (CM/S) | SYSTOLIC STRAIN (%) | STRAIN RATE ($S^{-1}$) | TISSUE TRACKING (cm) |
|---|---|---|---|
| Normal basal septum: 5.97 ± 1.14 | Normal basal septum: -17.5 ± 5.32 | Normal basal septum: 0.99 ± 0.49 | Normal basal septum: 1.2 ± 0.19 |

**SPECKLE TRACKING:** evaluation of the deformation of a structure; angle-independent, which allows measurement of longitudinal, radial or circumferential deformation (counterclockwise systolic movement of the apex and clockwise systolic movement of the base)

> **Global longitudinal strain (%):** relative length change of the LV myocardium between end-diastole and end-systole (normal peak GLS in the range of -20%)     +

# 1.5/ TRANSESOPHAGEAL ECHOCARDIOGRAPHY (TEE)

**EVALUATION:** mitral valve; aortic valve; prosthetic valve; endocarditis; LA; LAA - thrombus (pre-ECV); intracardiac mass; ASD; acute aortic syndrome; pulmonary venous return; perioperative; cardioembolic source; guidance of percutaneous procedures

**COMPLICATIONS:** < 1%; dental trauma; esophageal trauma; bronchospasm; laryngospasm; aspiration; respiratory depression; arrhythmias; methemoglobinemia (benzocaine)

## PREPARATION

> **Contraindications**: dysphagia; esophageal disease; recent esophageal symptoms; esophageal varices; history of radiotherapy to the neck
> **NPO:** minimum 6 hours before the examination ($H_2O$ allowed until 2 hours before the examination)
> Continuous ECG; IV route; O2; saturation and BP monitor; suction
   • Resuscitation trolley at hand
   • Flumazenil 0.2 mg IV PRN (benzodiazepine antagonist); Naloxone 0.1 to 0.4 mg IV PRN
> **Anesthesia:** topical (lidocaine); IV sedation (midazolam 0.075 mg/kg, i.e. 2-4 mg; fentanyl PRN); Meperidine PRN (anti-gag; 25-50 mg IV)

**POST-EXAMINATION:** NPO 2 hours post-examination; no driving for 12 hours

## 5 POSSIBLE MOVEMENTS

**1)** Advance - withdraw the probe
**2)** Rotation of the plane of section (0 degree = horizontal; 90 degrees = vertical)
**3)** Rotation of the hand piece: clockwise (R heart) or counterclockwise (L heart)
**4)** Anteflexion (bending of the tip of the probe toward the sternum) or retroflexion
**5)** Lateral flexion to the right or left (rarely used)

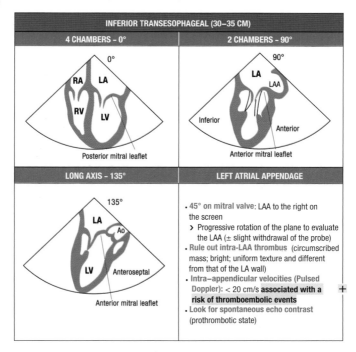

| INFERIOR TRANSESOPHAGEAL (30–35 CM) | |
| --- | --- |
| **4 CHAMBERS - 0°** | **2 CHAMBERS - 90°** |

**4 CHAMBERS - 0°**: 0°; RA, LA, RV, LV; Posterior mitral leaflet

**2 CHAMBERS - 90°**: 90°; LA, LAA; Inferior, Anterior; Anterior mitral leaflet

**LONG AXIS - 135°**: 135°; LA, Ao, LV, Anteroseptal; Anterior mitral leaflet

**LEFT ATRIAL APPENDAGE**

• **45° on mitral valve**: LAA to the right on the screen
  > Progressive rotation of the plane to evaluate the LAA (± slight withdrawal of the probe)
• **Rule out intra-LAA thrombus** (circumscribed mass; bright; uniform texture and different from that of the LA wall)
• **Intra–appendicular velocities (Pulsed Doppler)**: < 20 cm/s **associated with a risk of thromboembolic events**
• **Look for spontaneous echo contrast** (prothrombotic state)

## SUPERIOR TRANSESOPHAGEAL

| SHORT AXIS (AORTIC VALVE) – 45° | LONG AXIS – 135° |
|---|---|

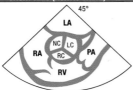

- **Coronary ostia:** 2 o'clock (left) and 6 o'clock (right)
- **Pulmonary valve and PA:** 100-130° ± counterclockwise rotation

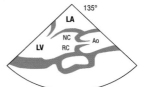

- NC = Non-coronary aortic leaflet
- RC = Right coronary aortic leaflet

| BICAVAL VIEW – 90° | PULMONARY VEINS – 90° |
|---|---|

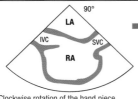

- Clockwise rotation of the hand piece
- Longitudinal interatrial septum
- **Rule out shunt:** Color Doppler (Nyquist 30-40 cm/s); agitated saline (± Valsalva)
- Pacemaker lead; central catheter

- On the bicaval view → clockwise rotation of the hand piece
- Counterclockwise rotation of the hand piece: left pulmonary veins (adjacent to the LAA)

### LEFT PULMONARY VEINS

- **LSPV:** position the probe over the LAA (next to LSPV); slight withdrawal of the probe + anteflexion + counterclockwise rotation of the hand piece (± rotation of the plane)
- **LIPV:** after having localized the LSPV, look for the LIPV by counterclockwise rotation of the hand piece and/or progressive rotation of the plane

### TRANSGASTRIC

| SHORT-AXIS LV (MITRAL PAPILLARY MUSCLES) 0–30° | 2 CHAMBERS – 90° |
|---|---|

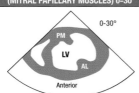

Mitral valve, short axis: slightly withdraw the probe + slight anteflexion + 10-20°

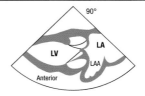

110–135°: long axis (LVOT - Ao valve)

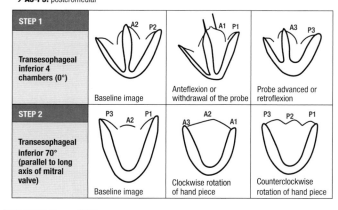

| 5 CHAMBERS (DEEP TRANSGASTRIC) – 0 to 20° | |
|---|---|
| 0 to 20° ↗<br>LV<br>Ao  LA | • Maximum anteflexion<br>• Evaluation of LVOT |

**DESCENDING THORACIC AORTA**

- Counterclockwise rotation of the hand piece
- 0°: short axis; 90°: long axis
- **Complex atherosclerosis**: plaque thickness ≥ 4 mm or mobile / pedunculated debris (= thrombus) or ulceration

## MITRAL REGURGITATION - NATIVE VALVE

**MECHANISM:** Carpentier classification (►►| Chapter 4 - Valvular heart disease); prolapse; eversion; restriction; annular dilatation; perforation

**IDENTIFICATION OF THE SEGMENTS INVOLVED**

> **A1-P1**: anterolateral
> **A3-P3**: posteromedial

| **STEP 1** | | | |
|---|---|---|---|
| **Transesophageal inferior 4 chambers (0°)** | A2 P2<br><br>Baseline image | A1 P1<br><br>Anteflexion or withdrawal of the probe | A3 P3<br><br>Probe advanced or retroflexion |
| **STEP 2** | | | |
| **Transesophageal inferior 70° (parallel to long axis of mitral valve)** | P3 A2 P1<br><br>Baseline image | A3 A2 A1<br><br>Clockwise rotation of hand piece | P3 P2 P1<br><br>Counterclockwise rotation of hand piece |

## MITRAL REGURGITATION - PROSTHETIC VALVE

**IDENTIFICATION OF THE SURGICAL QUADRANT:** transesophageal 4 chambers (0); rotation of the plane of section every 10° for 180°

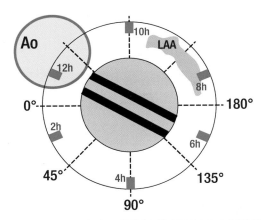

## 1.6/ STRESS ECHOCARDIOGRAPHY

**STRESS:** exercise (Bruce protocol) or Dobutamine

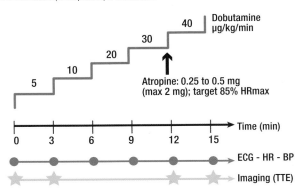

**INDICATIONS TO STOP DOBUTAMINE STRESS ECHOCARDIOGRAPHY:** > 85 % HRmax predicted for age; moderate *de novo* (or progressive) RWMA; significant arrhythmia; hypotension; severe HTN; intolerable symptoms

> **Antidote to dobutamine:** beta-blocker

**COMPLICATIONS (DOBUTAMINE):** angina; hypotension; VT (4%); supraventricular tachyarrhythmia / AF; VF or myocardial infarction (1 / 2,000 studies)

**CONTRAST AGENT:** ≥ 2 segments poorly visualized on baseline TTE

## STRESS-INDUCED ISCHEMIA

a) **RWMA (regional wall motion abnormality):** deterioration ≥ 1 grade of segmental wall motion (normokinetic or hypokinetic segment at rest); deterioration of endocardial excursion and/or segmental thickening

b) **Tardikinesia**: delayed and slow segmental contraction

c) **Chamber dilatation:** ↗ end-systolic LV volume

d) ↘ **LVEF:** deterioration of global systolic function

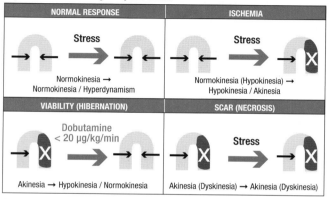

**SCAR**: regional wall motion abnormality unchanged by stress test (fixed deficit); thin < 6 mm and echodense (fibrotic) segment

**DECREASED PREDICTIVE VALUE:** target HR not achieved; LVH / concentric remodeling; imaging > 60 s post-stress; 1-vessel disease (particularly circumflex); LBBB; ventricular pacing

**FINDINGS IN REPORT:** type of stress protocol; result of stress test or dose of dobutamine used; maximum HR reached; test validity (> 85% HRmax); BP; reason for interruption; symptoms on stress test; ECG abnormalities; arrhythmias; ischemic threshold; segmental wall motion at rest and on stress test; LVEF and end-systolic LV volume at rest and on stress test

## FACTORS OF POOR PROGNOSIS

> **Resting LVEF:** < 35 %
> **Low ischemic threshold:** dobutamine ≤ 10 µg/kg/min or < 70% HRmax predicted or HR < 120 bpm
> **WMSI on effort:** > 1.4 to 1.7
> **Extensive ischemia:** ≥ 3 segments
> **Ischemia in several coronary territories (≥ 2 vessels)**
> **Deterioration of LVEF (< 45% or ↘ LVEF ≥ 10%) or LV dilatation on stress test**

**NEGATIVE STRESS ECHOCARDIOGRAPHY:** annual risk of cardiac event < 1% (exercise) or < 2% (dobutamine)

**VIABILITY:** improvement of the segmental wall motion (≥ 1 grade x ≥ 2 segments) with low-dose dobutamine (2.5 - 5 - 7.5 - 10 - 20 µg/kg/min)

> **Biphasic response**: improvement of wall motion at low-dose then deterioration at higher dose (up to 40 µg/kg/min); specific for improvement of wall motion post-revascularization
> **Sustained improvement**: viable but non-ischemic segment

# 1.7/ CHEST X-RAY

**QUALITY CONTROL: A)** Patient - Date; **B)** Adequate inspiration (right hemidiaphragm below the 6th rib anteriorly and below the 10th rib posteriorly); **C)** Patient centered - Absence of rotation (tracheal air column in the center of the vertebral bodies; spinous processes of vertebral bodies centered between clavicles); **D)** Adequate penetration (spinous processes of thoracic vertebral bodies visible); **E)** Compare with previous films

**SYSTEMATIC APPROACH:** Situs (gastric bubble and apex); Cardiothoracic index; Heart shadow and cardiac structures (RA; LA; RV; LV; Ao; PA); Calcifications; Pulmonary venous and arterial blood supply; Hila; Lung parenchyma; Pleura; Bone structures; Prosthetic material

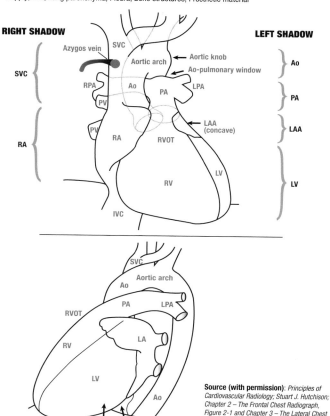

**RIGHT SHADOW**    **LEFT SHADOW**

**Source (with permission):** *Principles of Cardiovascular Radiology; Stuart J. Hutchison; Chapter 2 – The Frontal Chest Radiograph, Figure 2-1 and Chapter 3 – The Lateral Chest Radiograph, Figure 3-1; Copyright Saunders Elsevier; 2012.*

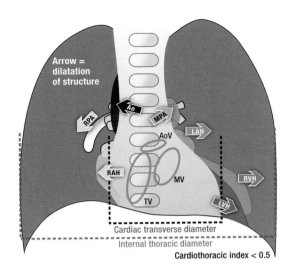

Arrow = dilatation of structure

Cardiac transverse diameter

Internal thoracic diameter

**Cardiothoracic index < 0.5**

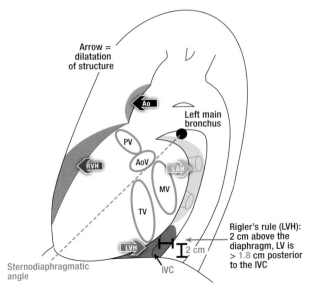

Arrow = dilatation of structure

Left main bronchus

Sternodiaphragmatic angle

Rigler's rule (LVH): 2 cm above the diaphragm, LV is > 1.8 cm posterior to the IVC

2 cm

**CARDIOTHORACIC INDEX (PA): < 0.5**

> **False-positive**: AP film; Obesity; Pregnancy; Pectus excavatum; Ascites; Scoliosis; Under-inspiration

**LA DILATATION**: convexity of the LAA (between LPA and LV); quadruple contour (Ao; PA; LAA; LV); elevation of left main bronchus (carina angle > 90°); right double contour; posterior dilatation on lateral film

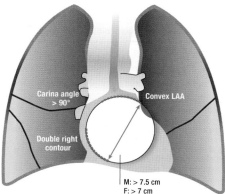

Carina angle > 90°

Convex LAA

Double right contour

M: > 7.5 cm
F: > 7 cm

**RA DILATATION**: right shadow shifted towards the right; ± dilatation of SVC - IVC - azygos vein secondary to ↗ CVP

**RV DILATATION: transverse displacement of the left shadow; RV > 1/3 of the distance between the cardiophrenic angle and the sternal angle (lateral film)**; ± PA dilatation

> **DDx of filling of retrosternal space**: post-sternotomy; lymphadenopathy; mediastinal mass (lymphoma; thymoma; thyroid); pulmonary trunk dilatation; aortic root dilatation; small antero-posterior diameter (pectus excavatum; scoliosis; kyphosis)

**LV DILATATION: prominent apex displaced downwards**; downward displacement of gastric bubble and posterior displacement of LV (> 1.8 cm with respect to IVC) on the lateral film

**PA DILATATION**: L→R shunt; post-stenotic dilatation (main PA and LPA); Pulmonary hypertension (venous or arterial); PR; idiopathic

> **RPA dilatation**: > **17 mm**

> **Main PA dilatation**: prominence between the aortic knob and the LAA

**ASCENDING AORTA DILATATION**: prominent right contour of mediastinum; prominent anterior contour of mediastinum on lateral film; distance between left lateral edge of tracheal air column and aortic knob > 35 mm

**NORMAL PULMONARY BLOOD SUPPLY**: peripheral attenuation (distal 1/3 not visible); vessels at base > vessels at lung apex

> **Venous congestion (venous PHT)**: redistribution to apices (cephalization); blurred peripheral vessels; Kerley B lines (1-3 cm long; 1 mm thick; horizontal; arising from pleura); interstitial edema; peribronchial edema; prominent and blurred hila; edema of fissure; pleural effusions; alveolar edema; PA dilatation

  • **Dilatation of azygos vein (>1 cm)**: Right heart failure (↗ CVP); SVC obstruction; Constrictive pericarditis; IVC interruption (venous return via azygos system); anomalous PV connection

> **Peripheral hypervascularization** (vessels visible below the diaphragm)
  a) **L→R shunt**: Dilated PA; branches of PA > associated bronchi; dilatation of heart chambers
  b) **High output state**: pregnancy; hyperthyroidism; anemia

> **Peripheral hypovascularization**
  a) **PHT**: RVH; PA - LPA - RPA dilatation; **early and marked attenuation of peripheral vessels**
  b) **RVOT obstruction**: post-stenotic LPA dilatation in the presence of PS; RVH

# 1.8/ CORONARY ANGIOGRAPHY

## PREPARATION

**BASIC WORK-UP:** CBC; ECG; electrolytes; creatinine-BUN; Clotting tests; target INR < 2.0

**DIABETES:** Discontinue metformin in the event of post-coronary angiography ARF

**PREVENTION OF CONTRAST NEPHROPATHY:** particularly if GFR < 60 mL/min or DM
  a) **Hydration with normal saline**: 1 mL/kg/h x 3-12 h before and 6-24 h after **angiography** (0.5 mL/kg/h if LVEF < 35% or NYHA III-IV)
  b) **Minimize the volume of contrast: < 300 mL or < 4 mL/kg; avoid a contrast volume (mL) / GFR ratio > 3.7**; avoid multiple procedures < 48-72 h
  c) **No benefit of N-acetyl-L-cysteine** (★ACT)
  d) **Avoid nephrotoxic medications** (NSAIDs; ACE inhibitors; ARB)
  e) **Preferred contrast agents: nonionic** (iso-osmolar or low osmolar)

**IODINE ALLERGY:** Prednisone 50 mg 12 h and 1 h before coronary angiography; Diphenhydramine 50 mg PO and Ranitidine 150 mg PO 1 h before coronary angiography

> **Urgent coronary angiography**: Methylprednisolone 125 mg IV + Diphenhydramine 50 mg

## VASCULAR ACCESS

**FEMORAL ACCESS:** use the common femoral artery; puncture site 3 cm below the inguinal ligament (anterior superior iliac crest to superior pubic ramus) but proximal to the femoral bifurcation (bifurcation distal to the middle third of the femoral head); risk of retroperitoneal bleeding if the artery is punctured too high; risk of pseudoaneurysm if the artery is punctured too low

> **Withdrawal of the introducer**: ACT < 180 s

**RADIAL ACCESS:** Allen's test before (color returns to normal < 10 seconds); intraarterial Verapamil; Heparin IV (bolus of 2000 to 5000 units); 4-6 F catheters (1 F = 0.3 mm)

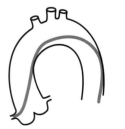 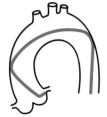

Right Judkins Catheter in the RCA          Left Judkins Catheter in the LCA

**RIGHT DOMINANCE**

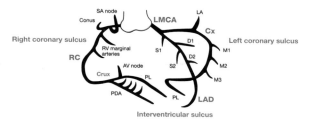

**LEFT DOMINANCE**         **CO-DOMINANCE**

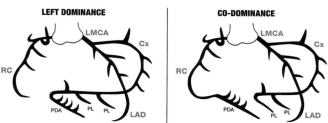

**Source (with permission):** *CathSource iPad application; Rocky Bilhartz, MD; http://ecgsource.com*

**RIGHT DOMINANCE**: 85% of patients; **PDA + ≥ 1 PL arise from the RCA**                +
> **Left dominance**: 7%; PDA and ≥ 1 PL arise from the circumflex; small RCA that does not perfuse the LV wall (ends before the crux cordis)
> **Co-dominance**: 7%; PDA arises from the RCA; all PL arise from the circumflex

**VEIN GRAFT**: adjacent to surgical clip
  a) **Bypass graft of the RCA**: 5 cm above the sinotubular junction; right anterolateral aspect of the Ao
  b) **Bypass graft of the LAD**: 7 cm above the sinotubular junction; anterior aspect of the Ao
  c) **Bypass graft of the circumflex**: 9 cm above the sinotubular junction; left anterolateral aspect of the Ao

## ANGIOGRAPHIC VIEWS

**OBTAIN AT LEAST 2 PERPENDICULAR VIEWS** for each vessel (to exclude eccentric lesions)
  1) **RAO versus LAO versus PA versus lateral**
  2) **Cephalic versus Caudal** (depending on the direction towards which the image intensifier above the patient is inclined); cephalic view → circumflex superior on the image; caudal view → LAD superior on the image

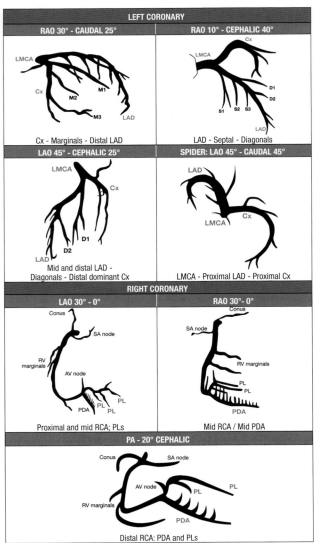

**LEFT CORONARY**

**RAO 30° - CAUDAL 25°**

LMCA

Cx

M2

M1

M3

LAD

Cx - Marginals - Distal LAD

**RAO 10° - CEPHALIC 40°**

Cx

LMCA

D1

D2

S1  S2  S3

LAD

LAD - Septal - Diagonals

**LAO 45° - CEPHALIC 25°**

LMCA

Cx

D1

D2

LAD

Mid and distal LAD -
Diagonals - Distal dominant Cx

**SPIDER: LAO 45° - CAUDAL 45°**

LAD

LMCA

Cx

LMCA - Proximal LAD - Proximal Cx

**RIGHT CORONARY**

**LAO 30° - 0°**

Conus

SA node

RV
marginals

AV node

PL

PDA  PL  PL

Proximal and mid RCA; PLs

**RAO 30° - 0°**

Conus

SA node

RV marginals

PL

PL

PDA

Mid RCA / Mid PDA

**PA - 20° CEPHALIC**

Conus

SA node

AV node

PL

PL

RV marginals

PDA

Distal RCA: PDA and PLs

Redrawn and expanded from (with permission): Uptodate 2015: Zimetbaum PJ, Josephson ME; Conduction abnormalities after myocardial infarction; www.uptodate.com; Post TW (Ed), UpToDate, Waltham, MA, March 2015.

# CORONARY ARTERY STENOSIS

| ANGIOGRAPHIC | HEMODYNAMIC | IVUS (INTRAVASCULAR ULTRASOUND) |
|---|---|---|
| ≥ 70 %<br>(LMCA: ≥ 50%) | FFR ≤ 0.80 | • LMCA: Area < 6 mm²<br>  (6 to 7.5 mm² → determine FFR)<br>• Other vessels: Area < 4 mm² |

Cardiac diagnostic assessment

| CHARACTERISTICS OF THE CORONARY LESION |||
|---|---|---|
| TYPE A: PCI WITH HIGH SUCCESS RATE (> 85%) AND LOW RISK | TYPE B: PCI WITH MODERATE SUCCESS RATE (60-85%) AND MODERATE RISK | TYPE C: PCI WITH LOW SUCCESS RATE (< 60%) AND HIGH RISK |
| • Short (10 mm)<br>• Concentric<br>• Only slightly calcified<br>• Not totally occluded<br>• Not ostial<br>• Easily accessible<br>• Not angulated (< 45°)<br>• Regular contours<br>• No branch lesion<br>• Absence of thrombus | • Tubular (10-20 mm)<br>• Eccentric<br>• Moderately calcified<br>• Total occlusion < 3 months<br>• Ostial<br>• Moderate tortuosities of proximal segment<br>• Moderate angulation (45-90°)<br>• Irregular contours<br>• Bifurcation<br>• Presence of thrombus | • Diffuse (> 20 mm)<br>• Severe tortuosities of proximal segment<br>• Extreme angulation (> 90°)<br>• Bifurcation with impossibility to protect a major branch<br>• Vein graft with friable lesions |

a) **Length**: short (< 10 mm) - tubular (10-20 mm) - diffuse (> 20 mm)
b) **Ostial**: < 3 mm from the ostium; aorto-ostial stenosis often fibrocalcified
c) **Bifurcation**: Medina's X, Y, Z classification
   > **X**: 0 if absence of stenosis or 1 if stenosis in the main proximal segment
   > **Y**: 0 if absence of stenosis or 1 if stenosis in the main distal segment
   > **Z**: 0 if absence of stenosis or 1 if stenosis in the daughter branch
d) **Calcification**: confers rigidity and non-compliance to the dilatation
e) **Angulation**: > 45° moderate; > 90° severe; makes stent placement more difficult and associated with a risk of late stent fracture
f) **Thrombus**: risk of distal microembolism
g) **Eccentricity**: variable stenosis according to angiographic view
h) **Irregularities**: ulcer; intimal flap; aneurysm; saw tooth irregularities (multiple successive irregular stenoses)
i) **Tortuosity of the proximal segment**: moderate (2 proximal curves > 75°) or severe (3 proximal curves > 75°)
j) **Presence of collaterals**: Rentrop classification
k) **TIMI flow**

| TIMI 0 | Total occlusion |
|---|---|
| TIMI 1 | Presence of a very faint anterograde flow beyond the stenosis; no opacification of the distal coronary bed |
| TIMI 2 | Opacification of the entire distal coronary bed, but sluggish flow (compared to vessels with normal flow) |
| TIMI 3 | Anterograde perfusion of all of the distal coronary bed; normal filling velocity |

**MICROVASCULAR EVALUATION**: myocardial "blush" score

## FRACTIONAL FLOW RESERVE (FFR)

**INDICATION**: **estimate the hemodynamic impact of an intermediate angiographic stenosis (50-70%)**

**CALCULATION**: Pressure distal to lesion (Pd) / Pressure proximal to lesion (Pa) ratio during maximum hyperemia (IV or intracoronary adenosine)

**CORONARY BLOOD FLOW DEPENDS ON**: **A)** DBP; **B)** Arteriolar resistance; **C)** Left intraventricular pressure; **D)** Degree of coronary stenosis

> **Abnormal FFR:** **≤ 0.80** (★FAME; ★FAME-2)                                        +

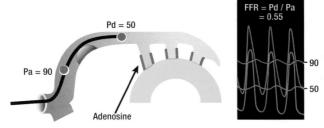

$$FFR = Pd / Pa = 0.55$$

## INTRAVASCULAR ULTRASOUND (IVUS)

**Transverse ultrasound section of the lumen and arterial wall**

**EVALUATION**: real dimensions of the lumen; abnormality of the arterial wall; degree of atherosclerotic infiltration; positive vascular remodeling (Glagov phenomenon)

**INDICATION**: **A)** Specify the severity of LMCA stenosis; **B)** Complex lesion (ostial; bifurcation; aneurysm; dissection); **C)** Bypass graft disease; **D)** Restenosis or intra-stent thrombosis; **E)** Guidance during PCI / evaluation of stent deployment

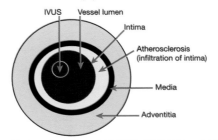

## COMPLICATIONS

**COMPLICATIONS**: **Major complications < 1%;** Death; MI; Contrast nephropathy; Stroke; Local vascular complication (thrombosis; distal embolism; dissection; hematoma; pseudoaneurysm; AV fistula); Arrhythmia; Allergy; Air embolism; Coronary artery dissection; Atheroembolism

**ANAPHYLAXIS:** epinephrine 1:10,000 - **1 mL IV every minute (0.1 mg every minute)**

**HEPARIN ANTIDOTE:** Protamine (1 mg for every 100 units of heparin; if IV infusion of heparine → 25-50 mg of protamine IV slowly); risk of allergy if the patient is treated with NPH insulin

> www.medicines.org.uk/emc/medicine/10807/spc

**RETROPERITONEAL HEMATOMA:** secondary to puncture above the inguinal ligament; hypotension / abdominal pain / back pain; CBC - clotting tests; CT scan; reverse anticoagulation; transfusion PRN; medical treatment in the majority of cases (or covered stent)

**PSEUDOANEURYSM:** pulsatile mass with systolic murmur; ultrasound diagnosis; good prognosis if diameter < 2 cm

> **Noninvasive percutaneous treatment**: ultrasound-guided compression or local injection of thrombin; follow-up US at 1 month
> **Surgery:** large or rapidly progressive pseudoaneurysm or infected or failure of noninvasive treatment

**AV FISTULA:** secondary to puncture below the femoral bifurcation; thrill or continuous murmur; surgical treatment in the majority of cases (risk of progression)

**RADIAL ACCESS COMPLICATIONS:** Hematoma; Arterial dissection or occlusion; Loss of radial pulse; Compartment syndrome; Spasm

**POST-CORONARY ANGIOGRAPHY ARF**

> **Contrast nephropathy**: Early and reversible ARF; Improvement by day 3 to 5

| RISK OF CONTRAST NEPHROTOXICITY POST-PCI | | |
|---|---|---|
| Hypotension | 5 points | **≤ 5 POINTS** |
| IABP | 5 points | • Contrast nephropathy: 7.5% |
| Heart failure | 5 points | • Dialysis: 0.04% |
| > 75 years | 4 points | **6-10 POINTS** |
| Anemia | 3 points | • Contrast nephropathy: 14% |
| Diabetes | 3 points | • Dialysis: 0.1% |
| Each 100 mL of contrast | 1 point | **11-16 POINTS** |
| Creatinine > 130 mmol/L or | 4 points or | • Contrast nephropathy: 26% |
| GFR 40-60 mL/m² | 2 points | • Dialysis: 1% |
| GFR 20-40 mL/m² | 4 points | **> 16 POINTS** |
| GFR < 20 mL/m² | 6 points | • Contrast nephropathy: 57% |
| | | • Dialysis: 13% |

*Mehran R, Aymong ED, Nikolsky E et al. JACC 2004; 44; 1393-1399.*

> **Atheroembolism: subacute ARF** (several days to several weeks); **eosinophilia / eosinophiluria; slightly active urinary sediment; hypocomplementemia; other micro atheroembolic lesions** (toes; livedo reticularis; petechiae; splinter hemorrhage; mesenteric or pancreatic ischemia; retinal Hollenhorst plaques); slight improvement of renal function

# 1.9/ HEMODYNAMIC ASSESSMENT

**INDICATIONS:** More refined assessment of heart disease when noninvasive evaluation is insufficient (heart failure; valvular heart disease; PHT; complicated myocardial infarction; congenital heart disease; intracardiac shunt; pericardial disease; cardiomyopathy; biopsy)

**COMPLICATIONS:** < 1%; death; MI; stroke; arrhythmia; access site complication; allergy to contrast agent; cardiac tamponade / perforation; RBBB during catheterization of RV and LBBB during catheterization of LV; pulmonary infarction; PA perforation

**RIGHT CARDIAC CATHETERIZATION**: RA - RV - PA - pulmonary capillary wedge pressures; cardiac output; search for a shunt; calculation of pulmonary vascular resistance

**LEFT CARDIAC CATHETERIZATION**: LA pressure (transseptal or estimated by wedge pressure) - LV - Ao pressures; coronary angiography; left ventriculography and aortography; calculation of systemic vascular resistance; evaluation of valvular heart disease

> **Transseptal**: verification of the correct position (LA) by atrial pressure curve - oxygen saturation - contrast injection
> **Left ventriculography**: RAO 30° ± LAO 45° (30-40 mL of contrast)

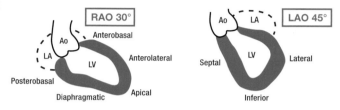

## HEMODYNAMIC DATA

**MEASUREMENTS: at the end of expiration**                                    +

|  | MEAN | NORMAL |
|---|---|---|
| **Cardiac output (L/min)** | 5 | 4 - 6 |
| **Cardiac Index (L/min/m²)** | 3.5 | 2.5 - 4.5 |
| **Aorta pressure (mmHg)** |  |  |
| Systole | 130 | 90-140 |
| End-diastole | 70 | 60-90 |
| Mean | 85 | 70-105 |
|  |  |  |
| Mean BP = 1/3 x SBP + 2/3 X DBP | | |
| **LV PRESSURE (mmHg)** |  |  |
| Systole | 130 | 90-140 |
| End-diastole | 8 | 5-12 |
| **LA pressure (v > a) (mmHg)** |  |  |
| Max | 12 | 6-21 |
| Mean | 8 | 2-12 |
| **PCWP (mmHg)** |  |  |
| Mean | 9 | 4-12 |
| **PAP (mmHg)** |  |  |
| Systole | 25 | 15-30 |
| End-diastole | 9 | 4-12 |
| Mean | 15 | 9-19 |
| Mean PAP = 1/3 x sPAP + 2/3 x dPAP | | |

| | MEAN | NORMAL |
|---|---|---|
| **RV pressure (mmHg)** | | |
| Systole | 25 | 15-30 |
| End-diastole | 4 | 1-7 |
| **RA (a > v) (mmHg)** | | |
| Max | 6 | 2-7 |
| Mean | 3 | 1-5 |
| **Resistance (dyn x s / cm⁵)** | | |
| Systemic vascular resistance | 1100 | 700-1600 |
| Pulmonary vascular resistance | 70 | 20-130 |

- $\Delta P = Q \times R$
- **Systemic vascular resistance (WU)** = Mean arterial pressure - Mean RA pressure / Systemic output
- **Pulmonary vascular resistance (WU)** = Mean PAP - Mean wedge pressure / Pulmonary output
- **Conversion:** 1 WU = 80 dyn x s / cm⁵

## CARDIAC OUTPUT

**FICK:** gold standard method

> - **Systemic cardiac output (L/min)** = $O_2$ consumption (mL/min) /
>   1.36 x Hb (g/L) x (Aortic $SaO_2$ - Mixed venous $SaO_2$)
> - **Pulmonary cardiac output (L/min)** = $O_2$ consumption (mL/min) /
>   1.36 x Hb (g/L) x (PV $SaO_2$ - PA $SaO_2$)

- **Estimation of $O_2$ consumption**: 125 ml/m² in young subjects; 110 mL/m² in elderly subjects
- **$SaO_2$:** expressed as a decimal (70% = 0.70)
- **Mixed venous $SaO_2$:** = 3/4 x SVC $SaO_2$ + 1/4 x IVC $SaO_2$
- **Caveats: A)** Estimation of $VO_2$ (instead of measurement of $VO_2$ by face tent); **B)** High output (attenuated arteriovenous $O_2$ difference)

**THERMODILUTION:** injection of a bolus of NaCl into the vena cava; detection of a change of temperature as a function of time in a distal port (pulmonary artery); **cardiac output is inversely proportional to the area under the curve**

- **Caveats: A)** Significant TR (underestimates cardiac output); **B)** Low output (< 2.5 L/m) in which case cardiac output is overestimated; **C)** Intracardiac shunt (cardiac output overestimated if L→R shunt)

**ANGIOGRAPHIC METHOD**

> - **Cardiac output** = (LV end-diastolic volume - LV end-systolic volume) x HR

- **Caveats: A)** Evaluation of cardiac output in a single cardiac axis; **B)** Less reliable in the presence of MR, AR or AF

## HEMODYNAMIC CURVES

Use the ECG to identify waves on the curves

**A) Polyphasic curves**: atrial recording; pulmonary capillary wedge pressure recording

**B) Monophasic curve**
- **Ventricular recording**: End-diastolic pressure > Early diastolic pressure
- **Arterial recording**: Early diastolic pressure > End-diastolic pressure

# ATRIAL RECORDING

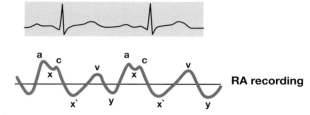

**RA recording**

A WAVE: atrial kick; **follows the P wave on the ECG**

> **Normally**: a > v in RA; v > a in LA
> **↗ a wave**: MS (or TS); ↘ ventricular compliance (LVH or RVH; LVOT or RVOT obstruction)
> **Canon a wave**: AV dissociation (AV block; ventricular pacemaker; VT; PVC; PAC)
> **Absent a wave**: AF or atrial flutter; severe atrial disease (Ebstein; rheumatic MS; cardiac amyloidosis)

X DESCENT: atrial relaxation; **after S1**

> **↗ x descent**: Tamponade; Constriction (W-M pattern)

C WAVE: protrusion of the AV valve into the atrium during isovolumic contraction of the ventricle

X' DESCENT: atrial relaxation + descent of AV valve during systolic ejection

V WAVE: passive atrial filling during ventricular systole in the presence of a closed AV valve; **at the end of the T wave on the ECG**

> **↗ v wave**: MR (or TR); VSD (or ASD on RA recording); rheumatic MS (↘ LA compliance); Heart failure

Y DESCENT: emptying of the atrium following opening of the AV valve (rapid ventricular filling); **after S2**

> **↗ y descent**: Constriction; RCM; MR (or TR)
> **↘ y descent**: Tamponade; MS (or TS)

PCWP: pulmonary capillary wedge pressure; similar curve to LA but delayed by 40-120 ms (pressure transmission delay) and slightly attenuated

> **Adequate wedge pressure**: oximetric confirmation ($SaO_2$ > 95 %); injection of contrast; respiratory variation of the curve
> **Inequality between wedge pressure and LA pressure**: PV obstruction; ↗ Pleural pressure; Catheter in non-dependent pulmonary zone (target West zone 3)
> **dPAP > Wedge**: Pulmonary disease; Pulmonary embolism; significant PHT

# VENTRICULAR RECORDING

SYSTOLE: **A)** Isovolumic contraction; **B)** Ejection; **C)** Reduced ejection then start of relaxation

DIASTOLE: **A)** Isovolumic relaxation; **B)** Rapid filling; **C)** Slow filling (diastasis); **D)** Atrial kick

> **End-diastolic pressure**: after atrial kick at point c (simultaneous with QRS)

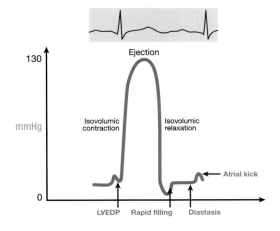

## ARTERIAL RECORDING

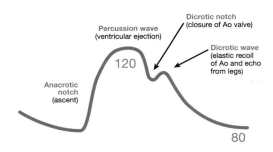

**PULSE PRESSURE**: reflects the stroke volume and compliance of the arterial system

> ↗ **pulse pressure: > 50 % of SBP** (or > 40 mmHg); HTN; Age; AR; patent ductus arteriosus; Ruptured aneurysm of the sinus of Valsalva; Fever; Anemia; Hyperthyroidism; Pregnancy; AV fistula; Paget's disease  +

> ↘ **pulse pressure**: **< 25% of SBP**; Tamponade; Heart failure; Cardiogenic shock; Aortic stenosis  +

**CAROTID PULSE**: similar to central aortic pulsation

| | | |
|---|---|---|
| **CORRIGAN'S PULSE (BOUNDING)** | Abrupt systolic ascent, followed by rapid collapse; increased pulse pressure | **DDx**: AR; patent ductus arteriosus; truncus arteriosus; fever; anemia; hyperthyroidism; pregnancy; exercise; AV fistula; Paget's disease; Beriberi; bradycardia in an elderly patient with non-compliant aorta |
| **PULSUS PARVUS ET TARDUS (ANACROTIC)** | | • **AS**<br>• **Tardus**: slow ascent<br>• **Parvus**: decreased amplitude<br>• ± Thrill |
| **PULSUS BISFERIENS (BIFID)** | 2 peaks during systole (percussion wave then tidal wave) | • **DDx**: AR; HCM; patent ductus arteriosus<br>• **Tidal wave**: echo from leg vessels<br>• **HCM: spike and dome** (rapid initial ascent then dynamic LVOT obstruction) |
| **DICROTIC PULSE** | 1 peak in systole and 1 peak in diastole | **DDx**: IABP; severe heart failure; tamponade; hypovolemia; sepsis |
| **PULSUS PARADOXUS** | **> 10 mmHg reduction** of systolic blood pressure on inspiration | **DDx**: Tamponade; constriction - effusion; RCM; COPD; Asthma; Pulmonary embolism; Pneumothorax; Hypovolemia; Obesity; Pregnancy<br>• **Reversed pulsus paradoxus**: HCM |
| **PULSUS ALTERNANS** | | **DDx**: Severe heart failure; bigeminy; tamponade; severe AR; tachypnea |

# AORTIC STENOSIS

**TRANSVALVULAR GRADIENT:** measurement of blood pressures in proximal Ao and LV

> **Mean gradient**: integral of the transvalvular gradient during systole
> **Peak-to-peak gradient**: not physiological as peaks not simultaneous
> **Pressure in femoral artery**: **underestimation** of transvalvular gradient (due to peripheral amplification of SBP)

**FIXED OBSTRUCTION: pulsus parvus et tardus** on aortic recording

**CARABELLO'S SIGN: > 10 mmHg** increase in SBP following withdrawal of the catheter from the LV towards the aorta (obstructive catheter in critical aortic stenosis)

---

**HAKKI FORMULA:** Aortic valve area = CO (L/min) / √ mean gradient (or peak-to-peak gradient)

**GORLIN FORMULA:** Aortic valve area = Stroke volume (mL/beat) / (44.3 x Systolic ejection period (s / beat) x √ Mean gradient mmHg)

---

**CAVEATS: A)** Concomitant AR: calculate cardiac output (or stroke volume) by the angiographic method; **B)** Aortic stenosis in the presence of low cardiac output (dobutamine challenge)

# MITRAL STENOSIS

**TRANSVALVULAR GRADIENT:** transseptal measurement of LA and LV pressures

> **LA pressure estimated by PCWP: overestimates the transvalvular gradient** (delayed transmission of pressure waves and attenuation of y descent)

---

**GORLIN FORMULA:** Mitral valve area = Stroke volume (mL/beat) / (37.7 x Diastolic filling period (s / beat) x √ mean gradient mmHg)

---

**CAVEAT:** Concomitant MR: calculate stroke volume by angiographic method

# VALVULAR REGURGITATION

**REGURGITANT VOLUME** = Angiographic stroke volume (end-diastolic volume - end-systolic volume) - Net anterograde stroke volume (Fick or Thermodilution)

**REGURGITANT FRACTION** = Regurgitant volume / Angiographic stroke volume

| SEMIQUANTITATIVE ANGIOGRAPHIC EVALUATION (ventriculography or aortography) | | |
|---|---|---|
| **GRADE** | **Regurgitant fraction** | **Opacification of the proximal chamber** |
| 1 | < 20 % | • Slight opacification<br>• Rapid elimination of contrast at each beat |
| 2 | 21-40 % | • Moderate opacification<br>• Density less than that of the proximal chamber<br>• Rapid elimination of contrast with subsequent beats |
| 3 | 41-60 % | • Intense opacification<br>• Similar density to that of the proximal chamber in 4-5 beats |
| 4 | > 60 % | • Intense and rapid opacification<br>• Density greater than that of the proximal chamber in ≤ 3 beats<br>• ± PV reflux in the presence of MR |

## INTRACARDIAC SHUNT

| Level of L→R shunt | Increased SaO$_2$ (step-up) | Example |
|---|---|---|
| **Screening** | PA SaO$_2$ - SVC SaO$_2$ ≥ 8% | Shunt at any level between the SVC and the PA |
| **Atrial** | RA SaO$_2$ - mixed venous SaO$_2$ ≥ 7% | ASD; Partial anomalous pulmonary venous connection; Ruptured aneurysm of the sinus of Valsalva; VSD + TR; Coronary fistula to RA |
| **Ventricular** | RV SaO$_2$ - RA SaO$_2$ ≥ 5% | VSD; Patent ductus arteriosus + PR; Primum ASD; Coronary fistula to RV |
| **Pulmonary artery** | PA SaO$_2$ - RV SaO$_2$ ≥ 5% | Patent ductus arteriosus; Aortopulmonary window; Palliative shunt (Pots; Waterston) |

**QP / QS**: Pulmonary blood flow / Total systemic blood flow

> **QP / QS** = Ao SaO$_2$ - mixed venous SaO$_2$ / PV SaO$_2$ - PA SaO$_2$
>
> **MIXED VENOUS SaO$_2$** = 3/4 x SVC SaO$_2$ + 1/4 x IVC SaO$_2$
>
> **PV SaO$_2$**: ≈ Ao saturation in the absence of R→L shunt

| Qp / Qs < 1.5 | Qp / Qs 1.5 - 2 | Qp / Qs > 2 |
|---|---|---|
| Small L→R shunt | Moderate L→R shunt | Large L→R shunt |

**OXIMETRIC RUN**: SVC (2 x); IVC (2 x); RA (3 x); RV (3 x); main PA; RPA; LPA; LV; Ao; ± PV and ± LA

**SCREENING OF R→L SHUNT**: Ao SaO$_2$ < 95% despite FiO2 = 100%

## 1.10/ NUCLEAR MEDICINE

### SPECT MYOCARDIAL PERFUSION IMAGING

**SPECT**: Single-Photon Emission Computed Tomography

**PRINCIPLE:** Injection of a radioisotope (at rest then on exercise) → extraction by viable perfused myocytes → **emission of photons proportional to myocyte perfusion**

**THREE STANDARD PERPENDICULAR PLANES: A)** Short axis (apex to base); **B)** Vertical long axis (septum to lateral wall); **C)** Horizontal long axis (inferior wall to anterior wall)

**ARTIFACTS / FALSE-POSITIVES: A)** Movement during acquisition; **B)** Extraction of radioisotope by visceral organs; **C)** LBBB (use pharmacological stress); **D)** Septal HCM (relative perfusion deficit in lateral wall compared to hypertrophied septum); **E)** Dilated cardiomyopathy or HCM (zones of fibrosis; endothelial dysfunction); **F)** Attenuation

> **Attenuation by interposed structure**: **A)** Breasts → anterior / anterolateral attenuation; **B)** Diaphragm → inferobasal attenuation (improvement when patient upright)
>   • **Rule out attenuation: A)** Raw cine mode (look for interposed structure); **B)** Ventricular function (real perfusion deficit unlikely if normal wall motion on stress test)
> **Normal variants**: Membranous basal septum (less perfused); Apical thinning; Lateral wall appears to be better perfused than the septum (closer to the camera)

|  | 201–Thallium | 99m Technetium |
|---|---|---|
| **Molecule** | Cation; similar properties to K+ | • Fat-soluble cationic compound<br>• Sestamibi and Tetrofosmin |
| **Photon energy** | 80 keV | 140 keV |
| **Half-life** | 73 h | 6 h |
| **First-pass myocardial extraction** | • 85 %<br>• Perfusion-dependent<br>• Via Na-K-ATPase pump | • 60 %<br>• Perfusion-dependent<br>• Passive myocardial extraction (radioisotope trapped in mitochondria) |
| **Myocardial redistribution** | • Imaging 3-4 h or 24 h post-injection<br>• Clearance of radioisotope is slower in ischemic myocardium ("differential washout") | Minimal (2 injections are therefore necessary: stress test and at rest) |
| **Protocol** | 1. **Detection of ischemia**: Injection on stress test with imaging #1; imaging #2 post-redistribution<br>2. **Viability study**: Injection at rest with imaging #1; imaging #2 post redistribution (re-injection at this time to improve sensitivity) | 1. **Same day**: injection at rest (8-10 mCi) with imaging #1; injection on stress test with imaging #2 (22-30 mCi)<br>2. **2 days**: injection at rest (20-30 mCi) with imaging #1; injection on stress test (20-30 mCi) with imaging #2<br>3. **Combined with Thallium**: Injection of Thallium at rest with imaging #1; imaging #2 4h pre-Technetium (redistribution; viability study); injection of Technetium on stress test with imaging #3 (to detect ischemia) |

**DIPYRIDAMOLE PHARMACOLOGICAL STRESS TEST**: ↗ intracellular adenosine → stimulation of smooth muscle cell adenosine A2a receptors → ↗ cAMP → coronary arteriolar vasodilatation → ↗ coronary blood flow

> **Dose**: 142 µg/kg/min x 4 min (then inject isotope 3 min later)
> **Adverse effects**: ↘ SBP and ↘ DBP (8-10 mmHg); reflex tachycardia (↗ **10-20 bpm**); minimal increase of double product (i.e. slightly ↗ $O_2$ demand); flushing; retrosternal chest pain; asthma; blocks; real ischemia (in 10% of cases; coronary steal in ischemic collateral vessels)
> **Antidote**: aminophylline 1-2 mg/kg

**REST**

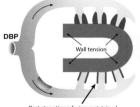

**Coronary perfusion depends on:**
* DBP
* Arteriolar resistance
* Wall tension
* Coronary stenosis

Post-stenotic perfusion maintained via arteriolar dilatation (autoregulation)

**STRESS TEST** (exercise; dipyridamole)

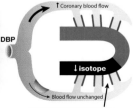

↑ Coronary blood flow

↓ isotope

Blood flow unchanged

Insufficient coronary flow reserve = relative perfusion defect

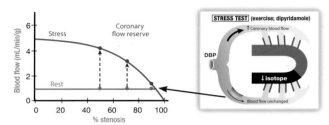

## HIGH RISK CRITERIA

> **Negative test:** 1-year risk of death or myocardial infarction < 1% (exercise) or < 2% (dipyridamole)
> **Resting LVEF:** < 35 %
> **Extensive perfusion abnormality during stress:** ≥ 10% of the myocardium or involving ≥ 2 vascular territories
> **Pulmonary uptake of** $^{201}$**Tl (during stress):** marker of severe CAD (↗ wedge pressure and ↘ LVEF during stress)
> **Transient LV dilatation (during stress):** ↗ ventricular chamber size; marker of severe CAD (↘ LVEF during stress and/or diffuse subendocardial ischemia)

**VENTRICULAR FUNCTION:** ECG-gated imaging → mean of hundreds of beats to obtain one cardiac cycle

## RADIONUCLIDE VENTRICULOGRAPHY (RVG)

### Evaluation of LVEF and RVEF

**EQUILIBRIUM (MUGA):** ECG gating; 99m Technetium-labeled RBC; mean of 1000 cycles; 3 standard views (anterior; LAO with optimal separation of RV and LV; lateral); evaluation of chamber dimension - regional wall motion - systolic function

> **Systolic function:** estimated on biplane mode by counting photon emissions in the ventricle (diastole - systole / diastole)
>   • **Systolic volume:** the count is proportional to ventricular volume (which can be estimated from a blood sample of a given volume and a given photon emission); measurement not influenced by ventricular geometry
> **Diastolic function:** curve of ventricular volume as a function of time

**FIRST-PASS:** rapid bolus of Technetium 99m-DTPA → RA - RV → Lungs → LA - LV; can distinguish the activity of right and left (**better evaluation of the RV and shunt**); RAO view

## POSITRON EMISSION TOMOGRAPHY

Quantitative evaluation of myocardial perfusion

**ADVANTAGES VERSUS SPECT:** better spatial resolution; better correction of attenuation; evaluates **absolute quantitative regional perfusion (mL/g/min) (unlike SPECT which evaluates relative regional perfusion);** better evaluation of balanced ischemia or microvascular disease

> **Disadvantages:** requires a cyclotron; short half-life (pharmacological stress test only)
> $^{82}$**Rubidium:** cation with similar properties to those of the potassium and thallium; transport via Na-KATPase pump; half-life 75 s; perfusion-dependent myocardial extraction
> [$^{13}$N]**ammonia:** passive diffusion or transport via Na-K-ATPase pump; half-life 10 min; perfusion-dependent myocardial extraction

**VIABILITY STUDY:** quantitative evaluation of myocardial metabolism (2-[$^{18}$F]FDG); **glucose extraction maintained in ischemic myocardium** (anaerobic glycolysis); **"mismatch" between myocardial perfusion and glucose metabolism in ischemic but viable (hibernating) myocardium**                                                      +

| MULTIMODAL EVALUATION OF VIABILITY | | | |
|---|---|---|---|
| **DOBUTAMINE ECHOCARDIOGRAPHY** | **THALLIUM** | **CARDIAC PET** | **GADOLINIUM ENHANCED CARDIAC MRI** |
| **Hibernating myocardium:** Biphasic response | **Hibernating myocardium:** Redistribution | **Hibernating myocardium:** Perfusion-metabolism discordance | **Late gadolinium enhancement** = scar (absence of viability) |

| | | | |
|---|---|---|---|
| Resting | Resting | Resting | Resting |
| Baseline RWMA | Relative perfusion deficit | Relative perfusion deficit | Late gadolinium enhancement = scar |
| Dobutamine 5 µg/kg/min | Redistribution | FDG metabolism | |
| Improvement | Differential washout | Glucose extraction maintained | |
| Dobutamine 20 µg/kg/min | | | |
| Deterioration | | | |

# 1.11/ CARDIAC MAGNETIC RESONANCE IMAGING (CARDIAC MRI)

**PHYSICAL PRINCIPLE:** detects electromagnetic signals of nuclei of hydrogen atoms following application of a specific sequence of magnetic fields

## PRECAUTIONS

**CONTRAINDICATIONS: ferromagnetic material** (stents and valve prostheses safe); **www.mrisafety.com**

> **Pacemaker and defibrillator (before new compatible generation):** contraindication to MRI; risk of arrhythmia; displacement of the device; inhibition; inappropriate shock; lead injury; battery depletion...

**GADOLINIUM:** risk of nephrogenic systemic fibrosis if **CrCl < 30 mL/min/1.73 m²**

## TISSUE CHARACTERIZATION

| T1 | **Fat content:** ARVD; myocardial mass |
|---|---|
| T2 | **Myocardial water content:** acute myocarditis; acute myocardial infarction (high-risk zone); graft rejection |
| T2* | **T2* < 20 msec:** (associated with LV dysfunction) compatible with iron overload cardiomyopathy (repeated transfusions; hemochromatosis) |
| T1 Gadolinium-enhanced | Visualization of intravascular (blood) and extravascular water (myocardium)<br>• **First pass:** myocardial perfusion<br>• **Early gadolinium enhancement (EGE):** sign of inflammation (myocarditis; acute myocardial infarction)<br>• **Late gadolinium enhancement (LGE):** 15 minutes post-redistribution; sign of fibrosis / myocardial necrosis |

| Ischemic heart disease | LGE: **subendocardial or transmural scar** | |
|---|---|---|
| Nonischemic cardiomyopathy | LGE: **non-subendocardial scar** | |
| HCM | **LGE:** scars in hypertrophied regions or in IV septum or close to the insertion of the RV | |
| Amyloidosis | • Rapid accumulation of contrast in the myocardium (rapid first-pass washout from blood)<br>• **LGE:** circumferential subendocardial enhancement; transmural patchy enhancement<br>• Late atrial enhancement | |
| Sarcoidosis Myocarditis | • **LGE:** intramural or subepicardial or epicardial scar, sparing the endocardium<br>• **Sarcoidosis:** anteroseptal and inferolateral walls often affected | |

## INDICATIONS

**CARDIOMYOPATHY / HEART FAILURE / MYOCARDITIS:** dimensions; systolic and diastolic functions; segmental wall motion; measurement of deformation (strain); tissue characterization (sarcoidosis; myocarditis; amyloidosis; hemochromatosis); viability - scars (LGE); HCM; ARVD; LV noncompaction; Chagas…

**CORONARY DISEASE:** scar - viability (LGE); congenital anomaly of coronary arteries; coronary fistula; segmental wall motion (at rest and with dobutamine); first-pass gadolinium perfusion study (at rest and with dipyridamole); acute myocardial infarction (T2)

**VALVULAR HEART DISEASE:** stenosis (phase contrast is used to measure transvalvular velocities); regurgitation (volumetric method comparing RV and LV stroke volumes; phase contrast is used to measure anterograde and retrograde transvalvular velocities to calculate the regurgitant volume); perivalvular mass (fibroelastoma; vegetation; thrombus); complication of endocarditis; prosthetic valve dysfunction

**CARDIAC MASSES:** intracardiac thrombus (**non-vascularized**; absence of gadolinium enhancement); primary and secondary tumors (metastases)

**PERICARDIAL DISEASE:** constriction (paradoxical movement of the interventricular septum; ventricular interdependence; IVC distension); congenital absence of pericardium

**CONGENITAL HEART DISEASE:** anatomical assessment; structure - dimensions - function of chambers; conduits; shunts; Ao and PA

**THORACIC AORTA:** aneurysm; ulcer; dissection; CoA; aortitis; post-surgery; intramural thrombus

# 1.12/ CARDIAC CT

## UNENHANCED CORONARY CALCIUM SCAN

This technique estimates the global coronary atherosclerotic burden; **very high sensitivity but low specificity for significant coronary stenosis**; independent predictor of coronary events (score of 0 associated with excellent prognosis)

> **INDICATIONS: asymptomatic patient with intermediate risk of cardiac events (10-20% at 10 years)**

> › **Agatston score:** score > 300 confers a 10-year risk of myocardial infarction or cardiovascular mortality of 28% (score of 100-399 increases the risk x 4 versus score < 100; score > 400 increases the risk x 6)

## CARDIAC CT ANGIOGRAPHY (CCTA)

**STRUCTURES EVALUATED:** heart chambers; ventricular function (R and L); coronary arteries; bypass grafts; aortic and pulmonary arteries; pericardium; other adjacent structures; congenital heart disease; congenital coronary artery anomalies; endocarditis; ARVD; prosthetic valve; cardiac mass / thrombus; pulmonary veins

**CORONARY CT ANGIOGRAPHY:** good spatial resolution (vessels > 1.5 mm); **excellent sensitivity for significant coronary stenosis (very high negative predictive value for CAD); stenosis identified is not necessarily hemodynamically significant** and is not necessarily associated with ischemia (FFR-CT under development); decreased specificity in the presence of significant calcifications (Agatston score > 400) or obesity or HR > 65 bpm or AF or stent; independent predictor of coronary events (negative CCTA associated with excellent prognosis); can be used to evaluate patency of coronary bypass grafts; no difference on clinical outcome between CCTA vs. Functional testing in patients with suspected CAD (★ PROMISE)

> **Indication: A)** Patient with no history of CAD presenting with retrosternal chest pain and intermediate pretest probability (especially when other noninvasive tests are inconclusive); **B)** Patient with low to moderate risk ACS (★ROMICAT-II); **C)** Rule out congenital anomaly of coronary arteries; **D)** Potential value for pre-op assessment before cardiac surgery when bypass graft is not planned (rule out significant CAD)

## 1.13/ CARDIOPULMONARY EXERCISE TESTING

**Global evaluation of the oxygen transport system**

INDICATIONS: **A)** Pre-transplantation assessment; **B)** Distinguish cardiac dyspnea from pulmonary dyspnea

PROTOCOL: Naughton; ↗ 1 MET every 2 min

FICK EQUATION

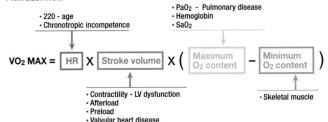

$$VO_2 \text{ MAX} = \boxed{HR} \times \boxed{\text{Stroke volume}} \times \left( \boxed{\substack{\text{Maximum} \\ O_2 \text{ content}}} - \boxed{\substack{\text{Minimum} \\ O_2 \text{ content}}} \right)$$

- 220 - age
- Chronotropic incompetence

- PaO$_2$ - Pulmonary disease
- Hemoglobin
- SaO$_2$

- Contractility - LV dysfunction
- Afterload
- Preload
- Valvular heart disease

- Skeletal muscle

PARAMETERS MEASURED: VO$_2$ (O$_2$ consumption); VCO$_2$ (CO$_2$ production); VE (minute ventilation); HR; BP; RR; SaO$_2$; PFTs; exercise ECG

> **Ventilatory anaerobic threshold (VAT):** value of VO$_2$ when the slope of VE (or the slope of VCO$_2$) increases disproportionately to the slope of VO$_2$ (↗ CO$_2$ to be expired secondary to anaerobic glycolysis with formation of lactate); often at 50-60% of VO$_2$max (point at which dyspnea is experienced); activities of daily living situated below the VAT

> **Respiratory exchange ratio (VCO$_2$/VO$_2$): ratio > 1.05 means that the patient has achieved adequate exertion**  +

> **VE/VCO$_2$ slope: slope > 35 associated with poor prognosis**; reflects hyperventilation secondary to V/Q abnormalities with ↗ dead space  +

> **Borg scale:** quantification of the exertion perceived by the patient; > 18 / 20 = maximum exertion; > 15-16 / 20 = anaerobic threshold reached

| | **VO$_2$ MAX** | **ANAEROBIC THRESHOLD** | **MAXIMUM CARDIAC INDEX** |
|---|---|---|---|
| **Heart failure with good prognosis** | > 18 mL O$_2$/kg/min | > 14 mL O$_2$/kg/min | > 8 L/min/m² |
| **High-risk heart failure (consider transplantation)** | < 10 mL O$_2$/kg/min (anaerobic threshold reached) | < 8 mL O$_2$ /kg/min | < 4 L/min/m² |
| **Gray zone** | VE/VCO$_2$ slope > 35 associated with poor prognosis | | |

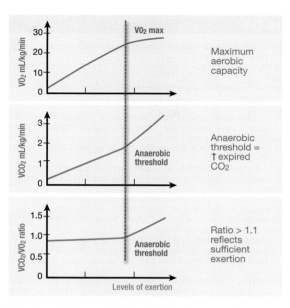

**VO₂ max** — Maximum aerobic capacity

**Anaerobic threshold** = ↑ expired $CO_2$

**Anaerobic threshold** — Ratio > 1.1 reflects sufficient exertion

Levels of exertion

## 1.14/ EXPOSURE TO RADIATION DURING CARDIAC EXAMINATIONS

| | |
|---|---|
| CXR (PA - lateral) | 0.1 mSv |
| Diagnostic coronary angiography | 7 mSv |
| PCI (or RF ablation) | 15 mSv |
| Coronary CT angiography | 5 mSv |
| Coronary calcium scan | 3 mSv |
| MibiP | 9.4 mSv |
| Thallium (stress - redistribution) | 41 mSv |
| FDG PET | 8 mSv |
| V/Q scintigraphy | 2.2 mSv |
| CT pulmonary angiography | 15 mSv |
| Radionuclide ventriculography (equilibrium) | 7.8 mSv |

- Bonow RO, Mann DL, Zipes DP, Libby P. *Braunwald's Heart Disease. A textbook of cardiovascular medicine.* Elsevier. 2012. 1961 p.
- Chizner MA. Cardiac Auscultation: Rediscovering the Lost Art. *Curr Probl Cardiol* 2008; *33* : 326-408
- AHA/ACCF/HRS Recommendations for the Standardization and Interpretation of the Electrocardiogram. Part II: Electrocardiography Diagnostic Statement List. *JACC* 2007; *49;* 1128-1135.
- AHA/ACCF/HRS Recommendations for the Standardization and Interpretation of the Electrocardiogram. Part III: Intraventricular Conduction Disturbances. *JACC* 2009; *53;* 976-981.
- AHA/ACCF/HRS Recommendations for the Standardization and Interpretation of the Electrocardiogram. Part IV: The ST Segment, T and U Waves, and the QT Interval. *JACC* 2009; *53;* 982-991.
- AHA/ACCF/HRS Recommendations for the Standardization and Interpretation of the Electrocardiogram. Part V: Electrocardiogram Changes Associated With Cardiac Chamber Hypertrophy. *JACC* 2009; *53;* 992-1002
- AHA/ACCF/HRS Recommendations for the Standardization and Interpretation of the Electrocardiogram. Part VI: Acute Ischemia/Infarction. *JACC* 2009; *53;* 1003-1011
- Exercise Standards for Testing and Training: A Scientific Statement From the American Heart Association. *Circulation* 2013; *128:* 873-934
- ACC/AHA 2002 Guideline Update for Exercise Testing. *Circulation* 2002; *106* :1883-1892
- Recommendations for Cardiac Chamber Quantification by Echocardiography in Adults: An Uptate from the American Society of Echocardiography and the European Association of Cardiovascular Imaging. *JASE* 2015; *28;* 1-39.
- Recommendations for the Evaluation of Left Ventricular Diastolic Function by Echocardiography. *JASE* 2009; *22;* 107-133. Guidelines for the Echocardiographic Assessment of the Right Heart in Adults: A Report from the American Society of Echocardiography. *JASE* 2010; *23;* 685-713.
- Echocardiographic Assessment of Valve Stenosis: EAE/ASE Recommendations for Clinical Practice. *JASE* 2009; *22;* 1-23.
- Wilkins GT, Weyman AE, Abascal VM et al. Percutaneous balloon dilatation of the mitral valve: an analysis of echocardiographic variables related to outcome and the mechanism of dilatation. *Br Heart J.* 1988; *60:* 299.
- Recommendations for Evaluation of the Severity of Native Valvular Regurgitation with Two-dimensional and Doppler Echocardiography. *JASE* 2003; *16;* 777-802.
- Recommendations for the echocardiographic assessment of native valvular regurgitation: an executive summary from the European Association of Cardiovascular Imaging. *EHJ - Cardiovas Imaging* 2013; *14;* 611–644
- Recommendations for Evaluation of Prosthetic Valves With Echocardiography and Doppler Ultrasound. *JASE* 2009; *22;* 975-1014.
- American Society of Echocardiography Recommendations for Performance, Interpretation, and Application of Stress Echocardiography. *JASE* 2007; *20;* 1021-1041.
- Guidelines for Performing a Comprehensive Transesophageal Echocardiographic Examination: Recommendations from the American Society of Echocardiography and the Society of Cardiovascular Anesthesiologists. JASE 2013; 26: 921-964
- Recommendations for Performing Transesophageal Echocardiography. *Eur J Echocardiography.* 2001; *2;* 8-21.
- Pibarot P; Dumesnil JG. Prosthesis-patient mismatch: definition, clinical impact, and prevention. *Heart* 2006; *92;* 1022-1029.
- Foster GP, Isselbacher EM, Rose GA. Accurate Localization of Mitral Regurgitant Defects Using Multiplane Transesophageal Echocardiography. *Ann Thorac Surg* 1998; *65* :1025-1031.

- ASE Guidelines for the use of echocardiography in the evaluation of a cardiac source of embolism. *JASE* 2016; *29;* 1-42.
- Otto, CM. *Textbook of clinical echocardiography.* Saunders Elsevier. 2009. 519 p.
- Hutchison, SJ. *Principles of Cardiovascular Radiology.* Elsevier Saunders. 2011. 464 pages.
- ACC/AHA/ASNC Guidelines for the Clinical Use of Cardiac Radionuclide Imaging. *Circulation* 2003; *108;* 1401-1418.
- 2011 ACCF/AHA/SCAI Guideline for Percutaneous Coronary Intervention. *JACC* 2011; *58;* e1-e81
- Guidelines on myocardial revascularization. *EHJ* 2010; *31;* 2501-2555.
- Mehran R, Aymong ED, Nikolsky E et al. A simple risk score for prediction of contrast-induced nephropathy after percutaneous coronary intervention: development and initial validation. *JACC* 2004; *44;* 1393-1399.
- Nishimura RA, Carabello BA. Hemodynamics in the Cardiac Catheterization Laboratory of the 21st Century. *Circulation* 2012, *125;* 2138-2150
- Ibrahim R, Matteau A, Piazza N. *Le bilan hémodynamique par cathétérisme cardiaque. Approche systématique.* Les Presses de l'Université de Montréal. 2009. 205 p.
- Baim DS. *Grossman's Cardiac Catheterization, Angiography and Intervention.* Seventh Edition. Lippincott Williams & Wilkins. 2006. 807 p.
- ACCF/ACR/AHA/NASCI/SCMR 2010 Expert Consensus Document on Cardiovascular Magnetic Resonance. *JACC* 2010; *55;* 2614-2662.
- Francis SA, Coelho-Filho OR. O'Gara PT et al. Classic Images in Cardiac Magnetic Resonance Imaging: A Case-based Atlas Highlighting Current Applications of Cardiac Magnetic Resonance Imaging. *Curr Probl Cardiol* 2009; *34* :303-322.
- West AM, Kramer CM. Cardiovascular Magnetic Resonance Imaging of Myocardial Infarction, Viability, and Cardiomyopathies. *Curr Probl Cardiol* 2010; *35:* 176-220
- ACCF/ACR/AHA/NASCI/SAIP/SCAI/SCCT 2010 Expert Consensus Document on Coronary Computed Tomographic Angiography; *JACC* 2010; *55;* 2663-2699.
- ACCF/AHA 2007 Clinical Expert Consensus Document on Coronary Artery Calcium Scoring By Computed Tomography in Global Cardiovascular Risk Assessment and in Evaluation of Patients With Chest Pain. *JACC* 2007; *49;* 378-402.
- Clinician's Guide to Cardiopulmonary Exercise Testing in Adults A Scientific Statement From the American Heart Association. *Circulation* 2010; *122;*191-225
- UpToDate 2015

**01**

Cardiac diagnostic assessment

# Coronary artery disease (CAD) & Myocardial infarction

**02**

| 2.1/ | Stable angina | 72 |
|---|---|---|
| 2.2/ | Biomarkers | 80 |
| 2.3/ | Myocardial infarction: Definition | 81 |
| 2.4/ | Unstable angina & NSTEMI | 83 |
| 2.5/ | STEMI | 88 |
| 2.6/ | Acute coronary syndrome: Adjuvant treatments | 95 |
| 2.7/ | Complications of myocardial infarction | 98 |
| 2.8/ | Revascularization - PCI | 103 |
| 2.9/ | Revascularization - Coronary artery bypass graft | 106 |
| 2.10/ | Prinzmetal angina (vasospastic angina) | 108 |
| 2.11/ | Cardiac syndrome X | 108 |

# 2.1/ STABLE ANGINA

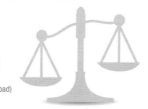

**O₂ DEMAND**
- HR
- Wall stress (preload; afterload)
- Contractility

**O₂ SUPPLY**
- Coronary perfusion pressure (DBP – LVEDP)
- Patent coronary arteries
- Blood O₂ content

## ANGINA: Clinical diagnosis ＋

| Constrictive retrosternal chest pain | On exertion (or emotions) | Relieved by rest (5–10 min) or nitrates |
|---|---|---|
| Typical chest pain = 3 | Atypical chest pain = 2 | Nonanginal chest pain = 1 |

**CLINICAL HISTORY**: Nature; Site; Radiation; Tempo; Duration; Modifiers; Associated symptoms (cardiovascular; respiratory; gastrointestinal)

## SEVERITY OF ANGINA

| CCS 1/4 | Ordinary activity does not cause angina | **≥ 7 METs**<br>• Angina occurs with strenuous or rapid or prolonged exertion only |
|---|---|---|
| CCS 2/4 | Slight limitation of ordinary activity | **5–7 METs**<br>• ≥ 2 flights of stairs<br>• Walking ≥ 3 blocks on the level (or walking uphill)<br>• Exertion after meals or in cold weather |
| CCS 3/4 | Marked limitation of ordinary activity | **2–5 METs**<br>• ≤ 1 flight of stairs<br>• Walking one or two blocks on the level |
| CCS 4/4 | Inability to carry out any physical activity without discomfort or angina at rest | **< 2 METs**<br>• Any activity<br>• Walking several steps |

**ANGINA EQUIVALENT:** Dyspnea; Tiredness

**CHARACTERISTICS NOT IN FAVOR OF CARDIAC CHEST PAIN**: Pleuritic; Abdominal; Localized; Reproduced on palpation; Reproduced on movement; Duration < several seconds or > several hours

**DDX**: Aortic dissection; Aortic stenosis; HCM; Secondary ischemia (anemia; hyperthyroidism; arrhythmia); Cocaine; Pericarditis; Myocarditis; Takotsubo; Cardiac syndrome X (Microvascular); Pulmonary embolism; Pneumothorax; Pneumonia; PHT (RV ischemia); Pleurisy; Ruptured esophagus (Boerhaave); Pancreatitis; Cholecystitis; Cholelithiasis; Peptic ulcer (perforated); GERD; Esophageal spasm; Musculoskeletal; Costochondritis; Neck pain; Shoulder tendinitis; Shingles; Psychiatric

**TWO OBJECTIVES**

**a) Confirm the diagnosis of CAD**
**b) Establish the prognosis of the patient's CAD**

**ISCHEMIC CASCADE**

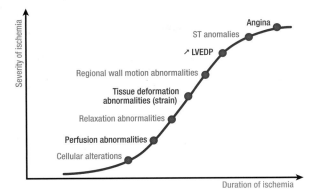

**PRETEST PROBABILITY OF SIGNIFICANT CAD** on coronary angiography in a patient with retrosternal chest pain

| AGE | NONANGINAL CHEST PAIN (≤ 1 CHARACTERISTIC) | | ATYPICAL CHEST PAIN (2 CHARACTERISTICS) | | TYPICAL CHEST PAIN (3 CHARACTERISTICS) | |
|---|---|---|---|---|---|---|
| | M | F | M | F | M | F |
| 30-39 | 4 % | 2 % | 34 % | 12 % | 76 % | 26 % |
| 40-49 | 13 % | 3 % | 51 % | 22 % | 87 % | 55 % |
| 50-59 | 20 % | 7 % | 65 % | 31 % | 93 % | 73 % |
| 60-69 | 27 % | 14 % | 72 % | 51 % | 94 % | 86 % |

*Diamond GA, Forrester JS. N Engl J Med 1979; 300:1350*

**BAYES' THEOREM**: the predictive value of a test depends on its sensitivity, specificity, and the pretest probability of the disease

> The diagnostic value of the test (when it is used to confirm the diagnosis of CAD) is maximal in patients with an **intermediate pretest probability of CAD (10-90%)**

## CHOICE OF NONINVASIVE STRATIFICATION MODALITY

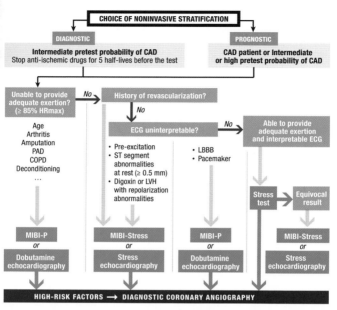

## SENSITIVITY AND SPECIFICITY OF DIAGNOSTIC TESTS TO PREDICT SIGNIFICANT CORONARY ARTERY STENOSIS ON CORONARY ANGIOGRAPHY

|  | SENSITIVITY | SPECIFICITY |
|---|---|---|
| Stress test | 68 % | 77 % |
| MIBI–Stress | 88 % | 72 % |
| MIBI–Dipyridamole | 90 % | 75 % |
| Stress echocardiography | 85 % | 81 % |
| Dobutamine echocardiography | 81 % | 79 % |
| Coronary CT angiography | 95 % | 83 % |

Coronary artery disease (CAD) & myocardial infarction

02

**02**

| **HIGH RISK (ANNUAL MORTALITY OR MYOCARDIAL INFARCTION > 3%)** | • **LVEF**: < 35% at rest (coronary cause)<br>• **LVEF**: LV dysfunction during stress with LVEF at peak stress < 45% or ↘ LVEF ≥ 10%<br>• **LV dilatation during stress**<br>• **Stress test:** Duke score ≤ -11<br>• **Stress test:** ST depression ≥ 2 mm (at low workload or persisting during recovery) or ST elevation or VT/VF on exercise<br>• **Echocardiography:** regional wall motion abnormality during stress involving ≥ 3 segments and/or ≥ 2 vascular territories<br>• **Echocardiography:** regional wall motion abnormality occurring at a low dose of Dobutamine (10 µg/kg/min) or at low HR (< 120 bpm)<br>• **MIBI:** perfusion abnormality at rest involving ≥ 10% of the myocardium (in the absence of a history of MI)<br>• **MIBI:** perfusion abnormality on stress involving ≥ 10% of the myocardium (or involving ≥ 2 vascular territories)<br>• **Agaston score (non-contrast CT):** > 400<br>• **Coronary CT angiography:** multiple vessel disease (stenosis ≥ 70%) or LMCA involvement (stenosis ≥ 50%) |
|---|---|
| **INTERMEDIATE RISK (ANNUAL MORTALITY OR MI: 1-3%)** | • **LVEF**: 35-49% at rest (coronary cause)<br>• **Stress test:** Duke score: -10 to +4<br>• **Stress test**: ST depression ≥ 1 mm + symptoms on exertion<br>• **Echocardiography:** regional wall motion abnormality during stress on 1-2 segments (involving 1 vascular territory)<br>• **MIBI:** perfusion abnormality at rest involving 5 to 9.9% of the myocardium (in the absence of a history of MI)<br>• **MIBI:** perfusion abnormality on stress involving 5 to 9.9% of the myocardium (involving 1 vascular territory)<br>• **Agaston score (non-contrast CT)**: 100-399<br>• **Coronary CT angiography**: 1 vessel with stenosis ≥ 70% (or ≥ 2 vessels with 50-69% stenosis) |
| **LOW RISK (ANNUAL MORTALITY FROM MI < 1%)** | • **Stress test:** Duke score ≥ +5 (or absence of ST abnormalities and symptoms with exercise achieving 85% of predicted HRmax)<br>• **Echocardiography**: normal or limited regional wall motion abnormality at rest and unchanged during stress<br>• **MIBI:** normal or small perfusion defect at rest or on stress involving < 5% of the myocardium<br>• **Agaston score (non-contrast CT):** < 100<br>• **Coronary CT angiography:** absence of stenosis > 50% |

## MANAGEMENT

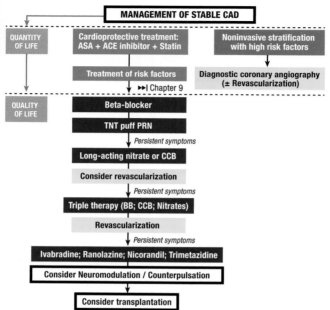

**MANAGEMENT OF STABLE CAD**

QUANTITY
OF LIFE

**Cardioprotective treatment:
ASA + ACE inhibitor + Statin**

**Noninvasive stratification
with high risk factors**

**Treatment of risk factors**
▸▸I Chapter 9

**Diagnostic coronary angiography
(± Revascularization)**

QUALITY
OF LIFE

**Beta-blocker**

**TNT puff PRN**
*Persistent symptoms*

**Long-acting nitrate or CCB**

**Consider revascularization**
*Persistent symptoms*

**Triple therapy (BB; CCB; Nitrates)**

**Revascularization**
*Persistent symptoms*

**Ivabradine; Ranolazine; Nicorandil; Trimetazidine**

**Consider Neuromodulation / Counterpulsation**

**Consider transplantation**

## CARDIOPROTECTIVE TREATMENT

**TREATMENT IMPROVING SURVIVAL**: **A)** ACE inhibitors; **B)** ASA; **C)** Statin

**ASA** (★ Antithrombotic Trialists' Collaboration); Plavix if allergy (★ CAPRIE)

**ACE INHIBITORS**: ★ HOPE; ★ EUROPA; cardioprotective effect; particularly beneficial if LV dysfunction / DM / HTN / CRF

**TREATMENT OF RISK FACTORS**: ▸▸I **Chapter 9**; HTN; Dyslipidemia (statins); DM; Smoking; Exercise program; Target healthy weight; Balanced diet

## ANTI-ANGINAL TREATMENT

**BB**: **first-line**; antagonist of catecholamine adrenergic receptors; **negative inotropic and negative chronotropic agent** (↗ duration of diastole → ↗ coronary perfusion); anti-anginal; antihypertensive; antiarrhythmic    +

> **Intrinsic sympathetic activity (ISA):** partially beta-agonist at rest

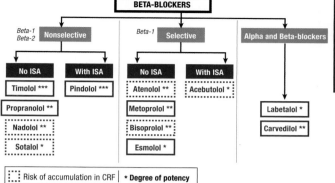

**NITRATES**: converted into NO in the cell → ↗ intracellular cGMP → smooth muscle relaxation (by decreasing intracellular Ca$^{2+}$); **veinodilatation** (↘ preload); **coronary vasodilatation** (↗ perfusion); **systemic arterial vasodilatation** (↘ afterload)

**CALCIUM CHANNEL BLOCKERS**

> **Dihydropyridines**: Nifedipine (★ ACTION); Amlodipine (★ CAMELOT); **systemic arterial vasodilatation** (↘ afterload); **coronary vasodilatation** (↗ perfusion)
> **Nondihydropyridines**: Verapamil; Diltiazem; **negative inotropic and negative chronotropic agent; systemic and coronary arterial vasodilatation**

**IVABRADINE (PROCORALAN):** sinus node I$_f$ channel inhibitor; ↘ **HR** (↗ duration of diastole → ↗ coronary perfusion); ★ INITIATIVE; ★ ASSOCIATE; ★ SIGNIFY: no effect on CV death or MI (but ↗ primary end point among patients with angina of CCS class ≥ 2/4)

**RANOLAZINE (RANEXA):** ↘ **myocyte calcium overload by I$_{Na}$ inhibition**; anti-anginal (★ CARISA; ★ ERICA; ★ MERLIN-TIMI 36)

**NICORANDIL:** 3 mechanisms: **A)** Opening of potassium channels of ischemic cells **(mimics ischemic preconditioning); B)** Opening of potassium channels allowing **systemic and coronary arterial vasodilatation; C)** Similar properties to Nitrates

> ★ **IONA:** Stable CAD; ↘ primary outcome with Nicorandil (cardiovascular mortality - MI - hospitalization)

**TRIMETAZIDINE (VASTAREL): fatty acid oxidation inhibitor;** ★ TRIMPOL II

**EXTERNAL COUNTERPULSATION:** 35 one-hour treatments for 7 weeks; cuffs on lower limbs that inflate in early diastole and deflate in pre-systole; ↗ **collateral circulation and/or angiogenesis and/or improvement of endothelial function**

> **Contraindications:** active DVT; PAD; Aortic aneurysm; Aortic stenosis; Aortic regurgitation; Uncontrolled HTN; Decompensated heart failure

**NEUROMODULATION:** Spinal cord stimulation (T1-T2); ↘ **nociceptive transmission to CNS**

**LASER MYOCARDIAL REVASCULARIZATION DURING CARDIAC SURGERY (THERAPEUTIC ANGIOGENESIS): create subendocardial channels** by left intraventricular laser; consider during refractory angina in the presence of a nonrevascularizable ischemic territory; used exceptionally

| ANTI–ANGINAL | DOSES | ADVERSE EFFECTS |
|---|---|---|
| BETA-BLOCKERS | **Target resting HR 50-60 bpm**<br>**Maintenance dose**<br>• Metoprolol: 50 - 100 mg bid<br>• Bisoprolol: 2.5 - 10 mg qd<br>• Carvedilol: 3.125 - 50 mg bid<br>• Atenolol: 50 - 100 mg qd<br>• Propranolol LA: 80 - 320 mg qd<br>• Nadolol: 40 - 240 mg qd<br>• Esmolol: Bolus IV 500 µg/kg;<br>infusion 50 - 200 µg/kg/min | Bradycardia - Blocks; Negative inotropic agent (heart failure); Bronchospasm; Depression / Tiredness; Nightmares; Erectile dysfunction; masked symptoms of hypoglycemia (prefer Bisoprolol or Metoprolol); rebound ischemia after sudden discontinuation; Possible exacerbation of PAD or Raynaud or Prinzmetal (unopposed alpha stimulation); ↗ TG and ↘ HDL (nonselective BBs) |
| NITRATES | • Sublingual: 0.4 mg/puff every 5 min x 3<br>• Patch: 0.2 - 0.8 mg/h; 8:00 a.m. to 8:00 p.m.<br>• Isosorbide 5-mononitrate (Imdur): 30 to 240 mg qd<br>• Isosorbide dinitrate: 10 - 40 mg tid<br>• IV: 5 - 200 µg/min | Headache; Flushing; Hypotension; Tolerance (prevention by 12-hour period without TNT each day); Methemoglobinemia; Interaction with PDE5 inhibitors; Avoid in the presence of aortic stenosis or HCM |
| DIHYDROPYRIDINE CCBS | • Nifedipine SR (long-acting): 30 - 60 - 90 mg qd<br>• Amlodipine: 2.5 - 10 mg qd | Headache; Faintness; Hypotension; Flushing; Leg edema |
| NONDIHYDRO-PYRIDINE CCBS | **Diltiazem**<br>• PO: 30 - 90 mg tid-qid<br>• CD: 120 - 360 mg qd<br>• Bolus: 0.25 mg/kg IV<br>• Infusion: 5 - 15 mg/h<br>**Verapamil**<br>• PO: 80 - 120 mg tid-qid<br>• SR: 120 - 480 mg qd<br>• Bolus: 0.075 - 0.15 mg/kg | Block; Bradycardia; Heart failure (negative inotropic agent); Hypotension; Flushing; Headache; Leg edema; Drug interactions |
| IVABRADINE | • 5 to 7.5 mg bid | Bradycardia; Phosphenes |
| NICORANDIL | • 10-20 mg bid | Ulcers; Nausea; Hypotension; Headache; Weakness; Flushing |
| TRIMETAZIDINE | • 20 mg tid or 30 mg bid | Nausea; Vomiting; Parkinsonism |
| RANOLAZINE | • 500 to 1000 mg bid | Drug interactions; Nausea; Weakness; ↗ QT (but ↘ delayed after-depolarizations) |

## REVASCULARIZATION

**2 OBJECTIVES**
a) Improve quantity of life (prognosis)
b) Improve quality of life (symptoms)

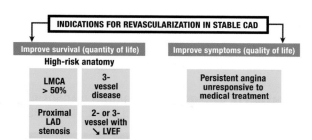

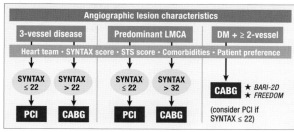

**FACTORS AFFECTING THE PATIENT'S PROGNOSIS**

a) Markers of high risk on noninvasive stratification   +
b) Significant ischemia (> 10% of LV)
c) LV dysfunction
d) Anatomical extent of CAD / Number of vessels involved

**BENEFITS OF CABG VERSUS MEDICAL TREATMENT ON SURVIVAL**: **A) LMCA;**   +
**B) 3 vessels; C) 2 vessels with proximal LAD** (★ Yusuf; ★ VA Cooperative; ★ CASS; ★ ECSS)

**PCI VERSUS MEDICAL TREATMENT**: ★ **COURAGE** → Stable CAD (30% with proximal LAD)   +
→ PCI vs medical treatment; similar survival and infarction rates; ↘ angina with PCI

**CABG VERSUS PCI**: **similar mortality and infarction rates (in patients eligible**   +
**for both procedures)**; ↗ reintervention with PCI; ↗ Procedural stroke with CABG (★ EAST;
★ BARI; ★ ARTS; ★ SOS; ★ BEST)

★ **SYNTAX**: 3-vessel CAD or LMCA (eligible for both procedures) → CABG vs PCI; **similar**   +
**mortality**; ↗ MI and ↗ reintervention with PCI

| SYNTAX score ≤ 22 | SYNTAX score 23–32 | SYNTAX score ≥ 33 |
|---|---|---|
| Similar primary outcome with CABG and PCI | ↗ adverse events with PCI | ↗ adverse events with PCI   + |

**CABG VERSUS PCI FOR LMCA**: ★ SYNTAX subgroup **(patients eligible for both
procedures)**: ↗ reintervention with PCI; ↗ Procedural stroke with CABG

## 2.2/ BIOMARKERS

**Released following myocyte necrosis (myocyte injury)**

**TROPONINS T AND I (CTNT AND CTNI):** very sensitive and specific for myocyte necrosis
**but not very specific for myocardial infarction (ischemic myocyte necrosis)**     +

> **MYOCYTE NECROSIS = LABORATORY DIAGNOSIS**
> **MYOCARDIAL INFARCTION = CLINICAL DIAGNOSIS**

| DIFFERENTIAL DIAGNOSIS OF ELEVATED TROPONIN | | |
|---|---|---|
| • Infarction | • Aortic dissection | • Significant PHT |
| • Heart failure | • Coronary vasospasm | • Severe anemia |
| • Bradyarrhythmia or | • Endothelial dysfunction | • Respiratory failure |
| Tachyarrhythmia | without CAD | • Intense physical exercise |
| • Myocarditis | • PCI | • Cardiotoxic chemotherapy |
| • Pulmonary embolism | • Cardiac surgery | • Cardiotoxins |
| • Aortic valve disease | • Balloon valvuloplasty | • Subarachnoid hemorrhage |
| • Myocardial contusion | • ECV / Defibrillation | • Acute brain syndrome |
| • Takotsubo | • Electrophysiological ablation | • Rhabdomyolysis |
| • Infiltrative cardiomyopathy | • Graft rejection | • Body burn (> 30% BSA) |
| • HCM | • Sepsis | • Scorpion venom |
| • Hypertensive crisis | • Renal failure | |

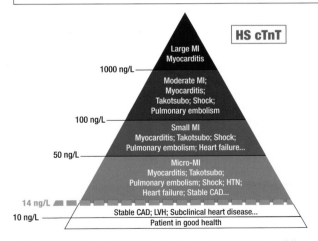

**HS cTnT**

- 1000 ng/L — Large MI / Myocarditis
- Moderate MI; Myocarditis; Takotsubo; Shock; Pulmonary embolism
- 100 ng/L — Small MI / Myocarditis; Takotsubo; Shock; Pulmonary embolism; Heart failure...
- 50 ng/L — Micro-MI / Myocarditis; Takotsubo; Pulmonary embolism; Shock; HTN; Heart failure; Stable CAD...
- 14 ng/L
- 10 ng/L — Stable CAD; LVH; Subclinical heart disease... / Patient in good health

**STANDARD TROPONIN:** obtain a baseline value on arrival in the emergency room (0 h)
and ≥ 1 value **> 6-9 h** after onset of chest pain     +

**HIGH-SENSITIVITY TROPONIN**: First troponin assay on arrival → sensitivity and specificity of 90% and NPV of 97%

> **If hs-cTn negative on arrival (0 h) and 3-6 h after arrival with no significant difference +
> between the two tests (< 20%) → NPV of 99%**

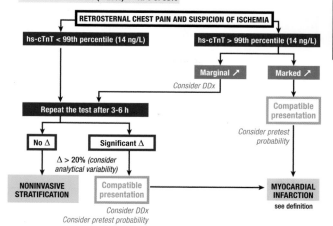

**REINFARCTION**: assay Troponin at 0h - 3h - 6h; **diagnosis of reinfarction if ↗ ≥ 20%** +
(when cTn > 99th percentile pre-reinfarction but with stable or ↘ level)

|  | **INITIAL ELEVATION** | **PEAK** | **RETURN TO NORMAL** |
|---|---|---|---|
| **CK-MB** | **3-12 h** | **24 h** | **48-72 h** |
| **Troponin I** | **3-12 h** | **24 h** | **5-10 d** |
| **Troponin T** | **3-12 h** | **12 h-48 h** | **5-14 d** |
| **Myoglobin** | **1-4 h** | **6-7 h** | **24 h** |

# 2.3/ MYOCARDIAL INFARCTION: DEFINITION

**NECROSIS OF THE MYOCARDIUM IN THE PRESENCE OF MYOCARDIAL ISCHEMIA**

## DIAGNOSTIC CRITERIA

| Detection of ↗ and/or ↘ of a cardiac biomarker (preferably cTn) with ≥ 1 value > 99th percentile (coefficient of variation of the test ≤ 10%) in the presence of myocardial ischemia **+** ≥ 1 of the following elements | • **Symptoms** compatible with **ischemia** +<br>• Δ **ECG changes** compatible with **ischemia** (Δ ST-T abnormalities) or *de novo* LBBB<br>• *De novo* pathological **Q waves**<br>• **Imaging:** loss of viable myocardium or *de novo* RWMA<br>• Intracoronary **thrombus** (on coronary angiography or at autopsy) |
|---|---|

# CLASSIFICATION

| TYPE 1 | **Acute coronary syndrome: primary coronary event**<br>• Plaque rupture / erosion / ulceration; Coronary dissection |
|---|---|
| TYPE 2 | **Infarction secondary to $O_2$ supply and demand imbalance**<br>• Anemia; Hypoxemia; Arrhythmia; HTN; Hypotension; Cocaine; Coronary spasm; Endothelial dysfunction; Coronary embolism |
| TYPE 3 | **Cardiac arrest / Sudden death**<br>• Symptoms suggestive of ischemia +<br>• $\Delta$ ECG changes compatible with ischemia or *de novo* LBBB +<br>• No biomarker assays |
| TYPE 4a | **Infarction secondary to PCI**<br>• Symptoms suggestive of ischemia or ischemic ECG changes or angiographic findings compatible with procedural complication or imaging compatible with loss of viable myocardium or *de novo* RWMA +<br>• Positive biomarkers<br>  a) ↗ cTn ≥ **5 x upper limit of normal** (> 99th percentile) when baseline cTn normal (< 99th percentile) or<br>  b) ↗ cTn > **20 %** when baseline value elevated (> 99th percentile) but stable |
| TYPE 4b | **Infarction secondary to stent thrombosis** |
| TYPE 5 | **Infarction secondary to CABG**<br>• ↗ cTn ≥ **10 x upper limit of normal** (> 99th percentile) when baseline cTn normal (< 99th percentile) +<br>• *De novo* Q waves or de novo LBBB or new coronary (or CABG) occlusion on coronary angiography or imaging compatible with loss of viable myocardium or *de novo* RWMA |

# CAUSES OF INFARCTION IN THE ABSENCE OF ATHEROSCLEROSIS

**$O_2$ SUPPLY/DEMAND IMBALANCE**: AS; AR; CO poisoning; Hyperthyroidism; Prolonged hypotension; Hypertensive crisis; Sepsis - Fever; Anemia; Respiratory failure; AV fistula; HCM; Tachyarrhythmia; Cocaine; Endothelial dysfunction

**CORONARY EMBOLISM**: Endocarditis (infective or non-infective); MVP; Intracardiac thrombus; Prosthetic valve; Myxoma; Iatrogenic; Paradoxical embolism; Fibroelastoma; Valvular calcification

**ARTERITIS**: Syphilis; SLE; Takayasu (coronary ostium); PAN; Kawasaki; RA; Ankylosing spondylitis; Giant cell arteritis; Scleroderma

> **SLE**: Arteritis; endothelial dysfunction; thrombosis (antiphospholipid syndrome); accelerated atherosclerosis; coronary aneurysm

**TRAUMA**: Laceration; Iatrogenic; Radiotherapy; Contusion

**INFILTRATIVE / PROLIFERATIVE**: Hurler's; Homocysteinuria; Fabry; Amyloidosis; Pseudoxanthoma elasticum

**CONGENITAL**: ALCAPA; Anomalous coronary origin; Coronary fistula; Coronary aneurysm

**HEMATOLOGICAL (*IN SITU* THROMBOSIS)**: Hyperviscosity; Polycythemia; Thrombocytosis; Hypercoagulable state - Antiphospholipid syndrome; TTP; DIC

**OTHER**: Prinzmetal; Aortic dissection; Coronary dissection (pregnancy; Marfan; Ehlers-Danlos; Cocaine); Takotsubo; Thrombosis then spontaneous thrombolysis; Medications; Myocardial bridge

# 2.4/ UNSTABLE ANGINA & NSTEMI

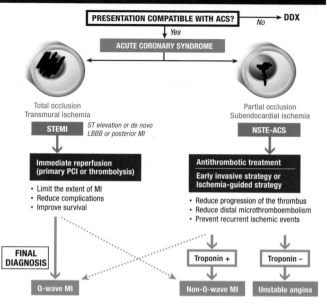

**IN-HOSPITAL MORTALITY** of STEMI is 50% higher than that of NSTEMI

> **Similar one-year mortality for STEMI and NSTEMI** (high risk of recurrent events after NSTEMI)    +

**PATHOPHYSIOLOGY: Rupture / Erosion of an unstable and friable atherosclerotic plaque with exposure of the subendothelial matrix then activation of primary and secondary hemostasis and thrombus formation**

## ASSESSMENT

| SYMPTOMS OF ACS | UNSTABLE NATURE |
|---|---|
| **Retrosternal chest pain \*** <br> • **Nature:** Constrictive - Tightness <br> • **Radiation:** Neck - Jaw - Upper limb <br> • **Associated symptoms:** Dyspnea; Nausea; Vomiting; Diaphoresis <br> \* Atypical presentation / Anginal equivalent in elderly - DM - women | **Any one of the following:** <br> • **De novo angina** < 2 months after presentation with CCS ≥ 3/4 <br> • **Crescendo angina:** more frequent or longer or on less exertion (with CCS ≥ 3/4) <br> • **Angina at rest** (often lasting > 20 min) < 1 week after presentation |

**CLINICAL FEATURES:** Diaphoresis; Cold skin; Sinus tachycardia; PVCs; ± Hypotension; S3 or S4; Ischemic MR murmur; Crackles

## ECG

| ST depression | • Horizontal or descending<br>• ≥ 0.5 mm (≥ 2 contiguous leads) | **+** |
|---|---|---|
| T–wave inversion | • ≥ 1-2 mm (≥ 2 contiguous leads)<br> > Leads with R/S > 1 | |

| NSTE–ACS AND UNSTABLE ANGINA | | |
|---|---|---|
| **HIGH RISK**<br>(≥ 1 CRITERION) | **INTERMEDIATE RISK**<br>(≥ 1 CRITERION) | **LOW RISK** |
| **Unstable atherosclerotic plaque; Urgent evaluation** | | **Outpatient stratification possible** |
| • Accelerated angina < 48 h<br>• Prolonged and persistent retrosternal chest pain at rest (> 20 min)<br>• Ischemic pulmonary overload<br>• *De novo* MR murmur<br>• S3 or Crackles<br>• Hypotension or Bradycardia or Tachycardia<br>• Age > 75 years<br>• Angina at rest with transient ST changes > 0.5 mm<br>• *De novo* bundle branch block<br>• Sustained VT<br>• Significant elevation of troponins | • History: myocardial infarction or PAD or cerebrovascular disease or history of CABG<br>• Treatment with ASA<br>• Prolonged retrosternal chest pain at rest (> 20 min) but resolved<br>• Prolonged retrosternal chest pain (> 20 min), but resolved with rest or TNT<br>• Nocturnal angina<br>• CCS III or IV angina (*de novo* or progressive) < 2 weeks without prolonged retrosternal chest pain at rest (> 20 min)<br>• Age > 70 years<br>• T wave abnormalities<br>• Pathological Q waves or ST depression at rest < 1 mm on multiple leads<br>• Marginal elevation of troponins | • More frequent or more severe or more persistent angina<br>• Angina induced by a lower workload<br>• *De novo* angina: between 2 weeks to 2 months before presentation<br>• Normal ECG<br>• Normal troponin |

| TIMI SCORE | GRACE SCORE |
|---|---|
| 1) Age > 65 years<br>2) ≥ 3 risk factors for CAD<br>3) Known stenosis > 50%<br>4) ASA < 7 days<br>5) ≥ 2 episodes of retrosternal chest pain x 24 h<br>6) ST depression ≥ 0.5 mm<br>7) Biomarkers<br><br>**Death / MI / Urgent revascularization within 14 days**<br>0-1 point...........4.7 %<br>2 points ............8.3 %<br>3 points ...........13.2 %<br>4 points ...........19.9 %<br>5 points ...........26.2 %<br>6-7 points.......40.9 % | www.gracescore.org<br>1) Age<br>2) SBP<br>3) HR<br>4) Killip Class<br>5) Heart failure<br>6) Cardiac arrest at presentation<br>7) ST segment depression<br>8) Biomarkers<br>9) Creatinine<br><br>**In–hospital mortality**<br>GRACE ≤ 108 points.............< 1 %<br>GRACE 109-140 points ........1-3 %<br>GRACE > 140 points ............> 3 % |

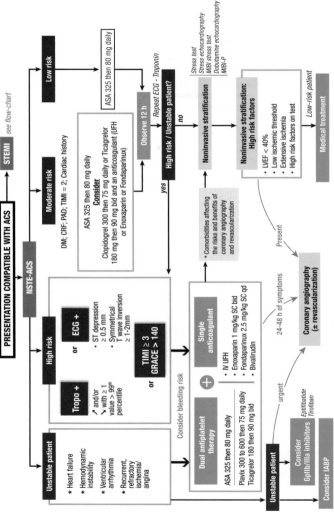

# PRESENTATION COMPATIBLE WITH ACS

**STEMI** *see flow-chart*

**NSTE-ACS**

## Low risk

ASA 325 then 80 mg daily

## Moderate risk

DM; CRF; PAD; TIMI = 2; Cardiac history

ASA 325 then 80 mg daily
**Consider**
Clopidogrel 300 then 75 mg daily or Ticagrelor 180 then 90 mg bid and an anticoagulant (UFH or Enoxaparin or Fondaparinux)

Observe 12 h

*Repeat ECG - Troponin*

**High risk / Unstable patient?**

no → Noninvasive stratification

yes →

## High risk

**Tropo +**
↗ and/or ↘ with ≥ 1 value > 99th percentile

**or**

**ECG +**
• ST depression ≥ 0.5 mm
• Symmetrical T wave inversion ≥ 1-2mm

**or**

**TIMI ≥ 3**
**or**
**GRACE > 140**

## Unstable patient

* Heart failure
* Hemodynamic instability
* Ventricular arrhythmia
* Recurrent, refractory ischemia/ angina

Consider bleeding risk

**Dual antiplatelet therapy**

ASA 325 then 80 mg daily
Plavix 300 to 600 then 75 mg daily
Ticagrelor 180 then 90 mg bid

**+**

**Single anticoagulant**
• IV UFH
• Enoxaparin 1 mg/kg SC bid
• Fondaparinux 2.5 mg/kg SC qd
• Bivalirudin

* Comorbidities affecting the risks and benefits of coronary angiography and revascularization

**Noninvasive stratification: High risk factors**
• LVEF < 40%
• Low ischemic threshold
• Extensive ischemia
• High risk factors on test

*Stress test*
*Stress echocardiography*
*MIBI stress test*
*Dobutamine echocardiography*
*MIBI-P*

Present →

*Low-risk patient*

**Medical treatment**

24-48 h of symptoms →

**Coronary angiography (± revascularization)**

urgent →

**Unstable patient**

**Consider GpIIb/IIIa inhibitors**

*Eptifibatide*
*Tirofiban*

**Consider IABP**

## INITIAL MANAGEMENT

**ARRIVAL IN THE EMERGENCY ROOM**: ECG within 10 min; IV lines; Monitor; ASA 325 mg; Sublingual TNT (except when contraindicated); $O_2$ (for SaO2 > 90%); ± Morphine 2.5 mg IV if persistent chest pain

## CHOICE OF STRATEGY

| EARLY INVASIVE STRATEGY | ISCHEMIA–GUIDED STRATEGY |
|---|---|
| ↘ Mortality; ↘ MI; ↘ Hospitalization (★ FRISC-II; ★ RITA-3; ★ TACTICS-TIMI 18) | According to non–invasive stress test (★ ICTUS) |
| • **Unstable patient** (urgent coronary angiography) <br> › Acute heart failure <br> › Hemodynamic instability <br> › Ventricular arrhythmia <br> › Recurrent and refractory angina/ischemia <br> • **Troponin +** <br> • **Positive ECG** (*De novo* ST depression) <br> • Patient at high risk of recurrent events <br> › **TIMI ≥ 3** <br> › **GRACE > 140** <br> • **PCI < 6 months** (rule out restenosis) <br> • **History of CABG** (multiple anatomical possibilities) | • **TIMI score 0-1** <br> • **GRACE < 109** <br> • **Risk of complications** associated with coronary angiography and/or revascularization <br> • **Comorbidities; Frailty** <br> • Patient's **preference** |

## DUAL ANTIPLATELET THERAPY

**ASA:** Irreversible inhibitor of COX-1 (and TXA synthesis)
> ★ **Antithrombotic Trialists**: ↘ all-cause mortality; ↘ recurrent ischemic events
> **Dose:** 325 mg then 80 mg qd (★ CURRENT-OASIS 7)

**CLOPIDOGREL:** Second-generation thienopyridine; irreversible ADP $P2Y_{12}$ receptor antagonist
> ★ **CURE**: ↘ recurrent ischemic events (**at 12 months**); ↗ major bleeding
> ★ **CURRENT-OASIS 7**: High-dose clopidogrel (600 mg then 150 mg qd for 6 days then 75 mg qd) versus standard doses (300 mg then 75 mg qd) → potential benefit in **the subgroup of patients undergoing PCI** (but ↗ bleeding risk)
> **Disadvantage: A)** Slow onset of action (requires 2 metabolism and activation steps); **B)** Genetic polymorphisms of the cytochrome P450 enzyme responsible for metabolism (and activation) of clopidogrel (some patients metabolize and activate the medication less effectively); **C)** Inhibits 50-60% of platelets

**TICAGRELOR:** Reversible direct $P2Y_{12}$ receptor antagonist; rapid onset of action
> ★ **PLATO**: Ticagrelor versus clopidogrel (**47% of patients had received clopidogrel prior to randomization**); Revascularization or medical treatment → ↘ **all-cause mortality**; ↘ recurrent ischemic events; ↗ major bleeding not related to CABG
> **Adverse effects**: Dyspnea; ↗ ventricular pauses; ↗ creatinine (reversible)
> **Contraindication**: History of intracranial bleeding; active bleeding; severe liver disease; potent CYP3A4 inhibitor
> ★ **PEGASUS**: Ticagrelor (60 or 90 mg bid) versus Placebo in patients with a myocardial infarction 1-3 years earlier; ↘ **CV death - MI - Stroke but** ↗ **major bleeding**

**PRASUGREL: no benefit** in ★ ACCOAST (upfront therapy) and ★ TRILOGY ACS (ischemia-guided strategy)

**GPIIB/IIIA INHIBITORS** : Block the formation of bridges between platelets (cross-links between GPIIb/IIIa receptors and fibrinogen)

> › ★ **EARLY-ACS: no benefit** of eptifibatide initiated routinely > 12 h before coronary angiography versus eptifibatide initiated on demand during PCI
> › **Consider the use of GPIIb/IIIa inhibitors** in patients treated with Ticagrelor (or Prasugrel): **during PCI for bailout situations / thrombotic complications**
>   · **Eptifibatide: A)** Bolus: 180 µg/kg IV then 2nd bolus of 180 µg/kg within 10 min; **B)** Infusion: 2 µg/kg/min (initiated after 1st bolus); decrease the dose by 50% if GFR < 50 mL/min
>   · **Tirofiban: A)** Bolus: 25 µg/kg IV; **B)** Infusion: 0.15 µg/kg/min; decrease the dose by 50% if GFR < 30 mL/min
>   · **Abciximab: A)** Bolus: 0.25 mg/kg IV; **B)** Infusion: 0.125 µg/kg/min (max 10 µg/min)
> › **Adverse effects**: thrombocytopenia; bleeding

## ANTICOAGULATION

Avoid crossover between antithrombins; stop anticoagulation after PCI (unless otherwise indicated)

### UNFRACTIONATED HEPARIN

> › ★ **Eikelboom meta-analysis** : ↘ mortality (before the age of dual antiplatelet therapy and early revascularization)
> › **Doses:** 60 IU/kg bolus then 12 IU/kg/h; PTT every 6 h; target PTT 50-70 s (1.5 to 2 x control)
>   · **During coronary angiography:** additional UFH as needed (2000-5000 U); **A)** Absence of GPIIb/IIIa inhibitors→ target ACT 250-300 s (HemoTec) or 300-350 s (Hemochron); **B)** Presence of GPIIb/IIIa inhibitors → target ACT 200-250 s
> › **Complications:** bleeding; HIT (consider Bivalirudin)

### ENOXAPARIN (LMWH): Xa inhibitor and weak thrombin inhibitor (factor IIa inhibitor)

> › ★ **SYNERGY**: Enoxaparin vs Unfractionated heparin → ↗ ↗ **bleeding** during early invasive strategy with enoxaparin
> › **Doses:** 1 mg/kg SC bid (reduce to once daily if GFR < 30 mL/min)
> › **PCI:** Last dose > 8 h → 0.3 mg/kg IV bolus

### FONDAPARINUX: indirect Xa inhibitor

> › ★ **OASIS-5**: Fondaparinux vs enoxaparin → ↘ bleeding; ↘ all-cause mortality; ↗ **catheter thrombosis during PCI** (as it does not act on already formed thrombin)
> › **Doses:** 2.5 mg SC once daily (avoid if GFR < 20 mL/min)
> › **PCI:** Add a bolus of unfractionated heparin (70-85 IU/kg; 50-60 IU/kg with concomitant GPIIb/IIIa inhibitors)

### BIVALIRUDIN: thrombin inhibitor (factor IIa inhibitor)

> › ★ **ACUITY**: Bivalirudin vs unfractionated heparin + GPIIb/IIIa inhibitors → non-inferiority for primary outcome; ↘ major bleeding
> › ★ **MATRIX**: ACS with PCI anticipated; Bivalirudin vs unfractionated heparin → no benefit
> › **Dose**: **A)** Bolus: 0.1 mg/kg; **B)** Infusion: 0.25 mg/kg/h
>   · **During PCI: A)** Bolus: 0.5 mg/kg; **B)** Infusion: 1.75 mg/kg/h

### RIVAROXABAN: oral Xa inhibitor

> › ★ **ATLAS ACS-TIMI 51:** Recent ACS on dual antiplatelet therapy; Rivaroxaban (2.5 or 5 mg bid; initiated an average of 4.5 days post-ACS) vs placebo; ↘ recurrent ischemic events; ↘ **all-cause mortality (2.5 mg bid)**; ↗ major bleeding
> › **Consider:** in combination with ASA and Clopidogrel (if Ticagrelor or Prasugrel are not available) in patients with high ischemic and low bleeding risks

Coronary artery disease (CAD) & myocardial infarction

| URGENT CORONARY ANGIOGRAPHY | EARLY INVASIVE STRATEGY (< 48 H) | ISCHEMIA–GUIDED STRATEGY |
|---|---|---|
| 1) ASA 325 mg<br>2) Ticagrelor 180 mg **or** Clopidogrel 600 mg<br>3) ± GpIIb/IIIa inhibitors (during PCI for bailout situations)<br>4) Unfractionated heparin | 1) ASA 325 mg<br>2) Ticagrelor 180 mg then 90 mg bid **or** Clopidogrel 300 mg then 75 mg qd (consider an additional 300 mg if PCI then 150 mg qd for 6 days then 75 mg)<br>3) Unfractionated heparin or Enoxaparin or Fondaparinux or Bivalirudin<br>  &gt; Stop after PCI in the absence of complications | 1) ASA 325 mg<br>2) Ticagrelor 180 mg then 90 mg bid **or** Clopidogrel 300 mg then 75 mg qd (consider an additional 300 mg if PCI then 150 mg qd for 6 days then 75 mg)<br>3) Unfractionated heparin (48 h or until PCI is performed) or Enoxaparin or Fondaparinux if bleeding risk (for the duration of hospitalization or until PCI is performed) |

- **Patient already on Clopidogrel:** another loading dose of 300 to 600 mg if PCI planned
- **Patient on Warfarin:** wait for INR < 2.0-2.5 before starting anticoagulant

## 2.5/ ST SEGMENT ELEVATION MYOCARDIAL INFARCTION (STEMI)

### ECG CRITERIA

| ST ELEVATION (FROM POINT J IN ≥ 2 CONTIGUOUS LEADS) | |
|---|---|
| V2 – V3 | • Male ≥ 40 years: ≥ 2 mm<br>• Male < 40 years: ≥ 2.5 mm<br>• Female: ≥ 1.5 mm |
| All other leads | ≥ 1 mm |
| V3R – V4R – V7 – V8 – V9 | ≥ 0.5 mm |

| DDX OF ST ELEVATION | | |
|---|---|---|
| Male ST pattern | • 90% of men < 35 years<br>• Concave ST elevation > 1 mm in V1 to V3 (especially V2) | 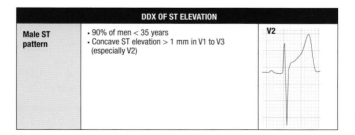 |

| | | |
|---|---|---|
| **Early repolarization** | • Large T waves (especially in V4)<br>• ST elevation in V2-V3-V4 (concave)<br>• Notch at point J<br>• PR segment depression | **V4** |
| **Juvenile T wave pattern and early repolarization** | • T wave inversion (juvenile T wave pattern) combined with early repolarization<br>• Short QT | **V3** |
| **LVH** | • Concave ST elevation in V1 to V3<br>• Positive voltage criteria | **V1** |
| **Post–MI with aneurysm** | • Persistent ST elevation (> 3 weeks post-MI) in the presence of Q waves | **V3** |
| **LBBB (or paced rhythm)** | • Concave ST elevation; the ST deviation is discordant with the QRS axis<br><br>**Sgarbossa criteria**<br><u>(infarction in the presence of LBBB)</u><br><br>1) **ST elevation ≥ 1 mm in leads with positive QRS (inappropriate concordance)**<br>  - Criterion with the best predictive value<br>2) ST depression ≥ 1 mm V1-V2-V3 (inappropriate concordance)<br>3) ST elevation ≥ 5 mm in leads with negative QRS (extreme discordance) | **V1** |
| **Acute pericarditis** | • Diffuse concave ST elevation (multiple anatomical territories)<br>• PR segment depression<br>• Reciprocal changes in aVR | **V5** |

Coronary artery disease (CAD) & myocardial infarction

| Brugada syndrome | • rSR' and ST elevation in V1 and V2 with descending slope and T wave inversion | V2 |
| Hyperkalemia | • Peaked and symmetrical T waves<br>• ST elevation<br>• Other signs: Wide QRS; decreased amplitude of P waves; blocks; asystole | V4 |
| Pulmonary embolism | • T wave inversion and ST elevation in right precordial and inferior leads<br>• S1 Q3 T3<br>• RBBB<br>• Sinus tachycardia | V1 |

## SITE OF INFARCTION ON ECG

| I<br>Lateral | aVR | V1<br>Antero-septal | V4<br>Anterior |
| II<br>Inferior | aVL<br>Lateral | V2<br>Antero-septal | V5<br>Antero-lateral |
| III<br>Inferior | aVF<br>Inferior | V3<br>Anterior | V6<br>Antero-lateral |

V3R-V4R
**Right heart**

V7-V8-V9
**Posterior**

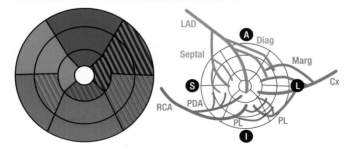

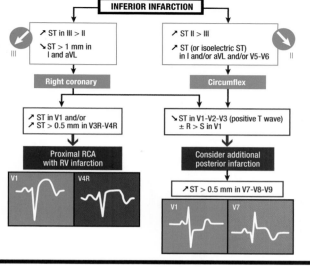

**INFERIOR INFARCTION**

| ↗ ST in III > II | ↗ ST II > III |
|---|---|
| ↘ ST > 1 mm in I and aVL | ↗ ST (or isoelectric ST) in I and/or aVL and/or V5-V6 |

**Right coronary** → **Circumflex**

↗ ST in V1 and/or ↗ ST > 0.5 mm in V3R-V4R

**Proximal RCA with RV infarction**

↘ ST in V1-V2-V3 (positive T wave) ± R > S in V1

**Consider additional posterior infarction**

↗ ST > 0.5 mm in V7-V8-V9

**ANTERIOR INFARCTION**

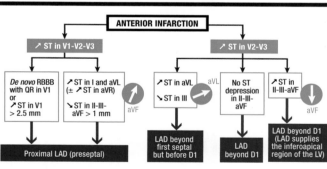

↗ ST in V1-V2-V3

- *De novo* RBBB with QR in V1 or ↗ ST in V1 > 2.5 mm
- ↗ ST in I and aVL (± ↗ ST in aVR) ↘ ST in II-III-aVF > 1 mm

**Proximal LAD (preseptal)**

↗ ST in V2-V3

- ↗ ST in aVL ↘ ST in III → **LAD beyond first septal but before D1**
- No ST depression in II-III-aVF → **LAD beyond D1**
- ↗ ST in II-III-aVF → **LAD beyond D1 (LAD supplies the inferoapical region of the LV)**

**UNSTABLE ANGINA**

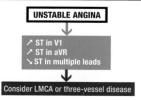

↗ ST in V1
↗ ST in aVR
↘ ST in multiple leads

**Consider LMCA or three-vessel disease**

02

Coronary artery disease (CAD) & myocardial infarction

A Practical Handbook / **91**

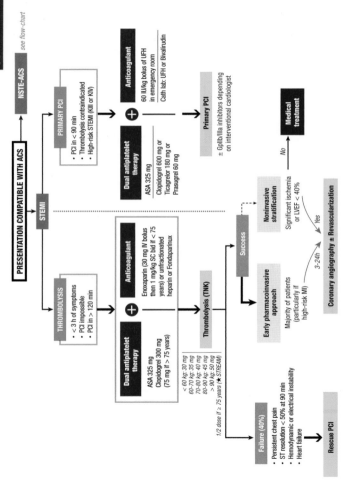

**PRESENTATION COMPATIBLE WITH ACS**

NSTE-ACS  *see flow-chart*

**STEMI**

**PRIMARY PCI**
- PCI in < 90 min
- Thrombolysis contraindicated
- High-risk STEMI (Kill or KIV)

**Dual antiplatelet therapy**
ASA 325 mg
Clopidogrel 600 mg or
Ticagrelor 180 mg or
Prasugrel 60 mg

**+**

**Anticoagulant**
60 IU/kg bolus of UFH
in emergency room
Cath lab: UFH or Bivalirudin

**Primary PCI**
± GpIIb/IIIa inhibitors depending
on interventional cardiologist

**THROMBOLYSIS**
- < 3 h of symptoms
- PCI impossible
- PCI in > 120 min

**Dual antiplatelet therapy**
ASA 325 mg
Clopidogrel 300 mg
(75 mg if > 75 years)

< 60 kg: 30 mg
60-70 kg: 35 mg
70-80 kg: 40 mg
80-90 kg: 45 mg
> 90 kg: 50 mg
1/2 dose if ≥ 75 years (★ STREAM)

**+**

**Anticoagulant**
Enoxaparin (30 mg IV bolus
then 1 mg/kg SC bid if < 75
years) or unfractionated
heparin or Fondaparinux

**Thrombolysis (TNK)**

**Failure (40%)**
- Persistent chest pain
- ST resolution < 50% at 90 min
- Hemodynamic or electrical instability
- Heart failure

**Rescue PCI**

**Success**

**Early pharmacoinvasive approach**
Majority of patients
(particularly if
high-risk MI)

**Noninvasive stratification**
Significant ischemia
or LVEF < 40%

**Medical treatment**

*No*

*Yes*

*3-24h*

**Coronary angiography ± Revascularization**

# INITIAL MANAGEMENT

**EMERGENCY ROOM**: ECG within 10 min; IV lines; Monitor; ASA 325 mg; Sublingual TNT (except when contraindicated); $O_2$ (for $SaO_2 > 90\%$); ± Morphine 2.5 mg IV if persistent chest pain

## KILLIP CLASSIFICATION

| Killip I | No crackles; No S3 |
|---|---|
| Killip II | Crackles (< 50% of lung fields) ± S3 |
| Killip III | Crackles > 50% of lung fields |
| Killip IV | Cardiogenic shock |

## TIMI SCORE IN STEMI

| CRITERIA | # POINTS | 30-DAY MORTALITY |
|---|---|---|
| Age 65-74 years or ≥ 75 years | 2 or 3 points | **0 : 0.8 %** |
| SBP < 100 | 3 points | **1 : 1.6 %** |
| HR > 100 bpm | 2 points | **2 : 2.2 %** |
| Killip II-III-IV | 2 points | **3 : 4.4 %** |
| History: DM or HTN or Angina | 1 point | **4 : 7.3 %** |
| < 67 kg | 1 point | **5 : 12.4 %** |
| Time to treatment > 4 h | 1 point | **6 : 16.1 %** |
| Anterior STEMI or LBBB | 1 point | **7 : 23.4 %** |
| | | **8 : 26.8 %** |
| | | **> 8 : 35.9 %** |

# IMMEDIATE REPERFUSION

| THROMBOLYSIS | PRIMARY PCI |
|---|---|
| **< 30 min after 1ˢᵗ medical contact\*** | **< 90 min after 1ˢᵗ medical contact\*** |
| ↘ **Mortality (vs Placebo)** (★ GISSI; ★ ISIS-2; ★ ASSET) | ↘ **Mortality (vs Thrombolysis)** ↘ **Recurrent infarction** ↘ **Risk of intracranial hemorrhage** |
| **Fibrinolysis less effective > 6 h after symptom onset** • Early presentation: < 3 h of symptoms • Significantly delayed PCI (1ˢᵗ medical contact until PCI **> 120 min**) • PCI impossible (cath lab not available; vascular access impossible) | • PCI available in < 90 min after 1ˢᵗ medical contact • > 3 h of symptoms • Contraindication to thrombolysis - Bleeding risk / Intracranial bleeding • High-risk STEMI • Doubtful diagnosis |

**\* Including paramedics**

# THROMBOLYSIS

**TENECTEPLASE (TNK):** < 60 kg → 30 mg; 60-70 kg → 35 mg; 70-80 kg → 40 mg; 80-90 kg → 45 mg; ≥ 90 kg → 50 mg; **if ≥ 75 years → half dose** (★STREAM)

> ★ **ASSENT-2:** Tenecteplase vs tPA → ↘ major bleeding with TNK

**TIME TO ADMINISTRATION**: maximum benefit on mortality < 2-3 h of symptoms    +

> ↘ **Response of thrombus** to thrombolysis after > 3 h of symptoms
> It is reasonable to perform thrombolysis up to 12-24 h after onset of symptoms in the presence of persistent ischemia (angina and ↗ ST on ECG) and significant infarction
>   • ★ LATE - ★ EMERAS: ↘ mortality between 6-12 h of symptoms

| ABSOLUTE CONTRAINDICATIONS | RELATIVE CONTRAINDICATIONS |
|---|---|
| • History of intracranial hemorrhage<br>• Structural CNS vascular disease<br>• Intracranial neoplasm<br>• Stroke < 3 months<br>• Suspicion of aortic dissection<br>• Active bleeding (excluding menstruation) or bleeding diathesis<br>• Significant facial / head trauma < 3 months<br>• Intracranial or spinal cord surgery < 2 months<br>• Severe refractory HTN | • SBP > 180 mmHg and/or DBP > 110 mmHg<br>• Stroke > 3 months or dementia or intracranial disease<br>• CPR > 10 min or traumatic<br>• Major surgery < 3 weeks<br>• Internal bleeding < 2-4 weeks<br>• Noncompressible vascular puncture<br>• Pregnancy<br>• Active peptic ulcer<br>• Oral anticoagulant |

• Risk of intracranial bleeding → **Prefer PCI if ≥ 2 criteria present**
**1)** > 65 years; **2)** BP > 160-170/95; **3)** M < 70 kg and F < 65 kg

## PRIMARY PCI: ADJUVANT TREATMENT

**ASA**: 325 mg then 80 mg qd

**CLOPIDOGREL:** 600 mg then 75 mg qd

**PRASUGREL**: Third-generation thienopyridine; irreversible inhibition of the P2Y$_{12}$ receptor; one-step activation (versus 2 steps for clopidogrel); metabolism not affected by genetic polymorphisms of cytochrome P450 enzymes

> ★ **TRITON-TIMI 38: thienopyridine-naive patients; known coronary anatomy** (except if primary PCI) → ↘ ischemic events; ↘ stent thrombosis; ↗ major bleeding
> **Avoid in patients**: > 75 years; < 60 kg; History of stroke - TIA    +

**TICAGRELOR**

> ★ **PLATO**: Clopidogrel-naive or non-naive patients; ↘ all-cause mortality; ↘ recurrent ischemic events; ↘ stent thrombosis; ↗ major bleeding not related to CABG

**GPIIB/IIIA INHIBITORS**: in the cath lab at **the interventional cardiologist's discretion** (significant thrombus; insufficient prior antiplatelet treatment; slow- or no-reflow; thrombotic complication)

> **Abciximab**: **A)** Bolus: 0.25 mg/kg IV; **B)** Infusion: 0.125 µg/kg/min

**UNFRACTIONATED HEPARIN**: 60 IU/kg bolus (max 4000 IU) then IV infusion with target aPTT of 50-70 s (12 IU/kg/h; max 1000 IU/h)

> **During coronary angiography**: **A)** Absence of GPIIb/IIIa inhibitors → target ACT 250-300 s (HemoTec) or 300-350 s (Hemochron); **B)** Presence of GPIIb/IIIa inhibitors → target ACT 200-250 s

**BIVALIRUDIN**: Thrombin inhibitor; used in cath lab

> ★ **HORIZONS-AMI**: Bivalirudin vs UFH + GPIIb/IIIa inhibitors; ↘ **all-cause mortality**; ↘ major bleeding
> ★ **MATRIX**: ACS (55% STEMI) with PCI anticipated; Bivalirudin vs UFH → no benefit with Bivalirudin
> **Dose**: **A)** Bolus: 0.75 mg/kg; **B)** Infusion: 1.75 mg/kg/h (decrease to 1 mg/kg/h if CrCl < 30 mL/min)

# THROMBOLYSIS: ADJUVANT TREATMENT

**ASA:** 325 mg then 80 mg qd (long-term); ★ ISIS-2

**CLOPIDOGREL:** 300 mg (75 mg if > 75 years) then 75 mg qd (14 days to 1 year);
★ CLARITY-TIMI 28 and ★ COMMIT

**ENOXAPARIN:** ★ EXTRACT-TIMI 25 → **Enoxaparin superior to Unfractionated heparin but** ↗ major bleeding
> **Bolus:** 30 mg IV (< 75 years)
> **Maintenance:** 1 mg/kg SC bid (max 100 mg for first 2 doses) (if > 75 years: 0.75 mg/kg SC bid; max 75 mg for first 2 doses)
> **GFR < 30 mL/min:** 1 mg/kg SC once daily
> **Duration:** until discharge from hospital (for one week or until revascularization)

**FONDAPARINUX:** 2.5 mg IV bolus then 2.5 mg SC once daily until discharge from hospital (or for one week or until revascularization); avoid if CrCl < 30 mL/min
> ★ **OASIS-6:** Fondaparinux vs Heparin; ↘ mortality; ↘ MI recurrence rate

**UNFRACTIONATED HEPARIN:** 60 IU/kg (max 4000 IU) then IV infusion for 48 h (or until revascularization) with target aPTT of 50-70 s (12 IU/kg/h; max 1000 IU/h)

**EARLY PHARMACOINVASIVE STRATEGY:** immediate transfer post-thrombolysis for coronary angiography ± revascularization within 3 to 24 h
> ★ **TRANSFER-AMI and** ★ **CARESS-in-AMI: ↘ recurrent ischemic events**                     +

**RESCUE PCI:** ★ REACT → ↘ recurrent MI; ↘ heart failure
> **Particularly beneficial if significant ischemic territory** (anterior MI; inferior infarction with RV involvement or with ST depression in V1-V3)

**INTRACRANIAL HEMORRHAGE**
a) Stop all agents potentially responsible
b) Brain imaging + Neurology / Neurosurgery consultation
c) 10 units of cryoprecipitate (fibrinogen and fVIII) + 2 units of FFP (fV and fVIII) + Protamine (1 mg for every 100 units of heparin over the last 4 hours) + Platelet transfusion (6-8 units)
d) ↘ Intracranial pressure (hyperventilation; Mannitol; head of bed to 30°; surgery)

# 2.6/ ACUTE CORONARY SYNDROME: ADJUVANT TREATMENTS

**NITRATES: venodilator** (↘ preload); **coronary vasodilator** (↗ perfusion); **arterial vasodilator** (↘ afterload)
> **Indications:** A) Ischemia / Recurrent angina; B) Significant HTN; C) Heart failure
> **Doses:** 0.4 mg sublingual every 5 min x 3 then IV infusion PRN (5-10 µg/min IV; increase by 10 µg/min every 5 min PRN up to a dose of 200 µg/min)
> **Contraindications:** SBP < 90 mmHg; HR < 50 bpm; HR > 100 bpm in the absence of heart failure; RV infarction; PDE-5 inhibitor (24 h for Sildenafil; 48 h for Tadalafil)

**BETA-BLOCKERS: negative inotropic / negative chronotropic agent;** ↘ $O_2$ demand
> ★ MIAMI - ★ ISIS-1 - ★ COMMIT → ↘ mortality; ↘ recurrent ischemic events; ↘ VF
> **Start orally within 24 h of presentation**
> **Contraindications:** Signs of heart failure; Low output state; Risk of cardiogenic shock (> 70 years; SBP < 120 mmHg; Sinus tachycardia > 110 bpm; HR < 60 bpm; Late presentation); PR > 0.24 s; 2nd or 3rd degree AV block; Active asthma
   · **Avoid BB with ISA**
   · **Short-acting BB:** IV Esmolol
   · **Verapamil or Diltiazem** as an alternative in the absence of contraindications and LV dysfunction

| AGENT | INDICATION | DURATION | CAUTION |
|---|---|---|---|
| ASA | • All patients with ACS (★ Antithrombotic Trialists' Collaboration) | **Long term** | ASA allergy Peptic ulcer |
| Clopidogrel (75 mg qd) | • Post-ACS (without Ticagrelor or Prasugrel) (★CURE) | • 1 year if DES<br>• Up to 1 year if BMS or medical treatment<br>• BMS: minimum 2-4 weeks | Clopidogrel allergy |
| Ticagrelor (90 mg bid) | • Post-ACS (without Clopidogrel or Prasugrel) (★PLATO)<br>• Consider > 1 year post MI in high-risk patients (★PEGASUS) | • 1 year if DES<br>• Up to 1 year if BMS or medical treatment | Dyspnea Ventricular pauses |
| Prasugrel (10 mg qd) | • Post-ACS (without Clopidogrel or Ticagrelor) (★TRITON-TIMI 38) | • 1 year if DES<br>• Up to 1 year if BMS | Avoid if weight < 60 kg or > 75 years or history of stroke - TIA |
| ACE inhibitor | • All patients with CAD (± HTN or DM or CRF) (★HOPE; ★EUROPA)<br>• Post-ACS with LVEF < 40% or heart failure (★TRACE; ★SAVE; ★AIRE) | **Start within 24 h of presentation**<br><br>**Long term** | ARF; Hyperkalemia; Cough; Angioedema<br><br>Contraindicated if SBP < 100 mmHg |
| ARB (Valsartan or Candesartan) | • Intolerance of ACE inhibitors with LVEF < 40% or heart failure (★VALIANT; ★CHARM-Alternative) | Long term | ARF; Hyperkalemia; Hypotension |
| Beta-blockers | • All patients post-myocardial infarction (★ Freemantle meta-analysis)<br>• Post-ACS with LVEF < 40% (★ CAPRICORN)<br>• Residual coronary stenosis (anti-anginal) | • **Long term** if LV dysfunction or as antianginal<br>• **Otherwise:** ≥ 3 years<br>• **Target HR 50-60 bpm; use BB without ISA** | Active heart failure AV block Asthma |
| Statines | • All patients with ACS (★PROVE IT-TIMI 22) | • **Long term**<br>• **High-dose statin** | Myopathy Myositis Transaminase |
| Eplerenone (25 mg then 50 mg qd) | • ACS with LVEF < 40% (with heart failure or DM) (★EPHESUS) | Long term | Hyperkalemia > 5 mmol/L GFR < 30 mL/min |
| TNT (Nitropuff) | • All patients with coronary disease | Long term | Avoid if hypotension or PDE-5 inhibitor |
| Warfarin | • LV thrombus<br>• Significant LV dysfunction with extensive regional wall motion abnormalities or LV aneurysm (class IIb recommendation) | **3 months then reevaluate**<br><br>Long term if mobile / pedunculated thrombus | **Target INR 2-2.5** in the presence of dual antiplatelet therapy Add PPI |

**GLYCEMIC CONTROL**: target blood glucose **< 10 mmol/L (180 mg/dL)** (★DIGAMI); avoid hypoglycemia (★NICE-SUGAR)

**PPI (PREFER PANTOPRAZOLE)**: patient on dual antiplatelet therapy with ≥ 1 risk factor:
**A)** History of upper GI bleeding / ulcer; **B)** > 60 years; **C)** Anticoagulant or Corticosteroids or NSAID; **D)** *H. pylori* - positive

**ANEMIA: target hemoglobin > 70-80 g/L**

**AVOID NSAID**
> **If unavoidable** (despite Acetaminophen; ASA; Narcotics) → **prefer nonselective NSAID** (Naproxen; Ibuprofen)

**AVOID HORMONE THERAPY**

**STRESS TEST BEFORE DISCHARGE FROM HOSPITAL**
> No angina / Heart failure / Arrhythmia for 48-72 h
> **Submaximal stress test (3-5 days):** stop if HR ≥ 120 bpm or ≥ 70% of predicted HRmax or ≥ 5 METs or Angina or Dyspnea or ↘ ST 2 mm or Hypotension or ≥ 3 consecutive PVCs
> **Stress test limited by symptoms (3 weeks):** not guided by HR or METs

## MANAGEMENT ON DISCHARGE FROM HOSPITAL

**MANAGEMENT OF RISK FACTORS**: ►►I Chapter 9

**ADMISSION TO CARDIAC REHABILITATION CENTER**

**SMOKING CESSATION**

**CONTROL OF LIPIDS**
> **Lipid profile** on day 1 of ACS (↘ TC and ↘ HDL within 24-48 h of ACS)
> **Target**: High-dose statin; **target ↘ > 50% LDL**

**BP CONTROL: < 140/90 mmHg** (< 140/85 mmHg in the presence of DM)

**DM CONTROL**: HbA1c < 7 %

**WEIGHT**: BMI: 18.5-24.9 kg/m2; waist < 102 cm (M) and < 88 cm (F)

**BALANCED DIET**

**PHYSICAL ACTIVITY**: **30 minutes of moderate exercise (rapid walking) 5 times a week**
> Pre-training stress test if necessary depending on risk factors

**INFLUENZA VACCINE** annually

**TREAT DEPRESSION** post-IM

**SICK LEAVE:** determined case by case; 2 weeks to 10 weeks

**SEXUAL ACTIVITY**: resume after 7-10 days (equivalent to one flight of stairs)

**PLANE TRAVEL**: ►►I Chapter 9

Coronary artery disease (CAD) & myocardial infarction

## CARDIOGENIC SHOCK

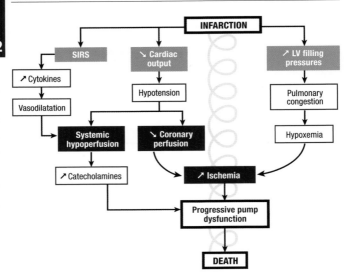

↘ Cardiac output with inadequate tissue perfusion (despite sufficient filling pressures)

### HEMODYNAMIC PARAMETERS

> Hypotension (SBP < 90 mmHg)
> Systemic hypoperfusion (cold extremities; altered level of consciousness; ↘ urinary output; $SVO_2 < 70$ %)
> ↘ Cardiac Index (< 2.2 L/min/m²)
> ↗ Filling pressures (Wedge pressure > 18 mmHg)

### ETIOLOGIES: Extensive infarction; Mechanical complication; RV infarction

> **DDx:** Hemorrhage; Pulmonary embolism; Tamponade; Sepsis; Myocarditis; Takotsubo; HCM; Endocarditis; Aortic dissection

### MANAGEMENT

> ★ **SHOCK:** ↘ mortality with early revascularization (< 75 years)                    +

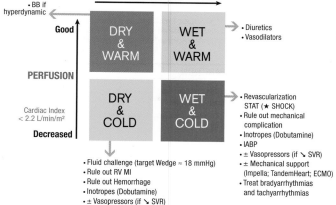

Wedge pressure > 18 mmHg

**CONGESTION** — No / Yes

• BB if hyperdynamic

**Good**

**PERFUSION**

Cardiac Index < 2.2 L/min/m²

**Decreased**

**DRY & WARM**

**WET & WARM**

**DRY & COLD**

**WET & COLD**

→ • Diuretics
• Vasodilators

→ • Revascularization STAT (★ SHOCK)
• Rule out mechanical complication
• Inotropes (Dobutamine)
• IABP
• ± Vasopressors (if ↘ SVR)
• ± Mechanical support (Impella; TandemHeart; ECMO)
• Treat bradyarrhythmias and tachyarrhythmias

↓ • Fluid challenge (target Wedge ≈ 18 mmHg)
• Rule out RV MI
• Rule out Hemorrhage
• Inotropes (Dobutamine)
• ± Vasopressors (if ↘ SVR)
• ± Mechanical support

## INTRA-AORTIC BALLOON PUMP

**INDICATIONS: A)** Cardiogenic shock; **B)** Refractory ischemia; **C)** Mechanical complication of MI; **D)** Support during a procedure at high risk of hemodynamic instability

**MECHANISM:** Inflation in diastole immediately after closure of the aortic valve (↗ **coronary perfusion**); deflation at systole just before opening of the aortic valve **(suction effect; ↘ afterload)**

› Increases cardiac output ≈ **10-15 %**
› Monitored by ECG and BP monitor
› ★ IABP-SHOCK II study: no benefit

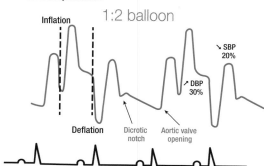

1:2 balloon

Inflation

Deflation

Dicrotic notch

Aortic valve opening

↗ DBP 30%

↘ SBP 20%

**CXR POSITION:** tip of the catheter **at the level of the carina** (> 4 cm below the aortic knob)  +

**CONTRAINDICATIONS**: Moderate to severe AR; Aortic dissection; Significant abdominal aortic aneurysm; severe PAD; Uncontrolled sepsis

**COMPLICATIONS:** Aortic lesion / perforation; Bleeding at site of introduction; Ischemia distal to introducer (target the common femoral artery during introduction); Thrombocytopenia; Hemolysis; Atheroembolism; Renal ischemia; Cerebral ischemia in the case of proximal migration of the balloon; Infection

## RIGHT VENTRICULAR INFARCTION

**RV very resistant to ischemia (thin myocardium)**
> **Excellent recovery of RV function post-MI**

**CLINICAL FEATURES:** Shock; ↗ CVP (↗ Y descent; mimics constrictive pericarditis); Kussmaul sign; Pulsus paradoxus; Clear lungs

**HEMODYNAMIC PARAMETERS:** Hypotension; ↗ RA pressure / ↗ RVEDP; ↘ RV systolic pressure; ↘ Wedge pressure; ↘ Cardiac index

**ECG: ST elevation > 0.5-1 mm V3R and/or V4R** (in the context of infarction of the inferior  + wall of the LV); ± ST elevation in V1-V2

**DDX**: Pulmonary embolism **(absence of RWMA in inferior wall of LV)**  +

**COMPLICATIONS**: R → L shunt (via PFO); Shock; Pulmonary embolism; Arrhythmia; AV block; Death

**MANAGEMENT**: **1)** Avoid TNT; **2)** Reperfusion; **3)** Bolus of normal saline to maintain adequate RV preload (attention to interdependence with LV; **avoid RVEDP > 15 mmHg); 4)** Target Wedge  + pressure 15-18 mmHg; **5)** Inotropes (Dobutamine); **6)** Decrease RV afterload (avoid hypoxia; minimize PEEP; NO); **7)** Maintain AV synchrony (to ensure good filling of the ischemic RV and to increase RV output); **8)** IABP; RVAD; Impella; Creation of an ASD when necessary

## LEFT VENTRICULAR FREE WALL RUPTURE

One to 14 days post-transmural infarction
> **Secondary to extension of the infarction**: thinning and dilatation of the necrotic zone
> Often anterior or lateral LV wall

**PRESENTATION**: Pleuritic pain; Hypotension; Shock; Sudden death (pulseless electrical activity)

**CLINICAL FEATURES**: JVD; Pulsus paradoxus; Shock

**TTE**: signs of tamponade; look for the site of rupture

## LEFT VENTRICULAR PSEUDOANEURYSM

Ventricular rupture contained by the pericardium and by thrombus / organized hematoma

**Narrow neck (<< diameter of the pseudoaneurysm)**

**High risk of rupture and hemopericardium**

## LEFT VENTRICULAR ANEURYSM

Thinning of myocardium (but no rupture, in contrast with pseudoaneurysm)

Dyskinesia with paradoxical systolic expansion (alters the geometry and efficacy of contraction; ↗ wall stress)

**Large neck (≥ 0.5 x diameter of the aneurysm)**

Low risk of rupture

**ECG**: persistent ST elevation

**COMPLICATIONS**: Embolism; Arrhythmia; Heart failure; Angina

## INTRAVENTRICULAR THROMBUS

↗ **RISK OF EMBOLIZATION**: Mobile; Protrusion into the ventricle; Visualized on several sections; Contiguous zones of akinesia and hyperkinesia

**MANAGEMENT**: Anticoagulant therapy for 3-6 months then re-evaluate

## VENTRICULAR SEPTAL RUPTURE

### SITE
> **Anterior infarction** → apical interventricular septum
> **Inferior infarction** → inferobasal interventricular septum (less favorable prognosis)

**PRESENTATION**: Hypotension - Shock; Acute pulmonary edema; R and L heart failure; Blocks

**CLINICAL FEATURES**: Shock; **Prominent holosystolic murmur ± thrill; S3;** Pulmonary edema; Signs of right heart failure

**TTE**: L→R shunt; RV insufficiency

**CARDIAC CATHETERIZATION**: $O_2$ step-up between RA and RV; Prominent V wave

**TREATMENT**: Nitroprusside; IABP; Inotropes; Surgery vs percutaneous closure

## PAPILLARY MUSCLE RUPTURE

**Posteromedial papillary muscle** (inferior infarction; supplied by PDA) >> anterolateral papillary muscle (double blood supply by LAD and circumflex)

**PRESENTATION**: Hypotension; Shock; Acute pulmonary edema; **Systolic murmur, often minor** (early systolic equalization of transvalvular pressures)

**TTE (± TEE)**: Rupture of a papillary muscle or chorda tendineae; Leaflet eversion; Severe MR on Doppler; Hyperdynamic LV; PHT

**CARDIAC CATHETERIZATION: Prominent V wave; ↗ PAP** (± contaminated by V wave)

**TREATMENT**: Nitroprusside; IABP; Inotropes; Mechanical ventilation; Urgent surgery

## PERICARDITIS

**EARLY:** pericardial extension of transmural MI
> **Presentation:** Pleuritic pain radiating to the trapezius; **Pericardial friction rub; Localized ECG changes**
> **Management:** Caution with anticoagulants (risk of hemorrhagic pericarditis; monitor by TTE); ASA 650 mg PO every 4-6 h; Colchicine

**LATE (> 7 DAYS)**: Dressler's syndrome; Immune phenomenon

**02**

**PVC**: BB; Correct electrolyte disorders; No benefit of AAD (★ CAST; ★ SWORD)

**MONOMORPHIC VT**: Correct electrolyte disorders; BB; AAD; ECV; **ICD if > 48 h (probable permanent arrhythmogenic substrate)**

**POLYMORPHIC VT**: Rule out ischemia; Rule out ↗ QT; BB; Correct electrolyte disorders

**VF: Rule out ischemia**; BB; AAD (Lidocaine; Amiodarone); ICD if > 48 h

**AIVR**: Ventricular rhythm 60-100 bpm; **Specific marker of reperfusion; Observation**; ↗ Sinus rhythm PRN (Atropine; Atrial pacing)

**SINUS BRADYCARDIA**: often associated with inferior STEMI (**Bezold-Jarish reflex**); Atropine; Atrial pacing

### AV BLOCK AND INTRAVENTRICULAR BLOCKS

| INFERIOR INFARCTION | ANTEROSEPTAL INFARCTION |
|---|---|
| **RCA 90%; Circumflex 10%** | **Proximal LAD (± septal branches)** |
| • Mechanism: ↗ **Vagal tone** (< 6h; Bezold-Jarish) and/or **AV node ischemia** | • Mechanism: **Extensive necrosis of the septum and conduction tissue** (His-Purkinje system) |
| **Bradyarrhythmias**<br>• Sinus bradycardia<br>• **Intranodal** AV block<br>   1st degree AV block or 2nd degree Mobitz I AV block or sometimes 3rd degree intranodal AV block | **Bradyarrhythmias**<br>• **Infranodal** AV block<br>   2nd degree Mobitz II AV block or 3rd degree infranodal AV block<br>• ↗ PR secondary to slowing of His-Purkinje conduction |
| • Progressive onset of AV block | • Sudden onset of AV block (< 24 h); often preceded by RBBB ± LAHB |
| • **Jonctional escape rhythm** (His); narrow QRS; 40-60 bpm | • **Escape rhythm distal to His bundle**<br>• Wide QRS; unstable; risk of asystole |
| • **Often benign and transient (5-7 days)** | • **Often associated with extensive infarction** |
| • Atropine within the first 24 h (vagal hypertonia)<br>• Permanent pacemaker rarely indicated (reversible conduction disorder) | **Temporary pacemaker**<br>• 2nd degree Mobitz II or 3rd degree AV block<br>• Alternating RBBB with LBBB<br>• Acute bifascicular block or *de novo* LBBB<br>• RBBB with ↗ PR<br><br>**Permanent pacemaker**<br>• 2nd degree intra- or infrahisian AV block with alternating branch block<br>• 3rd degree intra- or infrahisian AV block<br>• Persistent 2nd or 3rd degree AV block with symptoms<br>• High-grade transient infranodal 2nd degree or 3rd degree AV block with associated branch block (except for isolated left anterior hemiblock) |

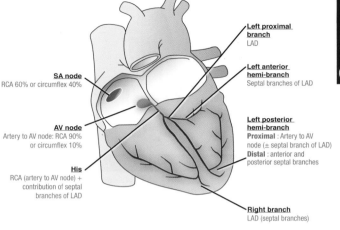

**SA node**
RCA 60% or circumflex 40%

**Left proximal branch**
LAD

**Left anterior hemi-branch**
Septal branches of LAD

**AV node**
Artery to AV node: RCA 90%
or circumflex 10%

**Left posterior hemi-branch**
**Proximal** : Artery to AV node (± septal branch of LAD)
**Distal** : anterior and posterior septal branches

**His**
RCA (artery to AV node) +
contribution of septal
branches of LAD

**Right branch**
LAD (septal branches)

## 2.8/ REVASCULARIZATION - PCI

### SIGNIFICANT STENOSIS

| ANGIOGRAPHIC | HEMODYNAMIC | IVUS (INTRAVASCULAR ULTRASOUND) |
|---|---|---|
| ≥ 70% (LMCA: ≥ 50%) | FFR ≤ 0.80 | • LMCA: Area < 6 mm² (6 to 7.5 mm² → determine FFR) • Other vessels: Area < 4 mm² |

### TECHNIQUES

**BALLOON ANGIOPLASTY (PTCA)**: stretches / tears / redistributes the atherosclerotic plaque in order to enlarge the coronary lumen; risk of dissection or abrupt closure; risk of restenosis

**STENT**: treats the dissection associated with PTCA and ↘ the risk of abrupt closure; ↘ risk urgent CABG; ↘ restenosis

> **One-year clinical restenosis rate: PTCA 30%; BMS 10-15%; DES 3-5%**
>  · **Clinical restenosis**: during the **first 6-9 months** post-PCI
> **DES**: ↘ restenosis and ↘ reintervention; ↗ very late stent thrombosis (> 1 year) (risk markedly decreased with new generation DES)
>  · **New generation DES:** thin-strut platform; limus-based antiprolferative drug; polymer with improved biocompatibility; improved safety compared to early-generation DES; should be considered by default in all clinical conditions and lesion subsets

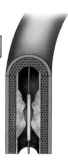
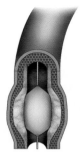
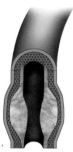

BALLOON ANGIOPLASTY

| PREFER DES | CONSIDER BMS |
|---|---|
| • LMCA<br>• Small vessels (< 2.5 mm diameter)<br>• Long lesion (> 20 mm)<br>• DM<br>• In-stent restenosis<br>• Bifurcation<br>• Vein graft<br>• Chronic total occlusion | • Dual antiplatelet therapy for 3-6 months impossible<br><br>• Probable surgery < 6 months<br><br>• Bleeding risk<br><br>• Anticoagulation (Warfarin or DOAC) required |

**FFR (Fractional flow reserve): to determine whether an intermediate stenosis (50-70%) is hemodynamically significant**

> **Quantify the trans-stenotic pressure gradient**

> ★ **FAME**: angioplasty guided by fractional flow reserve (FFR) determination **associated with improvement of primary outcome** (death; MI; reintervention)

**IVUS (Intravascular ultrasound): A)** Determines the severity of a stenosis on the LMCA; **B)** Determines the mechanism of stent restenosis or thrombosis; **C)** Guidance during complex PCI; **D)** Follow-up of cardiac allograft vasculopathy

**MANUAL ASPIRATION THROMBECTOMY:** aspiration of intra-coronary thrombus; ↘ distal embolism (no benefit in ★ TASTE and ★ TOTAL)

**ROTATIONAL ATHERECTOMY:** Grinding of calcified atherosclerotic plaque; facilitates passage and deployment of the balloon and stent; risk of coronary perforation

## SPECIFIC LESIONS

**IN-STENT RESTENOSIS**: DES implantation or drug-coated balloons; intracoronary imaging

**CHRONIC TOTAL OCCLUSION (CTO)**: revascularization in the presence of significant viability and a significant ischemic territory

> **Percutaneous revascularization**: complex technique via an anterograde approach (± subintimal dissection and re-entry) and/or retrograde approach (via collateral pathways)

**PCI ON VEIN GRAFT**: ↗ risk of periprocedural MI and no-reflow (atheroembolism); use an embolic protection device

### BIFURCATION: 2 strategies

a) PCI with stent in the main vessel only (angioplasty and/or stent in the branch if necessary)
(★ Nordic-Baltic Study IV and ★ TRYTON)

b) PCI with stenting of both vessels (especially if complex bifurcation with large branch
and significant risk of occlusion); terminate the operation with simultaneous inflation of a
balloon in each vessel ("kissing")

| T technique | Culotte | Crush | Kissing |
|---|---|---|---|

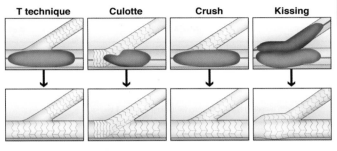

**LEFT MAIN CORONARY ARTERY**: percutaneous revascularization possible if low risk of procedural complications (proximal LMCA; SYNTAX ≤ 32) or high surgical risk

## COMPLICATIONS OF PCI

### RISK OF COMPLICATIONS DURING PCI ACCORDING TO THE TYPE OF LESION

| | |
|---|---|
| **TYPE I:**<br>**Low risk** | 1. Patent Lesion<br>2. Does not meet the criteria for a type C lesion |
| **TYPE II** | 1. Patent Lesion<br>2. Meets one of the criteria of a type C lesion<br>   > Diffuse lesion (> 20 mm long)<br>   > Severe proximal tortuosities<br>   > Extreme angle (> 90°)<br>   > Impossible to protect a major branch<br>   > Vein graft with friable lesions |
| **TYPE III** | • Occluded lesion<br>• Does not meet the criteria for a type C lesion |
| **TYPE IV:**<br>**High risk** | • Occluded lesion<br>• Meets one of the criteria of a type C lesion |

**COMPLICATIONS**: Death (0.7% elective PCI); MI; Stroke (0.2%); TIA; Vascular access site
complication; Coronary perforation (± tamponade); Coronary dissection (abrupt closure); No-reflow
(↘ anterograde flow in the absence of epicardial stenosis secondary to distal microembolism /
vasospasm / endothelial dysfunction; management with Adenosine or intracoronary Verapamil or
GPIIb/IIIa inhibitors); Branch occlusion; Urgent CABG (0.4%); ARF; Hemorrhage

> **Femoral or radial access complications**: ▶▶| Chapter 1 - Coronary angiography
> **Post-coronary angiography ARF**: ▶▶| Chapter 1 - Coronary angiography

**EARLY CHEST PAIN POST-PCI**: Stent thrombosis; Residual dissection / Abrupt closure; No reflow; Distal embolism; Branch occlusion

**STENT THROMBOSIS**: 1% at 1 year; Mortality 20-45%
> **BMS: during first 30 days** (rare after 30 days due to complete neo-endothelialization)  +
> **DES: can occur after 1 year** (very late thrombosis due to incomplete neo-endothelialization); decreased risk with new generation DES  +
> **Risk factors:** acute myocardial infarction; Nonadherence with P2Y12 inhibitor; Resistance to Clopidogrel; DM; Long segment; Small vessels (diameter < 2.5 mm); Bifurcation; Incomplete stent apposition; Dissection at the stent margin; Overlapping stents
> **Treatment:** emergency PCI; Prasugrel or Ticagrelor; IVUS or OCT to detect mechanical problems

## ADJUVANT TREATMENT - ELECTIVE PCI

▶️| Chapter 1 - Coronary angiography

**ASA**: 325 mg then 80 mg qd (long term)

**CLOPIDOGREL: 600 mg loading dose for elective stenting (★ ARMYDA-2) then 75 mg qd**
> **BMS with bleeding risk**: Clopidogrel for a **minimum of 2-4 weeks**
> **DES**: dual antiplatelet therapy for a minimum of **6 months (★ ISAR-SAFE)**
  • Strict minimum of 3-6 months with new generation DES
  • **★ DAPT**: 30 months of DAPT (vs 12 months) associated with ↘ stent thrombosis and MACCE but ↗ moderate or severe bleeding
  • **Prolonged dual antiplatelet therapy**: consider in the presence of a high risk of stent thrombosis (according to anatomy / procedure) or if late stent thrombosis would have major consequences (LMCA; bifurcation; ostium...)

**GPIIB/IIIA INHIBITORS**: at the interventional cardiologist's discretion

**UNFRACTIONATED HEPARIN: A)** Procedure without GPIIb/IIIa inhibitors: 70-100 U/kg targeting ACT 250-300 s (HemoTec) or 300-350 s (Hemochron); **B)** Procedure with GPIIb/IIIa inhibitors: 50-70 IU/kg targeting ACT 200-250 s

**STATIN PRE-PCI** ↘ risk of periprocedural MI (★ ARMYDA; ★ NAPLES II)

# 2.9/ REVASCULARIZATION - SURGERY

## ASSESSMENT OF PERIOPERATIVE RISK

**STS SCORE**: in-hospital or 30-day mortality, and in-hospital morbidity / http://riskcalc.sts.org

**EUROSCORE II**: in-hospital mortality / www.euroscore.org

## ADJUVANT TREATMENT

**ASA**: for all patients (to protect graft patency)

**P2Y12 INHIBITORS**: Stop Clopidogrel and Ticagrelor > 5 days pre-op; Stop Prasugrel > 7 days preop

**GPIIB/IIIA INHIBITORS**: Stop Eptifibatide / Tirofiban 2-4 h pre-op; Stop Abciximab > 12 h pre-op

**STATIN:** for all patients

**ACE INHIBITORS:** for all patients (start postoperatively when hemodynamic stability is achieved)

**BB: > 24h pre-op** (in the absence of contraindication) to prevent perioperative AF (continue post-op)

**GLYCEMIC CONTROL**: target perioperative blood glucose **< 10 mmol/L**

## ASSESSMENT OF CAROTID ARTERIES

**CAROTID DOPPLER IN HIGH-RISK PATIENTS**: > 65 years; LMCA; PAD; History of TIA - stroke; HTN; Smoking; DM

**INDICATIONS FOR PRE-CABG REVASCULARIZATION** (angioplasty / stent or endarterectomy)

a) History of TIA or stroke with 50-99% stenosis (class IIa recommendation)
b) Severe bilateral stenoses (70-99%) or severe unilateral stenosis (70-99%) with contralateral occlusion (class IIb recommendation)
  › Note: diverging indications according to the various guidelines
  › Assessment on an individual basis by a multidisciplinary team including a neurologist

## COMPLICATIONS

**COMPLICATIONS:** Death; Stroke (micro- or macroembolism; hypoperfusion); Cardiogenic shock; Tamponade (often localized over the RA); post-CPB cognitive deficits; ARF; post-CPB SIRS; Hemorrhage; Re-exploration; Prolonged mechanical ventilation; Sternal osteomyelitis / Mediastinitis; Perioperative myocardial infarction; AF; Pulmonary complications (ARDS; Pneumonia; Atelectasis; Phrenic nerve palsy); Intestinal ischemia

**MEDIASTINITIS / STERNAL INFECTION**

› **Risk factors**: DM; Obesity; COPD; Prolonged CPB; REDO; Prolonged intubation; Repeat surgical exploration
› **Management:** Antibiotics; Surgical debridement; Reconstruction (pectoralis muscle flap); VAC; Sternal plate

**VEIN GRAFT**: Early occlusion rate (before discharge from hospital): 10%;   1-year occlusion rate: 25%;   **10-year occlusion rate: 50%**                                                                          +

› **Arterial bypass graft**: **10-year patency rate > 90%**                                             +

## POSTOPERATIVE ATRIAL FIBRILLATION

**0-5 days post-op; Frequently resolves spontaneously in 6-12 weeks**
**PROPHYLAXIS: BB (1st choice)**; Amiodarone if BB contraindicated (400 mg PO bid x 6 days      +
preop and 6 days post-op)
› **Other options**: Sotalol; IV magnesium (1.5 g IV daily for 4 days post-op); Atrial overdrive; Colchicine (★ COPPS-POAF)

**MANAGEMENT**: rate control or rhythm control according to symptoms; anticoagulation if
**AF > 48 h**; review treatment at 12 weeks                                                             +

## MINIMALLY INVASIVE SURGERY

**BEATING HEART (OFF-PUMP):** requires sternotomy with cardiac stabilization device; theoretically avoids the disadvantages of CPB and clamping of the ascending aorta

› **No demonstrated benefit** to date (★ ROOBY, ★ GOPCABE, ★ CORONARY)

**MIDCAB**: left anterior mini-thoracotomy; beating heart internal mammary artery bypass graft to LAD; ventilation of only one lung

› **Hybrid procedure:** LIMA to LAD; PCI of other vessels; avoids sternotomy and clamping of the aorta

**ROBOTIC TOTAL ENDOSCOPIC BYPASS GRAFT**: with femoro-femoral CPB

## 2.10/ PRINZMETAL ANGINA (VASOSPASTIC ANGINA)

**Severe angina at rest with transient ST elevation**

> Worse between midnight and 8:00 am
> **Risk factors**: Smoking; Migraine; Raynaud; 5-fluorouracil; Cyclophosphamide; Hyperventilation; Cold

**COMPLICATIONS**: MI; VT; VF; AV block; Asystole; Sudden death

**STRESS TEST**: 1/3 negative; 1/3 with ST elevation; 1/3 with ST depression

**CORONARY ANGIOGRAPHY**: Coronary spasm; RCA > LAD; Multiple spontaneous spasms on multiples vessels possible

> **Provocation test rarely performed**
>   - **Ergonovine provocation test**: 0.05 to 0.2 mg IV
>   - **Acetylcholine provocation test**: 10-25-50-100 µg intracoronary; focal spasm during Prinzmetal angina

**MANAGEMENT**: Smoking cessation; CCB (combination of dihydropyridine and nondihydropyridine PRN); Nitrates; Prazosin (alpha-blocking agent) and Nicorandil if necessary; Avoid nonselective BB (risk of unopposed alpha stimulation); Avoid ASA (inhibits prostacyclin synthesis); PCI if associated stenosis; $Mg^{2+}$ supplement; Statins may be beneficial; Defibrillator for secondary prevention (especially if ischemia persists despite treatment)

## 2.11/ CARDIAC SYNDROME X

**More or less typical retrosternal chest pain with ischemia documented on noninvasive test (ST depression and/or perfusion abnormality) in the absence of any significant epicardial CAD**

**Associated with increased CARDIOVASCULAR RISK**

**MECHANISM**: probable microvascular endothelial dysfunction with decreased vasodilatation reserve; ± hypersensitivity to pain

> **40-50% of the resistance to coronary flow is derived from the microvasculature**; an insufficient vasodilatation reserve decreases coronary perfusion on exertion

**MANAGEMENT**: ACE inhibitors and Statins (improve endothelial dysfunction); Nitrates; BB; CCB; Treatment of risk factors; Regular exercise

> **Persistent retrosternal chest pain**: Nicorandil; Imipramine or Amitriptyline; Aminophylline; Neurostimulation (spinal cord); External counterpulsation; Psycho-intervention...

# /SOURCES

- Bonow RO, Mann DL, Zipes DP, Libby P. *Braunwald's Heart Disease. A textbook of cardiovascular medicine.* Elsevier. 2012. 1961 p.
- 2014 ACC/AHA/AATS/PCNA/SCAI/STS Focused Update of the Guideline for the Diagnosis and Management of Patients With Stable Ischemic Heart Disease. *JACC* 2014; *64;* 1929-1949.
- 2012 ACCF/AHA/ACP/AATS/PCNA/SCAI/STS Guideline for the Diagnosis and Management of Patients With Stable Ischemic Heart Disease. *JACC* 2012; *60;* e44-e164. 2013
- ESC guidelines on the management of stable coronary artery disease. *EHJ* 2013; *34;* 2949-3003.
- Parker JD, Parker JO. Stable Angina Pectoris: The Medical Management of Symptomatic Myocardial Ischemia. *CJC* 2012; *28;* S70-S80.
- Management of Patients With Refractory Angina: Canadian Cardiovascular Society/Canadian Pain Society Joint Guidelines. *CJC* 2012; *28;* S20-S41.
- Twerenbold R, Jaffe A, Reichlin T et al. High-sensitive troponin T measurements: what do we gain and what are the challenges? *EHJ* 2012; *33;* 579-586
- Morrow DA. Clinical Application of Sensitive Troponin Assays. *NEJM* 2009; *361;* 913-916.
- ACCF 2012 Expert Consensus Document on Practical Clinical Considerations in the Interpretation of Troponin Elevations. *JACC* 2012; *60;* 2427-2463.
- Third Universal Definition of Myocardial Infarction. *Circulation* 2012; *126;* 2020-2035.
- Fitchett DH, Theroux P, Brophy JM et al. Assessment and Management of Acute Coronary Syndromes (ACS): A Canadian Perspective on Current Guideline-Recommended Treatment - Part 1: Non-ST-Segment Elevation ACS. *CJC* 2011; *27;* S387 - S401.
- Fitchett DH, Theroux P, Brophy JM et al. Assessment and Management of Acute Coronary Syndromes (ACS): A Canadian Perspective on Current Guideline-Recommended Treatment - Part 2: ST-Segment Elevation Myocardial Infarction. *CJC* 2011; *27;* S402 - S412.
- 2013 ACCF/AHA Guideline for the Management of ST-Elevation Myocardial Infarction. *Circulation* 2013; *127;* e362-425.
- 2009 Focused Updates: ACC/AHA Guidelines for the Management of Patients With ST-Elevation Myocardial Infarction (Updating the 2004 Guideline and 2007 Focused Update) and ACC/AHA/SCAI Guidelines on Percutaneous Coronary Intervention (Updating the 2005 Guideline and 2007 Focused Update). *JACC* 2009; *54;* 2205-2241.
- 2007 Focused Update of the ACC/AHA 2004 Guidelines for the Management of Patients With ST-Elevation Myocardial Infarction. *JACC* 2008; *51;* 210-247.
- ACC/AHA Guidelines for the Management of Patients With ST-Elevation Myocardial Infarction. *JACC* 2004; *44;* e1-e211
- Morrow DA, Antman EM, Charlesworth A, et al. TIMI risk score for ST-elevation myocardial infarction: a convenient, bedside, clinical score for risk assessment at presentation: an intravenous nPA for treatment of infarcting myocardium early II trial substudy. *Circulation.* 2000; *102:* 2031–2037.
- 2014 AHA/ACC Guideline for the Management of Patients With Non–ST-Elevation Acute Coronary Syndromes. *JACC* 2014; *64;* e139-e228.
- 2015 ESC Guidelines for the management of acute coronary syndromes in patients presenting without persistent ST-segment elevation. *EHJ* 2016; *37;* 267-315.
- Antman EM, Cohen M, Bernink PJ, et al. The TIMI risk score for unstable angina/non-ST elevation MI: a method for prognostication and therapeutic decision making. *JAMA* 2000; *284:* 835–842
- ACCF/ACG/AHA 2010 Expert Consensus Document on the Concomitant Use of Proton Pump Inhibitors and Thienopyridines. *JACC* 2010; *56;* 2051-2066.
- The Use of Antiplatelet Therapy in the Outpatient Setting: Canadian Cardiovascular Society Guidelines. *CJC* 2011; *27;* S1-S59.

Coronary artery disease (CAD) & myocardial infarction

- Reynolds HR, Hochman JS. Cardiogenic Shock: Current Concepts and Improving Outcomes. *Circulation* 2008; *117;* 686-697
- Wang K, Asinger RW, Marriott HL. ST-Segment Elevation in Conditions Other Than Acute Myocardial Infarction. *NEJM* 2003; *349;* 2128-35.
- Zimetbaum PJ, Josephson ME. Use of the Electrocardiogram in Acute Myocardial Infarction. *NEJM* 2003; *348;* 933-940.
- AHA/ACCF/HRS Recommendations for the Standardization and Interpretation of the Electrocardiogram; Part VI: Acute Ischemia/Infarction. *JACC* 2009; *53;* 1003-1011.
- ACC/AHA/HRS 2008 Guidelines for Device-Based Therapy of Cardiac Rhythm Abnormalities. *JACC* 2008; *51;* e1-e62
- 2011 ACCF/AHA/SCAI Guideline for Percutaneous Coronary Intervention. *JACC* 2011; *58;* e1-e81
- Stefanini GG, Holmes DR. Drug-Eluting Coronary-Artery Stents. *NEJM* 2013; *368:* 254-65.
- 2011 ACCF/AHA Guideline for Coronary Artery Bypass Graft Surgery. *JACC* 2011; *58;* e123-210.
- 2014 ESC/EACTS Guidelines on myocardial revascularization: the Task Force on Myocardial Revascularization of the European Society of Cardiology (ESC) and the European Association for Cardio-Thoracic Surgery (EACTS). *EHJ* 2014; *35;* 2541-2619.
- Canadian Cardiovascular Society Atrial Fibrillation Guidelines 2010: Prevention and Treatment of Atrial Fibrillation Following Cardiac Surgery. *CJC* 2011; *27;* 91-97.
- Mehran R, Aymong ED, Nikolsky E. A Simple Risk Score for Prediction of Contrast-Induced Nephropathy After Percutaneous Coronary Intervention. *JACC* 2004; *44:*1393-1399
- Stern S, Bayes de Luna A. Coronary Artery Spasm: A 2009 Update. *Circulation* 2009; *199;* 2531-2534.
- Arthur HM, Campbell P, Harvey PJ et al. Women, Cardiac Syndrome X, and Microvascular Heart Disease. *CJC* 2012; *28;* S42-S49
- Haïat R, Leroy G. *Prescription guidelines in cardiology,* 5th edition. Éditions Frison-Roche. 2015. 350 p.
- UpToDate 2015

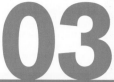

# Heart failure

3.1/ Heart failure: assessment 112
3.2/ Systolic heart failure: management 115
3.3/ Diastolic heart failure (preserved LVEF) 123
3.4/ Decompensated heart failure 125
3.5/ Heart transplantation 130
3.6/ Long-term ventricular assist device 133
3.7/ Right heart failure 136
3.8/ Palliative care 136

# 3.1/ HEART FAILURE: ASSESSMENT

**DEFINITION**: Complex clinical syndrome secondary to a functional or structural abnormality of the heart which impairs the capacity of the ventricle to eject blood (and perfuse tissues) or to be adequately filled

> **This clinical syndrome leads to typical symptoms and signs**                    +

| SYSTOLIC HEART FAILURE | HEART FAILURE WITH PRESERVED LVEF |
|---|---|
| **1. Typical symptoms**<br>**2. Typical signs**<br>**3. ↘ LVEF** | 1. Typical symptoms<br>2. Typical signs<br>3. Normal or slightly decreased LVEF; non-dilated LV<br>4. Structural heart disease (LVH; LAH) and/or diastolic dysfunction |

**LVEF = stroke volume (end-diastolic volume – end-systolic volume) / end-diastolic volume**

> **When LVEF is decreased: stroke volume is maintained by increasing end-diastolic volume** (eccentric LVH)

| SYMPTOMS | SIGNS |
|---|---|
| · Dyspnea<br>· **Orthopnea**<br>· **PND** (1-2 h after going to bed; resolution in 15-30 min)<br>· **↘ Exercise tolerance**<br>· Tiredness<br>· Lower limb edema<br>· **Peripheral edema**<br>· **Nocturnal cough**<br>· Wheezing<br>· Weight gain<br>· Loss of appetite<br>· RUQ pain<br>· Nocturia | · Cachexia<br>· Hypotension; OH; Narrow pulse pressure<br>· Pulsus alternans; ↘ Pulse amplitude<br>· **Tachycardia**<br>· Tachypnea<br>· Cheyne-Stokes breathing<br>· **JVD** ; HJ reflux<br>· Lateralized and widened apex<br>· Left parasternal heave / Signs of PHT<br>· Decreased S1<br>· **S3** - S4 (± palpable)<br>· AV valve regurgitation<br>· **Crackles**<br>· Wheezing<br>· **Signs of pleural effusion**<br>· **Hepatomegaly (± pulsatile)**<br>· **Peripheral edema** (leg edema; scrotum; presacral; ascites)<br>· Cold extremities<br>· Confusion / Decreased level of consciousness |

+

## NYHA FUNCTIONAL CLASS

| NYHA I | No limitation in ordinary physical activity (no tiredness, dyspnea or palpitations) | **≥ 7 METs**<br>· Climbing one flight of stairs with a bag of groceries<br>· Shoveling snow<br>· Bicycling; Skiing; Jogging/walking (8 kph) |
|---|---|---|

| NYHA II | Slight limitation during physical activity; ordinary physical activity causes symptoms (tiredness, dyspnea, palpitations) | **5-7 METs**<br>• Climbing one flight of stairs without stopping<br>• Walking briskly on level ground (6.5 kph)<br>• Gardening; Dancing |
| **NYHA III** | Marked limitation during physical activity; comfortable at rest; less than ordinary activity causes symptoms (tiredness, dyspnea, palpitations) | **2-5 METs**<br>• Showering without a break<br>• Getting dressed without a break<br>• Walking briskly on level ground (4 kph)<br>• Making a bed<br>• Bowling; Golf |
| **NYHA IV** | Inability to carry on any physical activity without discomfort ± symptoms at rest | **< 2 METs**<br>• Unable to perform the activities of NYHA III |

## ETIOLOGIES

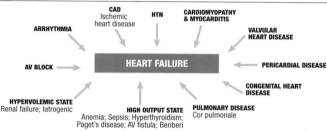

**ARRHYTHMIA**

**CAD** Ischemic heart disease

**HTN**

**CARDIOMYOPATHY & MYOCARDITIS**

**VALVULAR HEART DISEASE**

**AV BLOCK** ⟶

**HEART FAILURE**

⟵ **PERICARDIAL DISEASE**

**CONGENITAL HEART DISEASE**

**HYPERVOLEMIC STATE** Renal failure; Iatrogenic

**HIGH OUTPUT STATE** Anemia; Sepsis; Hyperthyroidism; Paget's disease; AV fistula; Beriberi

**PULMONARY DISEASE** Cor pulmonale

## PATHOPHYSIOLOGY

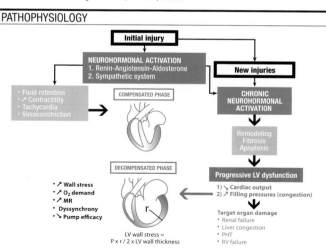

**Initial injury**

**NEUROHORMONAL ACTIVATION**
1. Renin-Angiotensin-Aldosterone
2. Sympathetic system

**New injuries**

• Fluid retention
• ↗ Contractility
• Tachycardia
• Vasoconstriction

COMPENSATED PHASE

**CHRONIC NEUROHORMONAL ACTIVATION**

Remodeling
Fibrosis
Apoptosis

DECOMPENSATED PHASE

**Progressive LV dysfunction**

1) ↘ Cardiac output
2) ↗ Filling pressures (congestion)

• ↗ Wall stress
• ↗ O₂ demand
• ↗ MR
• ↘ Dyssynchrony
• ↘ Pump efficacy

Target organ damage
• Renal failure
• Liver congestion
• PHT
• RV failure

LV wall stress = P x r / 2 x LV wall thickness

# ASSESSMENT

**WORK-UP**: CBC; Electrolytes (including $Ca^{2+}/Mg^{2+}$); Creatinine - BUN; LFTs; Blood glucose; HbA1c; TSH; Urinalysis; Lipids

> **If necessary**: CK; Iron assessment; HIV; ANA; RF; Urine metanephrines; SPEP - UPEP; Uric acid; CRP; Troponin; Polysomnography

**ECG**: Sinus tachycardia; arrhythmia (AF; PVCs; NSVT); Conduction disorder / LBBB; LVH; LAH; Q waves; ischemia; low voltage QRS

> **AV block**: Drug-induced; myocardial infarction; myocarditis; sarcoidosis; familial cardiomyopathy (LMNA; SCN5A); Lyme disease

**CXR**: prominent hila; Kerley B lines (fine horizontal linear opacities extending to the pleura); peribronchial edema; interstitial / alveolar edema; redistribution to apices; pleural effusion; fluid in the fissure; cardiomegaly; other cause of dyspnea

**TTE (± CONTRAST)**: chamber dimensions; LVH; systolic and diastolic function; LVEF (Simpson); valves; PAP; thrombus; cardiac output (LVOT VTI)

**RADIONUCLIDE VENTRICULOGRAPHY**: LVEF; RVEF

**CARDIAC MRI**: cardiac structure and function; LVEF; tissue characterization; evaluation of cardiomyopathy / myocarditis

**CORONARY ANGIOGRAPHY (± FFR)**: rule out significant CAD

> **Noninvasive evaluation** (MIBI-P; stress echocardiography; coronary CT angiography) possible if few risk factors / low pre-test probability / low impact of the result on management

**STRESS TEST / 6MWT / VO₂MAX**: **A)** Objective evaluation of functional class; **B)** Rule out ischemia; **C)** Pre-transplant (VO₂max); **D)** Prescription of exercise; **E)** Prognosis; **F)** Distinguish cardiac from pulmonary cause

> **VO₂max < 12 mL O₂/kg/min** associated with poorer survival than in patients with a heart transplant                                                                          +
> **6MWT**: normal > 600 m; < 350 m roughly equivalent to NYHA III

**BIOPSY**: ▶▶| Chapter 5

**BNP**: released by the failing heart or in response to hemodynamic stress; reflects wall stress and filling pressures

> Increases with age; decreases with obesity
> **DDx ↗**: CRF; arrhythmia; ACS; pulmonary embolism; severe COPD / PHT; sepsis; cirrhosis
> **Indications**: **A)** Identify the cause of dyspnea (cardiac versus non-cardiac); **B)** Prognosis
>   • BNP-guided management of heart failure remains controversial; studies report divergent results

| ACUTE HEART FAILURE UNLIKELY | NT-proBNP < 300 pg/mL (NPV 98 %) | BNP < 100 pg/mL |
|---|---|---|
| PROBABLE ACUTE HEART FAILURE | NT-proBNP > 450 pg/mL (< 50 years) > 900 pg/mL (50-75 years) > 1800 pg/mL (> 75 years) | BNP > 500 pg/mL |

> **Variation**: a change of > 30% in BNP level should call for more intesive follow-up / treatment

# PROGNOSIS

**SEATTLE HEART FAILURE MODEL:** http://depts.washington.edu/shfm

**HEART FAILURE SURVIVAL SCORE**

**PROGNOSTIC FACTORS:** Demographics; Etiology; Comorbidities; NYHA; Hemodynamics (LVEF; PAP; Wedge; Cardiac index; Transpulmonary gradient); Exercise stress test (BP; 6MWT; $VO_2$max; Anaerobic threshold; Ve/$VCO_2$ slope > 35); Anemia; Hyponatremia; QRS duration; BNP; Troponin...

# 3.2/ SYSTOLIC HEART FAILURE: MANAGEMENT

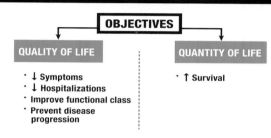

**OBJECTIVES**

**QUALITY OF LIFE**

- ↓ Symptoms
- ↓ Hospitalizations
- Improve functional class
- Prevent disease progression

**QUANTITY OF LIFE**

- ↑ Survival

PROGRESSIVE APPROACH

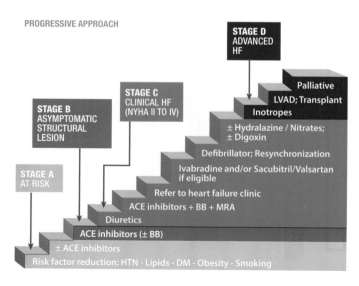

**STAGE D**
**ADVANCED HF**

Palliative

LVAD; Transplant

Inotropes

± Hydralazine / Nitrates; ± Digoxin

**STAGE C**
**CLINICAL HF (NYHA II TO IV)**

Defibrillator; Resynchronization

Ivabradine and/or Sacubitril/Valsartan if eligible

Refer to heart failure clinic

ACE inhibitors + BB + MRA

**STAGE B**
**ASYMPTOMATIC STRUCTURAL LESION**

Diuretics

ACE inhibitors (± BB)

**STAGE A**
**AT RISK**

± ACE inhibitors

Risk factor reduction: HTN - Lipids - DM - Obesity - Smoking

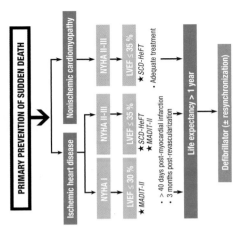

# PRIMARY PREVENTION OF SUDDEN DEATH

**Ischemic heart disease**

- NYHA I — LVEF ≤ 30 % ★ MADIT-II
- NYHA II-III — LVEF ≤ 35 % ★ SCD-HeFT ★ MADIT-II
  - · > 40 days post-myocardial infarction
  - · 3 months post-revascularization

**Nonischemic cardiomyopathy**

- NYHA II-III — LVEF ≤ 35 % ★ SCD-HeFT
  - · Adequate treatment

**Life expectancy > 1 year**

**Defibrillator (± resynchronization)**

---

# HEART FAILURE WITH LVEF < 40%

**Triple therapy**

**ACEi**
★ SOLVD ★ CONSENSUS
ARB if intolerant

**BB**
★ CIBIS ★ MERIT-HF ★ COPERNICUS

**MRA**
★ RALES ★ EMPHASIS-HF
LVEF ≤ 35 %; NYHA II to IV

Titrate to target doses / Maximum tolerated dose

**NYHA II to IV**

**Ivabradine**
★ SHIFT
LVEF ≤ 35%; HR ≥ 70 bpm (SR)

**Sacubitril/Valsartan** ★ PARADIGM-HF
↗ BNP; Replace ACEi or ARB

**Resynchronization - CRT (± ICD)** ★ COMPANION ★ CARE-HF ★ RAFT ★ MADIT-CRT
LVEF ≤ 35%; NYHA III-IV; QRS ≥ 120 ms; LBBB
LVEF ≤ 30%; NYHA II; QRS ≥ 130 ms; LBBB

**NYHA II to IV**

**Digoxin** ★ DIG

**Hydralazine / Nitrates** ★ V-HeFT ★ A-HeFT

**NYHA III to IV**

**Inotropes** **Transplant** **LVAD** **Palliative**

| | INITIAL DOSE (mg) | TARGET DOSE (mg) (to be reached whenever possible) |
|---|---|---|
| **ACE INHIBITORS - ANGIOTENSIN-CONVERTING ENZYME INHIBITORS** | | |
| Captopril | 6.25 tid | 50 tid |
| Enalapril | 1.25 bid | 10-20 bid |
| Lisinopril | 2.5 qd | 20-40 qd |
| Ramipril | 1.25 bid | 5 bid |
| Perindopril | 2.5 qd (2 qd in Canada) | 10 qd (8 qd in Canada) |
| Trandolapril | 0.5 qd | 4 qd |
| **BB - BETA-BLOCKERS** | | |
| Bisoprolol | 1.25 qd | 10 qd |
| Carvedilol | 3.125 bid | 25-50 bid |
| Metoprolol succinate XL | 12.5-25 qd | 200 qd |
| **ARB - ANGIOTENSIN RECEPTOR BLOCKERS** | | |
| Candesartan | 4 qd | 32 qd |
| Valsartan | 20-40 bid | 160 bid |
| **NEPRILYSIN INHIBITOR** | | |
| Sacubitril / Valsartan | 50 (24/26) - 100 (49/51) mg bid | 200 (97/103) mg bid |
| **I$_F$ CHANNEL INHIBITOR** | | |
| Ivabradine | 5 bid | 7.5 bid |
| **LOOP DIURETICS** | | |
| Furosemide | 20-40 qd or bid (adjusted to renal function) | max 600 /24h |
| Bumetanide | 0.5-1 qd or bid | max 10 /24h |
| **MRA - MINERALOCORTICOID RECEPTOR ANTAGONISTS** | | |
| Spironolactone or Eplerenone | **Eplerenone** CrCl > 50 mL/min: 25 mg qd; CrCl 30-49 mL/min: 25 mg every 2 days **Spironolactone** CrCl > 50 mL/min: 12.5 to 25 mg qd; CrCl 30-49 mL/min: 12.5 mg qd or every 2 days | **Eplerenone** CrCl > 50 mL/min: 50 mg qd; CrCl 30-49 mL/min: 25 mg qd **Spironolactone** CrCl > 50 mL/min: 25 mg qd or bid; CrCl 30-49 mL/min: 12.5 to 25 mg qd |
| **THIAZIDE DIURETICS** | | |
| Hydrochlorothiazide | 25 qd ou bid | max 200 /24h |
| Metolazone | 2.5-5 qd | max 20 /24h |
| Indapamide | 2.5 qd | max 5 /24h |
| **DIGOXIN** | | |
| Digoxin | 0.125 **Adjusted to renal function** Total loading dose of 1 mg PO per 24 h in 4 doses divided on the 1st day when rapid effect is required; adjusted to renal function | Plasma target: **0.5 to 0.9 ng/mL** (1 week after titration) |
| **HYDRALAZINE / NITRATES** | | |
| Hydralazine / Nitrates | Hydralazine: 10-25 tid Isosorbide dinitrate: 10 tid | Hydralazine: 75 tid Isosorbide dinitrate: 40 tid |

# ANGIOTENSIN-CONVERTING ENZYME (ACE) INHIBITORS

↘ Mortality; ↘ Hospitalization; Stabilizes remodeling; ↘ Symptoms

STUDIES: ★ CONSENSUS - ★ SOLVD; ★ SOLVD-Prevention (asymptomatic ↘ LVEF - NYHA I);
★ SAVE - ★ AIRE - ★ TRACE (myocardial infarction with heart failure and/or ↘ LVEF); ★ ATLAS
(low-dose vs high-dose Lisinopril)

ADVERSE EFFECTS: ARF; hyperkalemia; hypotension; cough (secondary to ↗ bradykinins);
angioedema

CONTRAINDICATIONS: angioedema; bilateral renal artery stenosis; pregnancy
> **Caution**: creatinine > 221 µmol/L (> 2.5 mg/dL) or GFR < 30 mL/min/1.73m²;
  hyperkalemia > 5.5 mmol/L; SBP < 90 mmHg
  · **< 30% rise in creatinine** or elevation of **K+ up to 5.5 mmol/L** is acceptable           +
> **Follow-up**: assessment 1 week after titration (creatinine; BUN; electrolytes)

# BETA-BLOCKERS (BB)

↘ Mortality; ↘ Hospitalization; ↘ Remodeling; ↘ Symptoms

STUDIES: ★ CIBIS (Bisoprolol) - ★ COPERNICUS (Carvedilol) - ★ MERIT-HF (Metoprolol
succinate XL); ★ SENIORS (Nebivolol; > 70 years); ★ COMET (Carvedilol vs Metoprolol tartrate);
★ B-CONVINCED (BB continued in the presence of decompensation); ★ CAPRICORN - ★ BEAT
(post-myocardial infarction)

ADVERSE EFFECTS: decompensated heart failure; bronchospasm; bradycardia / block;
hypotension; tiredness; depression; nightmares; erectile dysfunction; glucose intolerance

CONTRAINDICATIONS: **active decompensated heart failure** (continue BB if already used           +
predecompensation); shock - hypoperfusion; asthma; 2ⁿᵈ or 3ʳᵈ degree AV block; severe PAD
(ischemia at rest)

> **Treat congestion before initiating a BB; target euvolemia**                                  +
> **Titrate the dose every 2 weeks**
> **Caution**: HR < 60 bpm; recent decompensation; NYHA IV; SBP < 90 mmHg
> **COPD**: favor beta-1 selective BB (Bisoprolol; Metoprolol)

# MINERALOCORTICOID RECEPTOR ANTAGONISTS (MRA)

↘ Mortality; ↘ Hospitalization; ↘ Symptoms

STUDIES: ★ RALES (NYHA III-IV; LVEF < 35 %); ★ EMPHASIS-HF (NYHA II; LVEF < 30 % or < 35 %
with QRS > 130 ms; Recent hospitalization or ↗ BNP); ★ EPHESUS (myocardial infarction;
LVEF < 40%; heart failure or DM)

ADVERSE EFFECTS: hyperkalemia; ARF; gynecomastia - impotence - ↘ libido - menstrual
irregularities (Spironolactone)

CONTRAINDICATIONS: CRF **(creatinine > 221 µmol/L in males or > 177 µmol/L in**              +
**females or GFR < 30 mL/min); hyperkalemia > 5 mmol/L**

> Titration every 4-8 weeks
> **Follow-up**: assessment 1 week and 4 weeks after titration; at 8 weeks - 12 weeks;
  at 6 - 9 - 12 months; then every 4 months

# DIURETICS

↘ Symptoms

**Target dry weight; target lowest possible dose**

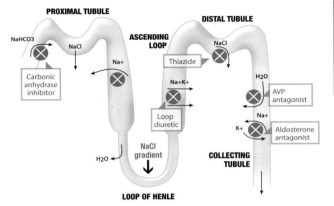

**PROXIMAL TUBULE**

NaHCO3

NaCl

Na+

Carbonic anhydrase inhibitor

**DISTAL TUBULE**

**ASCENDING LOOP**

NaCl

Thiazide

Na+K+

Loop diuretic

NaCl gradient

H2O

**LOOP OF HENLE**

H2O

AVP antagonist

Na+

K+

Aldosterone antagonist

**COLLECTING TUBULE**

**ADVERSE EFFECTS**: ARF; hypovolemia; hypokalemia; hyponatremia (thiazides); hypomagnesemia; metabolic alkalosis; hyperuricemia; ototoxicity

**CAUTION**: CRF; hypokalemia; hypotension

> **Follow-up:** assessment 1 week after titration (creatinine; BUN; electrolytes; $Mg^{2+}$)

> **Target K+ 4-5 mmol/L**

|  | SODIUM EXCRETION | DURATION OF ACTION | COMMENTS |
|---|---|---|---|
| **Loop diuretics** | 25 % | 4-8 h (furosemide) | • Inhibition of the ascending loop Na-K-2Cl pump<br>• **Secreted into the proximal tubule** (this secretion depends on renal perfusion and the bioavailability of the drug)<br>• **Dose−effect response** (a tubular concentration threshold must be reached to obtain an effect)<br>• Venodilator effect |
| **Thiazides** | 5-10 % | 6-12 h (HCTZ) 12-24 h (Metolazone) | • Inhibition of the distal tubule Na-Cl pump<br>• Less effective when GFR < 30 mL/min<br>• ↘ clearance of free water (risk of hyponatremia); ↗ $Ca^{2+}$ reabsorption |
| **Mineralo−corticoid receptor antagonists** | 1-2 % | 2-3 h | • Inhibition of the collecting tubule Na-K pump at the site of action of aldosterone<br>• **Antagonism of the harmful effects of aldosterone on the heart** |
| **Vasopressin antagonist** | 0 % | 24 h | • Free water diuresis (aquaretic)<br>• Action on collecting tubule (V2 receptors)<br>• Useful in the presence of hyponatremia; no benefit in ★EVEREST |

## DIURETIC RESISTANCE

> **Mechanisms: A)** Post-sodium excretion stimulation of RAA / sympathetic systems (rebound sodium absorption); **B)** ↘ Drug absorption (edema of intestinal wall); **C)** ↘ Cardiac output (↘ renal perfusion therefore ↘ tubular secretion of the diuretic); **D)** Hypertrophy of distal tubule; **E)** ARF or cardiorenal syndrome

> **Management**
  **a)** Strict water / NaCl restriction
  **b)** Increase the dose of the loop diuretic or increase the frequency of administration
  **c)** Addition of an mineralocorticoid receptor antagonist
  **d)** Combination of loop diuretic and metolazone (temporary measure; daily assessments)
  **e)** Continuous Lasix infusion (sustained sodium excretion):
  • 20-40 mg IV bolus then infusion 5-40 mg/h (400 mg/100 mL NS)
  **f)** Inotropes: Dopamine (renal effect) or Dobutamine or Milrinone
  **g)** Ultrafiltration: refractory patient (★UNLOAD: ↘ Hospitalization; no benefit in ★CARESS-HF); slow continuous veno-venous method

## ANGIOTENSIN RECEPTOR BLOCKERS (ARB)

INDICATIONS: **A)** Intolerance to ACE inhibitors (cough; angioedema); **B)** In combination with ACE inhibitors if intolerant to mineralocorticoid receptor antagonists and persistent symptoms

STUDIES

> **Intolerance to ACE inhibitors**: ★ CHARM-Alternative (Candesartan); ↘ Cardiovascular mortality; ↘ Hospitalization

> **ARB combined with ACE inhibitors**: ★ Val-HeFT (Valsartan) - ★ CHARM-ADDED (Candesartan); ↘ Cardiovascular mortality (Candesartan); ↘ Hospitalization; ↘ Symptoms

> **Post-myocardial infarction** (with heart failure and/or ↘ LVEF): ★ VALIANT (Valsartan vs Captopril vs Combinaison) → Valsartan non-inferior to Captopril

## NEPRILYSIN INHIBITOR

↗ Active natriuretic peptides

★ PARADIGM-HF: LVEF ≤ 35-40 %; NYHA II-IV; NTproBNP ≥ 600 pg/ml (or ≥ 400 pg/ml if hospitalized < 12 months); Sacubitril + Valsartan vs Enalapril → ↘ Mortality; ↘ Hospitalization; ↘ Symptoms; ↗ Hypotension; ↗ Angioedema

DOSING (SACUBITRIL/VALSARTAN): stop ACEi 36 h before; start with 50 (24/26) or 100 (49/51) mg bid; double the dose after 2-4 weeks; target dose of 200 (97/103) mg bid if tolerated

## IVABRADINE

Inhibits the sinoatrial node $I_f$ current channel

STUDIES: ★ SHIFT (LVEF ≤ 35 %; NYHA II-IV; HR ≥ 70 bpm; recent hospitalization); ↘ Hospitalization; ↘ Symptoms; ↘ Remodeling

ADVERSE EFFECTS: bradycardia; phosphenes

## DIGOXIN

Inhibits the Na-K-ATPase pump: ↗ intramyocyte $Ca^{2+}$ (positive inotropic agent); ↗ vagal tone

INDICATIONS: **A)** Persistent symptoms despite standard treatment; **B)** AF (rate control)

STUDIES: ★ DIG (NYHA II-IV; LVEF < 45 %) → ↘ Hospitalization; ↘ Symptoms

Adjustment according to renal function and serum digoxin levels

> **Target serum Digoxin level 0.5 to 0.9 ng/mL** +

ADVERSE EFFECTS: atrial / junctional / ventricular arrhythmias (especially in the presence of hypokalemia) combined with blocks; visual disorders; confusion; GI symptoms

CONTRAINDICATIONS: CRF; bradycardia - blocks

MULTIPLE DRUG INTERACTIONS

> ↗ **Serum Digoxin levels**: Amiodarone; Verapamil; Nifedipine; Diltiazem; Quinidine; Propafenone; Captopril; Carvedilol; Spironolactone; Cyclosporine; Macrolides

# HYDRALAZINE - ISOSORBIDE DINITRATE

↘ **Mortality in Afro-Americans;** ↘ Hospitalization; ↘ Symptoms

INDICATIONS: **A)** Intolerance to ACE inhibitors and ARB; **B)** Persistent symptoms despite BB - ACE inhibitors - MRA **(particularly in Afro-Americans)**

STUDIES: ★ V-HeFT-1 and 2; ★ A-HeFT (Afro-Americans)

ADVERSE EFFECTS: headache; hypotension; nausea; arthralgia; asymptomatic ↗ ANA; drug-induced lupus

# NON-PHARMACOLOGICAL TREATMENT

SELF-SURVEILLANCE OF WEIGHT

> Daily weight; on waking; before getting dressed; post-voiding → increase the dose of diuretics or notify if weight ↗ > 1.5-2 kg or 3-4 lbs (x 2-3 days)

SODIUM: < 2-3 g per day

FLUIDS: < 2 liters per day (especially if hyponatremia or refractory congestion)

VACCINATION: influenza (annually); pneumococcus (every 5 years)

TREATMENTS TO BE AVOIDED: **A)** Thiazolidinediones; **B)** Non-dihydropyridine CCBs; **C)** NSAIDs; **D)** Certain AAD: Dronedarone (★ ANDROMEDA); Class I AAD (★ CAST); **E)** Alpha-blockers

# EXERCISE

★ HF-ACTION → improves symptoms and functional capacity

Regular isotonic exercise (walking; stationary bike) after stress test (rule out ischemia - arrhythmia)

> **Prescription**: 3-5 times a week; 30-45 min; **60-70% of peak heart rate** (or peak VO$_2$) **or 4-5-6/10 on Borg's scale** (▶▶| Chapter 9)

# IMPLANTABLE CARDIAC DEFIBRILLATOR (ICD)

SECONDARY PREVENTION: defibrillator indicated

PRIMARY PREVENTION

> **Studies**: ★ SCD-HeFT (nonischemic cardiomyopathy or ischemic heart disease; NYHA II-III; LVEF ≤ 35% [mean = 25%]) and ★ MADIT-II (ischemic heart disease; LVEF ≤ 30%; NYHA I-III) → ↘ mortality

> **Avoid in NYHA IV (except when the patient is a candidate for transplant or mechanical + support) due to poor prognosis and death predominantly secondary to progressive heart failure**

# CARDIAC RESYNCHRONIZATION THERAPY (CRT)

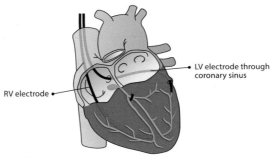

LV electrode through coronary sinus

RV electrode

## INDICATIONS

| ✓ AMBULANT, NYHA III OR IV<br>✓ LVEF ≤ 35 %<br>✓ LBBB – QRS ≥ 120 MS<br>✓ SINUS RHYTHM<br>✓ LIFE EXPECTANCY > 1 YEAR | ✓ NYHA II<br>✓ LVEF ≤ 30 %<br>✓ LBBB – QRS ≥ 120–130 MS<br>✓ SINUS RHYTHM<br>✓ LIFE EXPECTANCY > 1 YEAR |
|---|---|
| STUDIES: ★ CARE-HF - COMPANION<br>↘ Mortality; ↘ Hospitalization; ↘ Symptoms; Reverse remodeling | STUDIES: ★ RAFT - MADIT-CRT<br>↘ Mortality (★ RAFT); ↘ Hospitalization; ↘ Symptoms; Reverse remodeling |

### UNCERTAIN BENEFICIAL EFFECTS OF RESYNCHRONIZATION

a) **Permanent AF with above indications** (consider AV node blocking agents or AV node ablation to force resynchronization)
b) **Patient with systolic dysfunction and frequent RV pacing** (consider resynchronization if significant RV pacing > 40%)                     +

### PROCEDURAL SUCCESS: 90 %

> Minithoracotomy approach with epicardial lead PRN
> **Complications (14% in ★ RAFT)**: pneumothorax; pocket hematoma; pocket infection; lead migration; coronary sinus perforation / dissection (1%)

### PARAMETERS INFLUENCING THE RESPONSE TO RESYNCHRONIZATION: % biventricular pacing; baseline degree of asynchrony (QRS ≥ 150 ms); lead position (target = basal lateral branch of CS); lead pacing scar tissue; ischemic heart disease << nonischemic cardiomyopathy; CRT programming (AV delay; VV delay)

> **Non-responders**: 30 %

# ATRIAL FIBRILLATION

### RATE CONTROL: **non-inferior to rhythm control (★ AF-CHF)**                     +

> **A)** BB; **B)** Digoxin; **C)** Amiodarone to control HR as necessary (patient should be anticoagulated for 1 month because of the risk of CCV); **D)** AV node ablation + PPM; consider resynchronization

### RHYTHM CONTROL: patients with severe symptoms or reversible cause / precipitating factor

> **A)** ECV; **B)** Amiodarone or Dofetilide; **C)** ± PV isolation (benefit in ★ PABA-CHF and ★ AATAC-AF)

## WARFARIN - ANTICOAGULATION

INDICATIONS: **A)** AF; **B)** Thrombus; **C)** History of thromboembolic disease

No benefit in ★ WARCEF study (LVEF < 35% in SR; for thromboembolic primary prevention)

## SLEEP-DISORDERED BREATHING

**CENTRAL SLEEP APNEA - CHEYNE-STOKES (40%)**: hyperventilation followed by apnea
(≥ 10 s with no ventilatory effort); **associated with pulmonary congestion**; independent risk
factor of mortality

> **Diagnosis**: Polysomnography
> **Treatment**: Optimize management of heart failure; CPAP (no benefit in ★ CANPAP study);
> Adaptive servo-ventilation associated with ↗ mortality in ★ SERVE-HF

**OBSTRUCTIVE SLEEP APNEA (10%)**: Leads to hypoxemia / hypercapnia / intermittent
sympathetic stimulation

> Look for obesity / ↗ neck circumference; snoring; daytime sleepiness; apneas
> **Complications**: refractory HTN; nocturnal HTN; PHT; arrhythmias
> **Diagnosis**: Polysomnography (screening with nocturnal saturometry)
> **Treatment**: Weight loss; CPAP

## ANEMIA

Multifactorial

TREATMENT: Transfusions; IV iron (★ FAIR-HF; ★ CONFIRM HF); no benefit for EPO (★ RED-HF)

## ISCHEMIC LEFT VENTRICULAR SYSTOLIC DYSFUNCTION

**REVASCULARIZATION**: possible benefit in the presence of significant viability; highly controversial
topic (mixed results of ★ STICH study; ★ ISCHEMIA study ongoing)

## FUNCTIONAL MITRAL REGURGITATION

**Carpentier I and IIIb mechanisms**; maintains systolic dysfunction (which maintains MR)

**MVR OR MITRAL ANNULOPLASTY**: possible improvement in functional class; associated with
reverse remodeling; no convincing data on survival; MVR possibly superior (★ CTSN)

> Consider in severe secondary MR with: CABG or concomitant AVR (class IIa recommendation)
> or refractory NYHA III - IV (class IIb recommendation)

**MITRACLIP**: consider in the presence of significant MR with refractory symptoms in a patient
who is not a candidate for surgery

# 3.3/ DIASTOLIC HEART FAILURE (preserved LVEF)

**Secondary to abnormal active relaxation and/or ↗ passive rigidity**

**50% of patients with heart failure**

ALL-CAUSE MORTALITY similar to that of heart failure with ↘ LVEF

> Mortality is mostly due to non-cardiovascular causes

RISK FACTORS: Age; Female; HTN; LVH; Ischemia; DM; Obesity; RCM; HCM

FACTORS ASSOCIATED WITH DECOMPENSATION: uncontrolled / labile HTN; AF; Ischemia;
Volume overload; Extracardiac cause

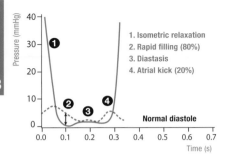

1. Isometric relaxation
2. Rapid filling (80%)
3. Diastasis
4. Atrial kick (20%)

**Normal diastole**

**DIASTOLIC DYSFUNCTION**

Abnormal relaxation
and/or ↑ passive rigidity

⬇

↑ Filling pressures

⬇

↑ LA pressure

**ETIOLOGIES OF**
**↓ RELAXATION VELOCITY**
- ↑ LV afterload
- Ischemia
- Age
- Systolic dysfunction
  (↓ recoil)
- LVH

**TTE**: LVH - concentric remodeling; diastolic pattern; filling pressures; LA dilatation; PAP; RV function; Rule out pericardial disease

> ↗ **Filling pressures**: E/e' > 15; E/A inversion with Valsalva; diastolic dominance (PV outflow); prolonged reversal of flow in PV during atrial kick; LA dilatation; PHT

**STRESS TEST**: Rule out exaggerated hypertensive response (which exacerbates diastolic dysfunction); Rule out chronotropic incompetence

**BNP**: less sensitive than in systolic heart failure

## MANAGEMENT

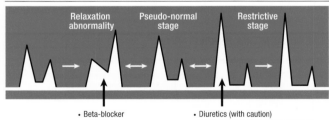

| Relaxation abnormality | Pseudo-normal stage | Restrictive stage |

- Beta-blocker
- ± Diuretics

- Diuretics (with caution)
- Avoid beta-blockers (cardiac output becomes rate dependent)

**No treatment proven to decrease morbidity or mortality**

> **No benefit in**: ★ CHARM-Preserved - ★ PEP-CHF - ★ I-Preserve - ★ TOPCAT - ★ NEAT-HFpEF

**DIURETICS**: symptoms / congestion control

**RISK FACTOR REDUCTION**: CAD; HTN (rule out renovascular syndrome in the presence of refractory HTN)

**REVASCULARIZATION**: if significant ischemia / symptoms

**RATE CONTROL** during AF (± rhythm control)

**CONSIDER**: ACE inhibitor or ARB; BB; MRA

# 3.4/ DECOMPENSATED HEART FAILURE

**Acute or subacute onset or modification of symptoms and signs of heart failure**

Decompensated chronic heart failure (80%) vs *de novo* heart failure (20%)

50% of patients have preserved LVEF

## PATHOPHYSIOLOGY

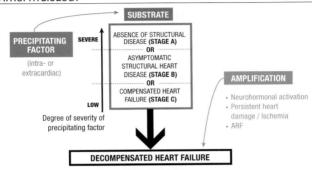

**↓ Cardiac output and/or ↑ Filling pressures**

---

## VARIOUS SCENARIOS

| TAS > 160; ACUTE PULMONARY EDEMA | NORMAL BP | HYPOTENSION (SBP < 90) |
|---|---|---|
| • LVEF often preserved<br>• Acute pulmonary edema<br>• **Treatment**: Vasodilators; Diuretics; BiPAP; Rule out renal artery stenosis | • Systemic congestion<br>• Subacute (often decompensated chronic heart failure)<br>• **Treatment**: Diuretics; ± Vasodilators | • Low output<br>• Renal hypoperfusion<br>• **Treatment**: Positive inotropes (Milrinone; Dobutamine); Vasopressors; Mechanical support |

| CARDIOGENIC SHOCK | MYOCARDIAL INFARCTION (KILLIP II OR III) | RIGHT HEART FAILURE |
|---|---|---|
| • Acute event (ACS; mechanical complication; fulminant myocarditis)<br>• **Treatment**: Reperfusion; Positive inotropes; Vasopressors; IABP; Mechanical support; Surgery | • Rapid onset<br>• Resolution with treatment of ischemia<br>• **Treatment**: Reperfusion; Nitrates; Ensure good coronary perfusion pressure | • RV infarction; PHT; Pulmonary embolism<br>• Hypotension / systemic congestion<br>• Interventricular dependence: RV dilatation induces ↘ LV filling<br>• **Treatment**: Diuretics; Inotropes; Reperfusion; Pulmonary vasodilators |

## PRECIPITATING FACTORS

| ACUTE DETERIORATION | SUBACUTE DETERIORATION |
| --- | --- |
| • Tachyarrhythmia<br>• Bradyarrhythmia - Blocks<br>• Acute coronary syndrome / Ischemia<br>• Mechanical complication of MI<br>• Valvular heart disease (e.g.: ischemic MR)<br>• Pulmonary embolism<br>• Hypertensive crisis<br>• Cardiac tamponade<br>• Aortic dissection<br>• Surgery<br>• Hemorrhage<br>• Endocarditis | • Infection<br>• COPD exacerbation / Asthma<br>• ARF<br>• Nonadherence to treatment<br>• Nonadherence to restrictions<br>• Drugs (NSAID; corticosteroids; Pregabalin)<br>• Arrhythmias - Blocks<br>• Uncontrolled HTN<br>• Hypothyroidism / Hyperthyroidism<br>• Alcohol - Illicit drugs<br>• Anemia<br>• LBBB<br>• Progression of heart disease |

## MANAGEMENT

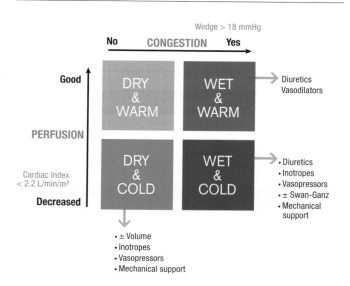

```
                                          • Monitor
                                          • Vital signs - SaO₂
┌─────────────────────────┐               • Urine output
│   ACUTE HEART FAILURE   │               • SVO₂
└─────────────────────────┘
```

```
┌──────────────────────────┐  and/or  ┌──────────────────────────┐
│ ↗ FILLING PRESSURES /    │ ◄──────► │ ↘ CARDIAC OUTPUT         │
│   CONGESTION             │          │   (< 2.2 L/min/m²)       │
│ (Wedge > 18 mmHg and/or  │          └──────────────────────────┘
│  CVP > 8 mmHg)           │
└──────────────────────────┘
```

```
• Diuretics (Lasix)                    ┌──────────────────────┐        • Cold skin
• Vasodilators (Nitrates)              │  TARGET ORGAN        │ ──►    • Urine output
• Morphine                             │  HYPOPERFUSION       │          < 20 mL/h
• O₂ (target SaO₂ > 92 %)              └──────────────────────┘        • SVO₂ < 70 %
• BiPAP or Mechanical ventilation                                      • Confusion
  if respiratory failure                                               • Ischemia
```

**Rule out reversible cause**

```
┌──────────────────────┐   ┌──────────────────────┐   ┌──────────────────────┐
│ Hemodynamic          │   │ Normal systemic      │   │ ↗↗ systemic vascular │
│ instability          │   │ vascular resistance  │   │ resistance           │
│ and/or               │   │ (1000 - 1200 dynes   │   │                      │
│ ↘ systemic vascular  │   │ x s/cm⁵)             │   │                      │
│ resistance           │   │                      │   │                      │
└──────────────────────┘   └──────────────────────┘   └──────────────────────┘
```

**Maintain perfusion of vital
organs (heart; CNS)**
• Vasopressors
  (Norepinephrine; Dopamine)
• Non-vasodilator inotropes

• Inotropes
• Vasodilators

• Vasodilators
• Inotropes

• Intra-aortic balloon pump
• Short-term percutaneous ventricular support (ECMO; Impella;
  TandemHeart) as "bridge to decision"

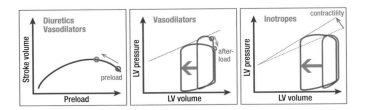

| VASODILATORS | | |
|---|---|---|
| Nitroglycerin | Dose: 10-20 µg/min up to 200 µg/min | • ↗ cGMP in smooth muscle cells (= vasodilatation)<br>• Venous vasodilator (↘ filling pressures) then arterial (↘ afterload; coronary vasodilatation) |
| | Standard dilution: 50 mg/250 mL D5% = 200 µg/mL | • Adverse effects: Tolerance during prolonged use; Hypotension; Headache |
| Nitroprusside | Dose: 0.3 µg/kg/min up to 5 µg/kg/min | • Balanced vasodilator<br>• Short half-life |
| | Standard dilution: 50 mg/250 mL NS = 200 µg/mL | • Used for hypertensive emergency or acute MR<br>• Adverse effects: Risk of cyanide toxicity; Hypotension |
| Nesiritide | • Bolus: 2 µg/kg<br>• Perfusion: 0.01-0.03 µg/kg/min | • Recombinant BNP<br>• Balanced vasodilator<br>• No benefit in ★ ROSE-AHF and ★ ASCEND-HF |

| INOTROPES | | |
|---|---|---|
| Dobutamine | Dose: 2-20 µg/kg/min | • Beta-1 and beta-2 agonist<br>• Supplementary alpha-1 effect at higher doses (neutralizing the beta-2 vasodilator effect) |
| | Standard dilution: 250 mg/ 100 mL D5% = 2500 µg/mL | • **Favor to Milrinone in the presence of significant hypotension** +<br>• Arrhythmogenic |
| Dopamine | • Renal effect (Dopamine) < 3 µg/kg/min<br>• Beta-1: 3-5 µg/kg/min<br>• Alpha-1 (and Beta-1): > 5 µg/kg/min (up to 20 µg/kg/min) | • Dose-dependent effect<br>• Positive inotrope and vasopressor (vasodilator at low doses)<br>• Norepinephrine precursor<br>• Arrhythmogenic |
| | Standard dilution: 400 mg / 250 mL D5% = 1600 µg/mL | • ↗ Mortality in cardiogenic shock (★ SOAP II) |
| Milrinone | • Bolus: 25-75 µg/kg x 10-20 min (optional; avoid if hypotension)<br>• Infusion: 0.375 - 0.75 µg/kg/min<br>• Adjustment to GFR | • Phosphodiesterase inhibitor (↗ intra-myocyte cAMP = ↗ intracellular Ca²⁺)<br>• Risk of hypotension (vasodilator)<br>• Caution in patients with CAD (hypotension can accentuate ischemia) |
| | Standard dilution: 10 mg/100 mL D5% = 90 µg/mL | • Effective despite BB<br>• Favor if BP preserved<br>• Less arrhythmogenic than dobutamine<br>• No benefit in ★ OPTIME-HF study |
| Levosimendan | • Bolus: 12 µg/kg x 10 min (optional; risk of hypotension)<br>• Infusion 0.05 - 0.2 µg/kg/min | • Calcium sensitizer<br>• Positive inotrope and vasodilator<br>• Equivalent to Dobutamine in ★ SURVIVE |

| Isuprel | Dose: 0.5 to 10 µg/min | • Beta-1 and beta-2 agonist |
| | Standard dilution: 1 mg / 250 mL D5% = 4 µg/mL | • Prominent positive chronotropic effect • Risk of hypotension (beta-2 effect) |

| VASOPRESSORS | | |
|---|---|---|
| Norepine-phrine | Dose: 0.2 -1 µg/kg/min | • Alpha-1 agonist • Beta-1 effect (but reflex bradycardia secondary to ↗ MAP) |
| | Standard dilution: 4 mg / 250 mL D5% = 16 µg/mL | |
| Epinephrine | • Bolus: 1 mg IV every 3-5 min (during resuscitation) • Infusion: 0.05 - 0.5 µg/kg/min | • Alpha-1, beta-1 and beta-2 agonist • Arrhythmogenic |
| | Standard dilution: 5 mg / 250 mL D5% = 20 µg/mL | |
| Phenylephrine | Dose: 40 - 60 µg/min | • Pure alpha-1 agonist |
| | Standard dilution: 10 mg / 250 mL NS = 40 µg/mL | |

MONITORING: Cardiac monitoring - Regular vital signs - $SaO_2$ - urine output; daily weight

LMNOP: **IV Lasix; Morphine if anxiety / distress (2.5-5 mg IV); Nitrates (avoid if hypotension); $O_2$; Position - PEEP**

> **Diuretic**: ★ DOSE study → bolus bid equivalent to IV infusion; low-dose IV (equal to usual oral doses) equivalent to high-dose IV (2.5 x usual oral doses)

> **BiPAP**: contraindicated in the presence of hypotension; Vomiting; Impaired level of consciousness; Uncooperative patient

INOTROPES (Dobutamine; Milrinone): **indicated in the presence of peripheral hypoperfusion**

> **Adverse effects**: Hypotension (vasodilator effect); Arrhythmogenic; ↗ $O_2$ demand; ↗ Long-term mortality

VASOPRESSORS (Norepinephrine): indicated in the presence of severe hypotension

> **Objective: redirect cardiac output to vital organs**                                    +

> **Adverse effects**: ↗ Afterload; ↗ $O_2$ demand; Arrhythmogenic

SWAN-GANZ: Indications → **A)** Cardiogenic shock despite inotropes / vasopressors;
**B)** Patient refractory to treatment; **C)** Uncertain hemodynamic parameters (filling pressures; SVR);
**D)** Hemodynamic assessment prior to transplant / mechanical support

> **Hemodynamic targets**

| WEDGE | CVP | BP | $SVO_2$ | SVR | CARDIAC INDEX |
|---|---|---|---|---|---|
| < 18 mmHg | < 8 mmHg | MAP > 60 mmHg SBP > 80 mmHg | > 70 % | 1000 to 1200 dynes x s/cm⁵ | > 2.2 L/min/m² |

MONITORING OF TREATMENT: improvement in symptoms / signs of congestion / peripheral perfusion; $SVO_2$; BP; weakness - OH; urine output; daily weight; CVP; BUN - creatinine - electrolytes

IDENTIFICATION AND TREATMENT OF REVERSIBLE CAUSES: Ischemia; Arrhythmia; Valvular heart disease; Other precipitating factors

DISCHARGE FROM HOSPITAL: congestion resolved; **dry weight achieved**; ACE inhibitors - BB - mineralocorticoid receptor antagonist initiated; stable dose of diuretics and stable labs for > 48 h; restrictions explained; registration in specialized clinic; follow-up < 1 month (vulnerable phase)

# SHORT-TERM AND MEDIUM-TERM MECHANICAL SUPPORT

**OBJECTIVE: Maintain adequate target organ perfusion** during acute treatment and/or while waiting for recovery and/or while waiting for heart transplant or long-term ventricular support

### SHORT-TERM PERCUTANEOUS MECHANICAL SUPPORT

> **IABP**: increases cardiac output **< 10-15 %**; increases coronary perfusion; contraindicated in the presence of AR or aortic dissection
> **Impella 2.5 and 5.0 L/min**: Femoral artery → Aortic valve
> **TandemHeart: A)** Filling cannula: femoral vein → transseptal → LA; **B)** Ejection cannula: femoral artery
  - **Disadvantages** (Impella and TandemHeart): lower limb ischemia; cannula displacement; difficult transport
> **ECMO**: complete cardiopulmonary support
  - **Disadvantages**: anticoagulation; lower limb ischemia; incomplete LV decompression; requires qualified personnel; activation of an inflammatory cascade

### MEDIUM-TERM MECHANICAL SUPPORT (LVAD OR RVAD OR PARACORPOREAL BIVAD)
Thoratec VAD; CentriMag; Abiomed BVS5000

## CARDIORENAL SYNDROME

Impaired renal function associated with heart failure

**MECHANISMS: A)** Low output; **B)** Venous congestion; **C)** Medications (ACE inhibitors; ARB; contrast agents); **D)** Intravascular hypovolemia (diuretics) = activation of RAA / sympathetic systems; **E)** Underlying renal disease (HTN; DM; PAD); **F)** ↗ Intra-abdominal pressure (ascites)

**RENAL PERFUSION PRESSURE** = MAP - CVP

| NORMAL RENAL FUNCTION | GFR > 90 mL/min/1.73 m² |
|---|---|
| STAGE II CRF | GFR 60 - 89 mL/min/1.73 m² |
| STAGE III CRF | GFR 30 - 59 mL/min/1.73 m² |
| STAGE IV CRF | GFR 15 - 29 mL/min/1.73 m² |
| STAGE V CRF | GFR < 15 mL/min/1.73 m² |

# 3.5/ HEART TRANSPLANTATION

### INDICATION

**Late-stage heart disease after optimal medical / surgical therapy, in presence of an unacceptable quality of life and a poor anticipated survival**
Late-stage heart failure; Severe refractory ischemic symptoms; Refractory life-threatening arrhythmias; Complex congenital heart disease...
- **Cardiopulmonary stress testing** to guide transplant listing (reach anaerobic threshold)
  > Peak VO₂ **≤ 12 mL/kg/min** (in the presence of a beta-blocker)
  > Peak VO₂ **≤ 14 mL/kg/min** (patients intolerant to beta-blockers)
  > Percent of predicted peak VO₂ ≤ 50% (in young patients)
- **Heart failure prognosis score** to guide transplant listing
  > Seattle Heart Failure Model: 1-year survival < 80%
  > Heart Failure Survival Score: High / Medium risk

# ASSESSMENT

**POTENTIAL DONOR**: cold ischemia time < 4 h; TTE; coronary angiography (depending on risk factors / age); donor size

**IMMUNOLOGICAL WORK-UP**: blood group; antibody screening; Panel reactive antibody (PRA); specific HLA antibodies (directed against human leukocyte antigens)

> **PRA > 10 %**: recipient patient sensitized; ↗ risk of humoral rejection
>  • **Management**: IV Ig; Rituximab; plasmapheresis

## CONTRAINDICATIONS

> **Fixed high pulmonary vascular resistances**
>  • **Pulmonary vascular resistances > 5 WU**
>  • **Transpulmonary gradient (mPAP – Wedge) > 16-20 mmHg**
>  • **Pulmonary vascular resistance index (TPG / CI) > 6**
>  • **Pulmonary vascular resistances > 2.5 WU in response to pharmacological challenge while maintaining SBP > 85 mmHg (NO; Nitroprusside; Prostanoids; Inotropes)**
>   • High risk of RV failure and mortality after cardiac transplantation
>   • Consider aggressive medical therapy (diuretics; inotropes; IV vasodilators; NO) and temporary mechanical support (IABP; LVAD) to improve these parameters

> **Others**: **A)** Irreversible renal dysfunction (GFR < 30 mL/min); **B)** Irreversible significant liver disease (biopsy PRN); **C)** Pre-existing cancer when the risk of tumor recurrence is significant; **D)** Active infection; **E)** Clinically severe symptomatic cerebrovascular disease; **F)** Peripheral arterial disease when it limits rehabilitation; **G)** DM with target organ damage or persistent poor glycemic control (HbA1c > 7.5%); **H)** Active mental illness / Nonadherence; **I)** Active smoking (previous 6 months) or active substance abusers (including alcohol); **J)** Obesity (BMI > 35 kg/m²); **K)** Age > 70 years old (consider selected patients); **L)** Frailty

# PRIORITY ALLOCATION SYSTEM

| | |
|---|---|
| **STATUS 4** | • Dependent on mechanical support (or mechanical ventilation) and in the intensive care unit |
| **STATUS 3.5** | • In-hospital inotrope-dependent (high doses or multiple agents)<br>• Highly sensitized patient<br>• Refractory life-threatening arrhythmia |
| **STATUS 3** | • Uncomplicated LVAD / without intensive care<br>• In-hospital on inotropes (low dose / only one agent)<br>• Congenital heart disease<br>  > arterial shunt-dependent<br>  > with SaO₂ < 65 %<br>  > complex with progressive arrhythmia<br>  > complex with systemic ventricle decline<br>• Heart-lung transplantation |
| **STATUS 2** | • In-patient<br>• Outpatient on inotropes<br>• Congenital heart disease<br>  > with SaO₂ 65-75 %<br>  > with Fontan and exudative enteropathy<br>• Multiple organ transplantation (other than heart-lung) |
| **STATUS 1** | • Other |

*Canadian Cardiac Transplant Network*

# IMMUNOSUPPRESSION

### INDUCTION
- **Anti-IL2 receptor antibodies** (Basiliximab) or **rATG** (antithymocyte immunoglobulins)
- **Precise indications**: high risk of rejection; risk of renal toxicity with calcineurin inhibitors

### CORTICOSTEROIDS
- Decrease lymphocyte activation (T cells and B cells)
- Tapering after 6 months
- **Adverse effects:** Cushing; HTN; dyslipidemia; weight gain; DM; ulcers; cataracts; avascular necrosis of the hip; osteoporosis; shingles

### CALCINEURIN INHIBITORS: CYCLOSPORINE OR TACROLIMUS
- Decrease T cell activation
- **Adverse effects:** Nephrotoxicity; HTN; DM; Neurotoxicity...

### PURINE SYNTHESIS INHIBITORS: AZATHIOPRINE OR MMF (MYCOPHENOLATEMOFETIL)
- Inhibit T cell and B cell proliferation
- **Adverse effects:** Bone marrow suppression; Granulocytopenia; Diarrhea; Interaction with Allopurinol (Azathioprine)

### M-TOR INHIBITORS: SIROLIMUS (RAPAMYCIN) AND EVEROLIMUS
- **Alternative to calcineurin inhibitors in the presence of renal toxicity**
- Block T cell (and B cell) activation
- Inhibit endothelial cell and fibroblast proliferation
  > **Decrease the risk of cardiac allograft vasculopathy**
- **Adverse effects:** Altered healing

# COMPLICATIONS

**TRANSPLANT:** bicaval anastomosis

**POST-TRANSPLANT HEART FAILURE:** optimize coronary perfusion; optimize RV preload (diuretics; UF; minimize transfusions); atrial pacing (junctional rhythm is common post-transplant); avoid hypercapnia - acidosis; inotropes (Milrinone; Dobutamine); pulmonary vasodilators (NO; Prostacyclins; Sildenafil); IABP - ECMO - RVAD - Impella

**CELLULAR REJECTION: Lymphocyte infiltrates (T cells)**; several weeks to several years post-transplant; 40% in the first year

> **Presentation: ranges from asymptomatic to cardiogenic shock**
> **Diagnosis**: weekly biopsy for 6 weeks - monthly for 6 months - every 3 months for 2 years - every 4 to 6 months
> **Risk factors**: Young age; female; CMV+; HLA incompatibility
> **Treatment:** corticosteroids; intensification of immunosuppression

| | |
|---|---|
| **GRADE 0 R** | Absence of rejection |
| **GRADE 1 R (MILD)** | Interstitial / Perivascular lymphocyte infiltration (≤ 1 zone of myocyte injury) |
| **GRADE 2 R (MODERATE)** | ≥ 2 zones of infiltration with myocyte injury |
| **GRADE 3 R (SEVERE)** | Diffuse infiltration; multiple zones of myocyte injury (± edema; ± bleeding; ± vasculitis) |

**HUMORAL REJECTION (ANTIBODIES): anti-donor HLA antibody or anti-endothelial antigen antibody**; absence of lymphocyte infiltrate; acute graft dysfunction ($\searrow$ LVEF)

> **Treatment**: Plasmapheresis; Corticosteroids; Rituximab

| CLINICAL | • Graft dysfunction; $\searrow$ LVEF; Wall thickening (edema) |
|---|---|
| HISTOLOGICAL (BIOPSY) | • Capillary endothelial congestion ($\pm$ interstitial edema)<br>• Macrophages in capillaries ($\pm$ neutrophils) |
| IMMUNO-PATHOLOGICAL | • Immunofluorescence: Immunoglobulins + complement (C3d / C4d / C1q) in capillaries<br>• Immunohistochemistry: CD68+ macrophages in capillaries or C4d in capillaries |
| SEROLOGICAL | • Anti-HLA class I or II antibodies or other anti-donor antibodies |

**CHRONIC REJECTION**: chronic humoral rejection $\pm$ cardiac allograft vasculopathy

**CARDIAC ALLOGRAFT VASCULOPATHY**: 50% at 10 years; **diffuse concentric neointimal proliferation; no angina (denervation)**

> **Complications**: MI; allograft heart failure; arrhythmia; sudden death
> **Risk factors:** number of episodes of rejection; HLA incompatibility; conventional risk factors for CAD; graft ischemia time; donor age; CMV+...
> **Screening**: Dobutamine echocardiography; MIBI-P; Coronary angiography / IVUS
> **Treatment**: Statins; Control of conventional risk factors; Intensification of immunosuppression; m-TOR inhibitors; PCI; re-transplantation

**INFECTION**: nosocomial (early); fungal (Aspergillosis; Candidiasis); CMV (fever; leukopenia; transaminase elevation); HSV; VZV; PCP; Toxoplasmosis; TB; Nocardiosis; Cryptococcosis; *L. monocytogenes*

> **Prophylaxis (6–12 months post-transplant)**: CMV (Acyclovir / Valganciclovir); *Pneumocystis carinii* and Toxoplasmosis (TMP/SMX); Antifungal agents (Voriconazole / Itraconazole)

**NEOPLASIA**: 30% at 10 years (lymphoma; cutaneous; solid organs)

**OTHER COMPLICATIONS**: HTN; Dyslipidemia; DM; CRF (calcineurin inhibitors); sinus tachycardia at rest (parasympathetic denervation); gout

> **Mean survival**: 10 years

# 3.6/ LONG-TERM VENTRICULAR ASSIST DEVICE

## INDICATIONS

| **ADVANCED HEART FAILURE\*** <br><br> • **NYHA IIIb – IV** and <br> • **≥ 2 of these elements:** | • LVEF < 25% and/or VO$_2$ max < 14 mL/kg/min (or < 50% predicted for age / gender / BSA)<br>• Inotrope dependence<br>• Progressive target organ dysfunction due to hypoperfusion<br>• Repeated hospitalizations (≥ 3 per year)<br>• Progressive discontinuation of beneficial medication (ACE inhibitors; BB) due to hypotension or ARF |
|---|---|

**\*Estimated one-year mortality > 50% on medical therapy** (Seattle Heart Failure Model; Heart Failure Survival Score)

| BRIDGE TO DECISION | Acute hemodynamic collapse; maintain the patient alive in order to evaluate other therapeutic options; **short-term / medium-term mechanical support** (percutaneous or paracorporeal) |
|---|---|
| BRIDGE TO RECOVERY | Maintain the patient alive until recovery of sufficient cardiac function to wean mechanical support (by reverse remodeling); acute fulminant myocarditis or sometimes DCM or peripartum cardiomyopathy or following cardiac surgery or myocardial stunning |
| BRIDGE TO TRANSPLANTATION | Maintain the patient alive while waiting for transplantation |
| BRIDGE TO CANDIDACY | Improve target organ function to potentially make the patient eligible for transplantation |
| DESTINATION THERAPY | Use of long-term mechanical support (patient not a candidate for transplantation, but satisfactory life expectancy) |

**INTERMACS** CLASSIFICATION

| | INTERMACS PROFILE | TIME TO MECHANICAL SUPPORT |
|---|---|---|
| 1 | CRASHING AND BURNING - Critical cardiogenic shock | Hours |
| 2 | PROGRESSIVE DECLINE - Positive inotrope-dependent; continuous deterioration | Days |
| 3 | STABLE BUT INOTROPE-DEPENDENT - Stable | Weeks |
| 4 | RECURRENT HEART FAILURE - Recurrent decompensation | Weeks - Months |
| 5 | EXERTION INTOLERANT - Comfortable at rest | Variable |
| 6 | EXERTION LIMITED - Fatigue with the slightest exertion | Variable |
| 7 | ADVANCED NYHA III - Comfortable at an acceptable level of exertion | Not a candidate |

## ASSESSMENT

**Refer the patient for assessment before significant irreversible target organ damage** +
**(RV dysfunction; Irreversible PHT; irreversible congestive liver disease; irreversible renal failure; coagulopathy; malnutrition)**

> **Target CVP < 15 mmHg** (decreases hepatic congestion; decreases the risk of post-LVAD right heart failure)
> **Right ventricular stroke work index (RVSWI)** = [(mPAP - CVP) x stroke volume] / BSA
> · **Target RVSWI > 300 mmHg x mL/m²**
> · **Mean PAP < 25 mmHg associated with low right ventricular reserve** +
> **Liver disease**: risk of bleeding and post-op transfusion (with deterioration of RV function due to secondary volume overload)

> **Assessments**: Target → BUN < 40 U/dL; creatinine < 221 µmol/L; GFR > 50 mL/kg/min; INR < 1.2; Hb > 100 g/L; Platelets > 150,000/mm³; Albumin > 30 g/L; Prealbumin > 15 g/L; ALT - AST < 2 ULN

> **Valvular heart disease**: correct AR ≥ 3/4 or moderate MS or TR ≥ 3/4 or mechanical AVR

## RISK OF POST-LVAD IN-HOSPITAL MORTALITY

| PARAMETERS | POINTS | |
|---|---|---|
| **Platelets < 148 000 / mm³** | **7** | |
| **Albumin < 33 g/L** | **5** | **POST-LVAD IN-HOSPITAL SURVIVAL** |
| **INR > 1.1** | **4** | • 0-8 points: 87.5 % |
| **Ongoing vasodilator therapy** | **4** | • 9-16 points: 70.5 % |
| **Mean PAP < 25 mmHg** | **3** | • 17-19 points: 26 % |
| **AST > 45 IU/mL** | **2** | • > 19 point: 13.7 % |
| **Hematocrit < 34 %** | **2** | **If ≥ 17 points: patient optimization** |
| **BUN > 51 U/dL** | **2** | **prior to LVAD** |
| **Absence of IV inotrope** | **2** | |

*Lietz K, Long JW, Kfoury AG, et al. Circulation. 2007;116:497-505*

## LEFT VENTRICULAR ASSIST DEVICE (LVAD)

**"DESTINATION THERAPY" STUDIES**: ★ REMATCH (HEARTMATE XVE) and ★ HEARTMATE II → ↘ Mortality compared to conventional medical therapy; Improvement in NYHA class and quality of life; Reverse remodeling

> **2-year survival (registries)**: 65 %

**SECOND-GENERATION LVAD PUMPS**: **non-pulsatile flow (continuous)**; HeartMate II; Jarvik 2000

> **Flow rate**: up to 10 L/min
> **Pump speed**: adjusted by TTE (LV and RV chambers; position of IV septum; Ao valve opening every 3 beats)
> **Anticoagulation**: Target INR 2 to 3 ± ASA 80 qd
> **BP monitoring (continuous flow pump)**: use sphygmomanometer and Doppler (target mean BP < 80 mmHg)

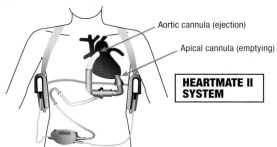

Aortic cannula (ejection)

Apical cannula (emptying)

**HEARTMATE II SYSTEM**

COMPLICATIONS: bleeding (acquired vWF deficiency; AV malformation); HIT; right heart failure; thromboembolism; stroke; infection; mechanical breakdown; fused aortic valve leaflets (leads to AR or AS); allosensitization; hemolysis; device thrombosis

THIRD-GENERATION PUMPS: HeartWare HVAD (intrapericardial)

MICROPUMPS: CircuLite Synergy (partial support up to 3 L/min; subclavian approach)

# 3.7/ RIGHT HEART FAILURE

## ETIOLOGIES

> Right heart failure secondary to left heart failure (most frequent)

> Precapillary PHT (including pulmonary embolism)

> Cardiomyopathy with RV involvement (including ARVD) (▶▶| Chapter 5 - Cardiomyopathies)

> RV infarction

> Right valvular heart disease

> Congenital heart disease (including ASD and intracardiac shunt)

> Right heart failure post-cardiac surgery

> Constrictive pericarditis (mimics right heart failure)

## SYMPTOMS AND SIGNS

> Fatigue; anasarca - edema; anorexia; nausea; RUQ pain

> Hypotension; JVD ± Kussmaul; left parasternal heave ; Harzer's sign; ± signs of PHT; right S3 (↗ inspiration); tricuspid regurgitation; hepatomegaly - pulsatile liver; systemic congestion (ascites; edema)

## ASSESSMENT

TTE; radionuclide ventriculography; cardiac MRI; V/Q scintigraphy; Right-Left catheterization

## MANAGEMENT

**Diuretics** (caution in the presence of normal Wedge pressure due to the risk of decreased LV preload); ± mineralocorticoid receptor antagonists

**Specific treatment of PHT; Specific treatment of LV HF**

**Surgical or percutaneous correction** of structural abnormality (valvular or congenital malformation)

# 3.8/ PALLIATIVE CARE

> Discussing the patient's wishes at the stage of advanced heart failure

> Good communication with the patient and family

> Desactivation of the defibrillator

> Analgesia

> ± IV diuretics; ± palliative IV inotropes

- Bonow RO, Mann DL, Zipes DP, Libby P. *Braunwald's Heart Disease. A textbook of cardiovascular medicine.* Elsevier. 2012. 1961 p.
- 2013 ACCF/AHA Guideline for the Management of Heart Failure. *JACC* 2013; *62*; e147-e239
- ESC Guidelines for the diagnosis and treatment of acute and chronic heart failure 2012. *Eur Heart J.* 2012; *33* :1787-847
- 2009 Focused Update: ACCF/AHA Guidelines for the Diagnosis and Management of Heart Failure in Adults. *JACC* 2009; *53*: 1343-1382.
- ACC/AHA 2005 Guideline Update for the Diagnosis and Management of Chronic Heart Failure in the Adult—Summary Article. *JACC* 2005; *46*; 1116-1143
- The 2011 Canadian Cardiovascular Society Heart Failure Management Guidelines Update: Focus on Sleep Apnea, Renal Dysfunction, Mechanical Circulatory Support, and Palliative Care. *CJC* 2011; *27*; 319-338
- The Canadian Cardiovascular Society Heart Failure Companion: Bridging Guidelines to Your Practice. *CJC* 2016; In press.
- Canadian Cardiovascular Society Consensus Conference guidelines on heart failure. update 2009: Diagnosis and management of right-sided heart failure, myocarditis, device therapy and recent important clinical trials. *CJC* 2009; *25*; 85-106
- Canadian Cardiovascular Society Consensus Conference guidelines on heart failure - 2008 update: Best practices fort the transition of care of heart failure patients and the recognition, investigation and treatment of cardiomyopathies. *CJC* 2008; *24*; 21-40
- Canadian Cardiovascular Society Consensus Conference recommendations on heart failure update 2007: Prevention, management during intercurrent illness or acute decompensation, and use of biomarkers. *CJC* 2007; *23*; 21-45.
- Canadian Cardiovascular Society consensus conference recommendations on heart failure 2006: Diagnosis and management. *CJC* 2006; *22*: 23-45
- 2012 ACCF/AHA/HRS Focused Update of the 2008 Guidelines for Device-Based Therapy of Cardiac Rhythm Abnormalities. *JACC* 2012; *60*; 1297-1313.
- Goldhaber JI. Hamilton MA. Role of Inotropic Agents in the Treatment of Heart Failure. *Circulation* 2010; *121*; 1655-1660.
- Haïat R, Leroy G. *Prescription guidelines in cardiology,* 5th edition. Éditions Frison-Roche. 2015. 350 p.
- The 2016 International Society for heart lung transplantation listing criteria for heart transplantation: a 10-year update. *J Heart Lung Transplant* 2016; *35*; 1-23.
- Listing Criteria for Heart Transplantation: International Society for Heart and Lung Transplantation Guidelines for the Care of Cardiac Transplant Candidates—2006. *J Heart Lung Transplant* 2006; *25*; 1024-42
- Canadian Cardiovascular Society Consensus Conference update on cardiac transplantation 2008: Executive Summary. *CJC* 2009; *25*; 197-205.
- 2001 Canadian Cardiovascular Society Consensus Conference on cardiac transplantation. *CJC* 2003; *19*; 620-654.
- Stewart S, Winters GL, Fishbein MC, et al. Revision of the 1990 working formulation for the standardization of nomenclature in the diagnosis of heart rejection. *J Heart Lung Transplant* 2005; *24*: 1710-20.
- Slaughter MS, Pagani FD, Rogers JG. Clinical management of continuous-flow left ventricular assist devices in advanced heart failure. *J Heart Lung Transplant* 2010; *29*; S1-S39.
- The 2013 International Society for Heart and Lung Transplantation Guidelines for Mechanical Circulatory Support: Executive Summary. *J Heart Lung Transplant* 2013; *32*: 157–187.
- Miller LW, Guglin M. Patient Selection for Ventricular Assist Devices. *JACC* 2013; *61*; 13 p.
- UpToDate 2015

# Valvular heart disease

04

| 4.1/ | Aortic stenosis | 140 |
|---|---|---|
| 4.2/ | Chronic aortic regurgitation | 145 |
| 4.3/ | Acute aortic regurgitation | 148 |
| 4.4/ | Mitral stenosis | 148 |
| 4.5/ | Chronic mitral regurgitation | 151 |
| 4.6/ | Acute mitral regurgitation | 155 |
| 4.7/ | Tricuspid stenosis | 156 |
| 4.8/ | Tricuspid regurgitation | 156 |
| 4.9/ | Pulmonary stenosis | 157 |
| 4.10/ | Pulmonary regurgitation | 157 |
| 4.11/ | Multivalvular heart disease | 158 |
| 4.12/ | Valvular prostheses | 158 |
| 4.13/ | Infective endocarditis | 160 |
| 4.14/ | Cardiovascular implantable electronic device infections | 167 |
| 4.15/ | Rheumatic fever | 168 |

# 4.1/ AORTIC STENOSIS

## ETIOLOGIES

**SENILE CALCIFIC AS**: Similar risk factors and pathophysiology to CAD and mitral annular calcification (MAC)

**BICUSPID AORTIC VALVE**
> 1-2% of the population
> **70-80%: fusion of right and left coronary leaflets**
  - 20-30%: fusion of right coronary and non-coronary leaflets
  - Fusion of non-coronary and left coronary leaflets is rare
> **TTE**: Demonstrates valve opening during systole with **only two commissures** (unicuspid valve: only one commissure)
> Screening TTE should be performed in 1st degree relatives
> **Associated aortopathy** (medial degeneration); **aneurysm; dissection**                           +
  • Imaging (TTE; CT angiography; MRI) annually if aorta > 45 mm
  • BB if aorta > 40 mm (in the absence of significant AR)
  • **Ascending aorta replacement if aorta > 55 mm (> 45 mm when AVR is also necessary) or > 50 mm with risk factors for dissection (family history or progression ≥ 5 mm/year)**

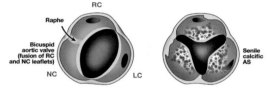

**RHEUMATIC**: fusion of commissures; triangular orifice; concomitant AR and AS; associated mitral valve disease in the majority of cases

**CONGENITAL AORTIC STENOSIS** (can be treated by balloon valvuloplasty)

**RHEUMATOID AORTIC STENOSIS** (rare)

**DDx**: Aortic sclerosis (calcification but **peak velocity < 2.5 m/s**); HCM (dynamic obstruction)
> **Supravalvular aortic stenosis: strong A2**; murmur radiates to the right carotid; BP right arm > BP left arm; associated with Williams syndrome
> **Subvalvular aortic stenosis**: membrane or tunnel; combined with AR; absence of systolic anterior motion (SAM) of mitral leaflet

## HEMODYNAMIC CONSEQUENCES

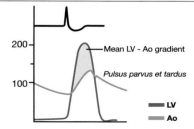

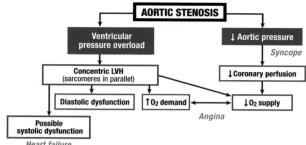

**SYSTOLIC DYSFUNCTION SECONDARY TO:**

1) ↘ **Intrinsic contractility** secondary to remodeling (only slight improvement with surgery)
2) **Mismatch between high afterload and insufficient concentric LVH** (afterload mismatch) (improved by surgery)

## SEVERITY

**NORMAL AREA:** 3-4 cm²

|  | MILD | MODERATE | SEVERE | CRITICAL |
|---|---|---|---|---|
| **Jet velocity (m/s)** | 2.6-2.9 | 3.0 - 4.0 | > 4.0 | > 5.0 |
| **Mean gradient (mmHg)** | < 20 | 20 - 40 | > 40 | > 60 |
| **Valve area (cm²)** | > 1.5 | 1.0 - 1.5 | < 1.0 | < 0.6 |
| **Indexed valve area (cm²/m²)** | > 0.85 | 0.6 - 0.85 | < 0.6 |  |
| **LVOT VTI / Ao valve VTI ratio** | > 0.50 | 0.25 - 0.50 | < 0.25 |  |

## SYMPTOMS AND SIGNS

**SYMPTOMS:** Heart failure / Dyspnea; Angina; Syncope

> Bleeding (destruction of von Willebrand factor; Heyde's syndrome)

**CAROTID:** *pulsus parvus* et *tardus* (slow ascent; late peak; low amplitude) (absent in the presence of arteriosclerosis); carotid thrill

**APEX:** sustained; lateralized if LV dysfunction; S4 sometimes palpable; **apical-carotid delay**

**AORTIC AREA:** look for **thrill**

**AUSCULTATION:** **crescendo - decrescendo murmur with late peak**; carotid radiation; radiation to apex in the case of Gallavardin phenomenon (high-pitched murmur); accentuation of murmur post-PVC; decrescendo diastolic murmur in the presence of associated AR

> **S2 with a single component: Inaudible A2** or delayed A2 and at same time as P2 with paradoxical expiratory splitting
> **S4**
> **Systolic ejection click** of bicuspid aortic valve disappears in the case of ↘ valve mobility

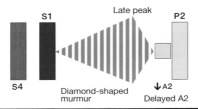

S4  S1  Diamond-shaped murmur  Late peak  ↓A2 Delayed A2  P2  ± AR murmur

## INVESTIGATIONS

**STRESS TEST**: To distinguish asymptomatic from symptomatic aortic stenosis; contraindicated if the patient presents symptoms of AS

> Look for symptoms - decreased exercise capacity (< 80% predicted) - abnormal BP response (↗ SBP < 20 mmHg)

### ECHOCARDIOGRAPHIC FOLLOW-UP

| MILD AS | MODERATE AS | SEVERE ASYMPTOMATIC AS |
|---------|-------------|------------------------|
| TTE every 3 to 5 years | TTE every 1 to 2 years | TTE every 6 months to 1 year |

### HEMODYNAMIC ASSESSMENT - INDICATIONS

a) Inconclusive noninvasive investigation
b) Discordance between clinical findings and noninvasive investigation

### PREOPERATIVE CORONARY ANGIOGRAPHY - INDICATIONS

> Angina; documented ischemia; LV systolic dysfunction; known CAD; Male > 40 years; postmenopause; cardiovascular risk factors
  • Consider coronary CT angiography in patients with low-to-moderate pretest probability of CAD
  • It is reasonable not to perform preoperative coronary angiography in a surgical emergency in the presence of acute valvular regurgitation, acute aortic syndrome or bacterial endocarditis (class IIa recommendation)

## OUTCOME

↘ Valve area by 0.1 cm² / year; ↗ Mean gradient by 7 mmHg / year

**Asymptomatic AS**: risk of sudden death < 1% / year

**Symptomatic AS**: ↘ survival (sudden death); **2 years in the presence of HF; 3 years in the presence of syncope; 5 years in the presence of angina**

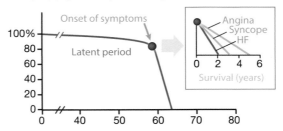

## LOW-FLOW LOW-GRADIENT AORTIC STENOSIS

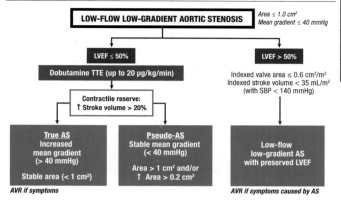

**LOW-FLOW LOW-GRADIENT AORTIC STENOSIS**

*Area ≤ 1.0 cm²*
*Mean gradient ≤ 40 mmHg*

**LVEF ≤ 50%**

**Dobutamine TTE (up to 20 µg/kg/min)**

**Contractile reserve:**
↑ Stroke volume > 20%

**True AS**
Increased
mean gradient
(> 40 mmHg)

Stable area (< 1 cm²)

*AVR if symptoms*

**Pseudo-AS**
Stable mean gradient
(< 40 mmHg)

Area > 1 cm² and/or
↑ Area > 0.2 cm²

**LVEF > 50%**

Indexed valve area ≤ 0.6 cm²/m²
Indexed stroke volume < 35 mL/m²
(with SBP < 140 mmHg)

**Low-flow
low-gradient AS
with preserved LVEF**

*AVR if symptoms caused by AS*

## MANAGEMENT

**MEDICAL**: Patient education - report all symptoms; avoid strenuous physical exertion; echocardiographic follow-up; low-dose diuretics; avoid BB; cautious use of vasodilators (fixed obstruction); treatment of cardiovascular risk factors

**SURGERY - INDICATIONS**

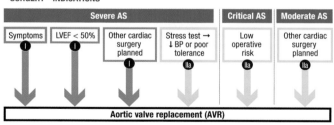

| Severe AS | | | | Critical AS | Moderate AS |
|---|---|---|---|---|---|
| Symptoms | LVEF < 50% | Other cardiac surgery planned | Stress test → ↓ BP or poor tolerance | Low operative risk | Other cardiac surgery planned |
| **I** | **I** | **I** | **IIa** | **IIa** | **IIa** |

**Aortic valve replacement (AVR)**

> **Complication of AVR**: mortality 1-3%; stroke 2%; prolonged ventilation 11%; thromboembolism; bleeding; prosthetic dysfunction

## PERCUTANEOUS BALLOON VALVULOPLASTY

Risk of major complications > 10%

Recurrent symptoms and restenosis at 6 months

**Does not constitute a medium-term or long-term alternative to AVR or TAVI**

**LIMITED INDICATIONS**: bridge to AVR or TAVI in a patient with severe symptoms
> Effective in adolescents / young adults with congenital AS in the absence of calcification

## TAVI (Transcatheter aortic valve implantation)

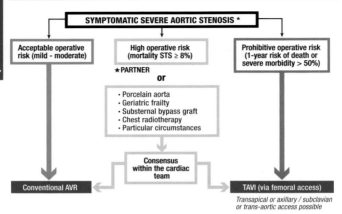

* Absence of futility: an operation will probably improve life span and/or quality of life; survival with treatment will probably be ≥ 1-2 years

**PRE-TAVI ASSESSMENT**: **A)** TTE; **B)** TEE: aortic annulus dimensions at insertion of leaflets on anteroposterior view (PLAX) and side-to-side (short-axis); **C)** CT angiography: Ao; aortic annulus dimensions; aortic-iliac-femoral PAD; distance between coronary ostia and aortic annulus; **D)** Coronary angiography - Aortography - Ventriculography

> Aortic annulus diameter: **> 18 mm and < 29 mm**
> Coronary ostia - aortic annulus distance ≥ **10-11 mm**
> Femoral vascular access: **femoral artery diameter > 6 mm** (to accommodate a 7 mm catheter); evaluate the degree of calcification and arterial tortuosities
> **Geriatric frailty:** increased risk of adverse events during major surgery; **5-meter walking time > 6 s**; Katz index of independence in ADL

**STEPS OF THE FEMORAL APPROACH**: **A)** Femoral access; **B)** Transvalvular guide; **C)** Delivery catheter; **D)** Pre-dilatation by valvuloplasty during rapid ventricular pacing (180-200 bpm); **E)** Positioning of the valve under fluoroscopic / angiographic guidance and/or by TEE (50% above and 50% below the plane of the aortic annulus); **F)** Valve deployment during rapid ventricular pacing (180-200 bpm) (Sapien valve); **G)** Identification and management of complications; **H)** Closure of access site

**LIMITED BENEFIT OF TAVI**: Life expectancy < 1 year;  2-year survival with estimated benefit < 25%;  STS > 15% (no benefit on survival in ★ PARTNER B);  advanced geriatric frailty (dependence for multiple ADL);  multiple comorbidities

**COMPLICATIONS**: 30-day mortality: 3-5%; stroke (6-7%); vascular complications (17%); valve embolization; coronary occlusion (due to migration of a leaflet or calcification); mitral valve disease; perivalvular regurgitation (incomplete apposition); tamponade; AV block requiring PPM (2-9% Sapien; 19-43% Corevalve); arrhythmias; bleeding; aortic rupture

**POST-TAVI MANAGEMENT**: Long-term ASA; Thienopyridine for 1 to 6 months (except when treated with warfarin); prophylactic antibiotics; annual clinical and TTE follow-up

### ETIOLOGIES

**VALVULAR: A)** Degenerative (calcification); **B)** Endocarditis; **C)** Leaflet prolapse (loss of support due to aortopathy); **D)** Bicuspid aortic valve; **E)** Rheumatic; **F)** VSD; **G)** Subaortic membrane; **H)** Iatrogenic (post-balloon valvuloplasty); **I)** Myxomatous proliferation; **J)** SLE - RA - ankylosing spondylitis

**AORTIC: A)** Aortic dilatation: degenerative / cystic medial necrosis (isolated; Marfan; bicuspid aortic valve); osteogenesis imperfecta; syphilis; Behçet; Takayasu; giant cell arteritis; spondyloarthropathies / ankylosing spondylitis / psoriatic arthritis; polychondritis; HTN; **B)** Dissection: leaflet prolapse following loss of support or presence of intravalvular flap or leaflet perforation by dissection; **C)** Traumatic

### HEMODYNAMIC CONSEQUENCES

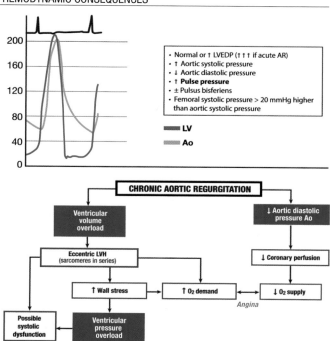

- Normal or ↑ LVEDP (↑↑↑ if acute AR)
- ↑ Aortic systolic pressure
- ↓ Aortic diastolic pressure
- ↑ **Pulse pressure**
- ± Pulsus bisferiens
- Femoral systolic pressure > 20 mmHg higher than aortic systolic pressure

**■ LV**
**■ Ao**

**CHRONIC AORTIC REGURGITATION**

Ventricular volume overload → Eccentric LVH (sarcomeres in series) → ↑ Wall stress → ↑ O₂ demand

↓ Aortic diastolic pressure Ao → ↓ Coronary perfusion → ↓ O₂ supply

*Angina*

Possible systolic dysfunction ← Ventricular pressure overload

*Heart failure*

*Mismatch between high afterload (wall stress) and insufficient wall thickness (Laplace law)*

## SEVERITY

| | MILD AR (1/4) | MODERATE AR (2 to 3/4) | SEVERE AR (4/4) |
|---|---|---|---|
| **Vena contracta (mm)** | < 3 | 3 - 5.9 | ≥ 6 |
| **Regurgitant volume (mL/b)** | < 30 | 2/4: 30 - 44 <br> 3/4: 45 - 59 | ≥ 60 |
| **Regurgitant fraction (%)** | < 30 | 30 - 49 | ≥ 50 |
| **Regurgitant orifice (cm²)** | < 0.10 | 2/4: 0.1 - 0.19 <br> 3/4: 0.2 - 0.29 | ≥ 0.30 |
| **Jet width (PLAX)** | Central; < 25% of LVOT | Intermediate | > 65% of LVOT |
| **Area of regurgitant jet (PSAX)** | < 5 % of LVOT area | Intermediate | > 60 % of LVOT area |
| **Pressure half-time (ms)** | > 500 | 200-500 | < 200 |
| **Diastolic reversal of descending Ao** | Brief; Early diastolic | Intermediate | Holodiastolic and prominent (end-diastolic velocity > 20 cm/s) |
| **LV dimensions** | Normal | | Dilatation |
| **Angiography** | 1+ | 2+ | 3-4+ |

**OTHER MARKERS OF SEVERITY**: Holodiastolic reversal of flow in proximal abdominal aorta

## SYMPTOMS AND SIGNS

**SYMPTOMS**: Heart failure - Dyspnea; Angina; Tiredness
> Poorly tolerated bradycardia (↗ regurgitation time)

**VITAL SIGNS**: ↗ pulse pressure (with ↘ DBP)

**PULSE**: bounding; *pulsus bisferiens* (more accurately assessed in brachial or femoral arteries); carotid thrill (↗ stroke volume)

**APEX**: large; hyperdynamic; lateralized; ± palpable S3

**AUSCULTATION**: **decrescendo diastolic murmur starting at A2**; more accurately assessed with the patient seated and leaning forward in forced expiration; duration correlated with severity
> Murmur increases with fists clenched
> **Radiation to left parasternal region indicates a valvular etiology; Radiation to right parasternal region indicates an aortic etiology**
> **Decreased A2** indicates a valvular etiology
> Systolic ejection click (abrupt distension of the aorta)
> **S3**
> **Systolic ejection murmur** (↗ stroke volume) ± thrill
> **Austin Flint murmur**: diastolic rumbling due to aortic reflux onto anterior mitral leaflet
> **Distinguish AR from PR**: AR → murmur starting at A2; peripheral signs; PR murmur ↗ during inspiration

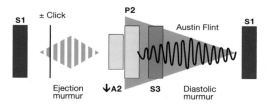

| Musset's sign | Systolic nodding of the head |
|---|---|
| Müller's sign | Systolic pulsation of uvula |
| Quincke's sign | Capillary pulsation (by pressing lightly on the tip of the nail) |
| Corrigan's pulse / Water hammer pulse | Abrupt distension with prominent pulse then rapid collapse (more accurately assessed in the radial artery with the arms raised) |
| Traube's sign (pistol shot) | Systolic and diastolic bruit in the femoral artery |
| Duroziez' sign | Systolic murmur in the femoral artery with proximal compression and diastolic murmur with distal compression (from the stethoscope) |
| Hill's sign | SBP in arms > 20 mmHg higher than SBP in legs |

## OUTCOME AND FOLLOW-UP

Survival rate declines markedly in the presence of symptoms or LV dysfunction

> **Mortality in the presence of symptoms**: > 10 % / year

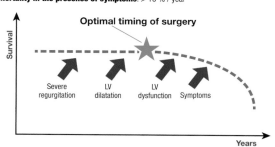

| NEWLY DIAGNOSED AR | MILD AR | MODERATE AR | SEVERE AR | SEVERE AR WITH LV DILATATION |
|---|---|---|---|---|
| TTE at 3 months to ensure stability | TTE every 3 to 5 years | TTE every 1 to 2 years | TTE every 6 to 12 months | TTE every 4 to 6 months |

## MANAGEMENT

**MEDICAL:** patient education - report all symptoms; avoid strenuous physical exertion / isometric exercises; echocardiographic follow-up; treat diastolic HTN (ACE inhibitors or Nifedipine); avoid bradycardia; ACE inhibitors and beta-blockers if poor candidate for surgery with severe AR with symptoms and/or LV dysfunction

**SURGERY:** AVR vs AVR + ascending aorta replacement (Bentall) vs Valve repair vs Ascending aorta replacement + valvular resuspension (David procedure) vs Ross procedure

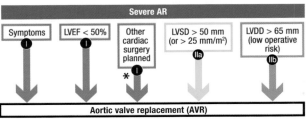

* IIa if moderate AR

# 4.3/ ACUTE AORTIC REGURGITATION

**ETIOLOGIES: A)** Endocarditis; **B)** Aortic dissection; **C)** Trauma; **D)** Prosthetic valve dysfunction

**HEMODYNAMIC CONSEQUENCES:** Regurgitant volume in poorly compliant LV → ↗↗ diastolic pressures → Congestive heart failure

> ↘ Anterograde flow → Systemic hypoperfusion / Shock
> Early mitral valve closure (restrictive diastolic filling pattern)

**PHYSICAL EXAMINATION:** Tachycardia; shock; pulmonary edema

> ↘ S1 (early mitral valve closure); S3 and S4
> **Brief diastolic murmur** (early pressure equalization on either side of the valve)
> **Austin Flint rumble**
> Systolic murmur (↗ stroke volume)
> Signs of PHT

**MANAGEMENT:** Urgent surgery

> Positive inotropic agent (Dobutamine) and/or vasodilator (Nitroprusside)

# 4.4/ MITRAL STENOSIS

## ETIOLOGY

**RHEUMATIC FEVER:** Leading cause of MS

> 25% of patients have isolated MS; 40% have MS and MR; 35% have concomitant aortic valve disease; 6% have concomitant tricuspid valve disease

**OTHER RARE CAUSES: A)** Congenital; **B)** Carcinoid with lung metastases or PFO; **C)** SLE; **D)** RA; **E)** Hunter-Hurler; **F)** Fabry; **G)** Whipple; **H)** Methysergide; **I)** Calcific MS (age related)

**DDX (LV INFLOW OBSTRUCTION):** LA tumor - Myxoma; LA thrombus; Obstructive vegetation; Cor triatriatum; Severe mitral annular calcification (age); Pulmonary vein stenosis

## SEVERITY

**NORMAL AREA:** 4-5 cm²

|  | MILD | MODERATE | SEVERE |
|---|---|---|---|
| **Valve area (cm²)** | > 1.5 | 1.0 - 1.5 | < 1.0 |
| **Mean gradient (mmHg)** | < 5 | 5 - 10 | > 10 |
| **sPAP (mmHg)** | < 30 | 30 - 50 | > 50 |
| **Pressure half-time (ms)** |  | 150 - 220 | > 220 ms |

Indices valid for heart rate between 60 and 90 bpm

## HEMODYNAMIC CONSEQUENCES

> ↗ LA pressure → pulmonary congestion / PHT / Right heart failure
> LA dilatation → risk of AF / atrial stasis / peripheral embolism
> Intolerance of tachycardia or loss of atrial kick
> Low output state

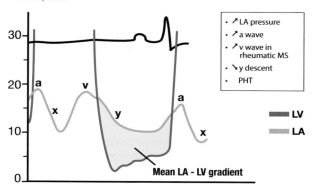

- ↗ LA pressure
- ↗ a wave
- ↗ v wave in rheumatic MS
- ↘ y descent
- PHT

**LV**
**LA**

**Mean LA - LV gradient**

## SYMPTOMS AND SIGNS

**SYMPTOMS:** Dyspnea; tiredness; poor exercise tolerance; OTP; PND
> **PHT:** Right heart failure; hemoptysis (rupture of bronchial veins; rupture of capillaries; pulmonary edema)
> Palpitations; peripheral embolism
> Recurrent laryngeal nerve compression by dilated LA (Ortner's syndrome)

**MITRAL FACIES:** secondary to systemic vasoconstriction; pink-purple plaques on cheeks

**JUGULAR:** JVD; prominent a wave (sinus rhythm)

**AUSCULTATION:** ↗ S1 when leaflets still pliable and only slightly calcified

**OPENING SNAP**: Heard more clearly with the diaphragm; absent during significant leaflet calcification

> **A2 - opening snap interval inversely proportional to the severity of MS (severe if < 80 ms)**

**DIASTOLIC RUMBLE**: Heard more clearly in left lateral supine position with the bell at the apex; look for thrill; murmur increased during tachycardia - exercise

**SIGNS OF PHT**: left parasternal heave; P2 increased (± palpable); ejection click (PA dilatation); TR murmur; Graham Steell murmur; right S3-S4

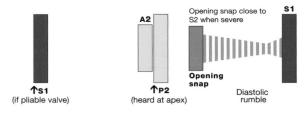

↑S1 (if pliable valve)

↑P2 (heard at apex)

Opening snap close to S2 when severe

Opening snap

Diastolic rumble

## INVESTIGATIONS AND OUTCOME

**TTE**: Rheumatic MS → thickening ± calcification of leaflets; hockey stick appearance of anterior mitral leaflet; LA dilatation; commissural fusion with "fish-mouth" mitral orifice (PSAX)

### ECHOCARDIOGRAPHIC FOLLOW-UP

| MILD MS | MODERATE MS | SEVERE MS |
|---|---|---|
| TTE every 3 to 5 years | TTE every 1 to 2 years | TTE annually |

**STRESS TEST**: Evaluate exercise capacity and symptoms

> Combined with TTE to evaluate PAP and mean gradient on exertion when there is a discordance between symptoms and TTE at rest

**OUTCOME**: Valve area ↘ by 0.09 cm²/year

> 5-year survival in patients with symptomatic severe MS without intervention: 44%

## MANAGEMENT

**MEDICAL:** prevention of recurrence of rheumatic fever (penicillin-based prophylactic antibiotics); avoid strenuous exertion; follow-up and decision to operate at the optimal time; aggressive treatment of AF and thromboembolic risk; diuretics PRN; avoid tachycardia

> **Indication for anticoagulation**: AF; Cardioembolic history; LA thrombus

**BALLOON MITRAL VALVULOPLASTY**: transseptal approach; TEE guidance; Inoue 23 to 25 mm balloon; inflation of the balloon inside the valve orifice in order to open commissures

> **Better results in a context of favorable anatomy**: Wilkins score (BVR) ≤ 8 points      +
> - **Success**: valve area > 1.5 cm² and LA pressure < 18 mmHg
> **Contraindications**: moderate to severe MR; LA thrombus (pre-procedure TEE); unfavorable anatomy
> **Complications**: mortality 1%; stroke - embolism 1-2%; cardiac perforation 1%; MR requiring surgery 2%; iatrogenic ASD; myocardial infarction < 1%

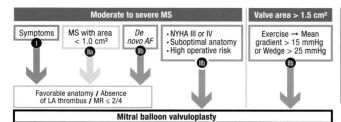

**SURGICAL APPROACH: A)** Closed commissurotomy (obsolete approach); **B)** Open commissurotomy ± mitral valve repair (under CPB); **C)** MVR

> Consider MAZE and LAA amputation during surgery (★ CTSN AF)

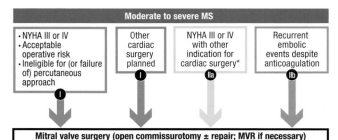

\* TR; CAD; aortic valve disease; aortic aneurysm, etc.

# 4.5/ CHRONIC MITRAL REGURGITATION

## ETIOLOGY

**DEGENERATIVE: MVP - Myxomatous disease**; Marfan; Ehlers-Danlos; Pseudoxanthoma elasticum; Mitral annular calcification

**INFLAMMATORY: Rheumatic disease**; SLE; Scleroderma; Hypereosinophilia syndrome

**INFECTIOUS: Endocarditis**

**STRUCTURAL: Ruptured chordae tendineae** (spontaneous - idiopathic; MI; trauma; MVP; endocarditis; rheumatic fever; acute LV dilatation)

**CONGENITAL:** Cleft mitral valve; parachute mitral valve (absence of mitral papillary muscle)

**FUNCTIONAL MR**: associated with LV dysfunction / LV dilatation; **structurally normal valve;**  +
MR secondary to: **A)** Mitral papillary muscle displacement (malcoaptation of leaflets; tenting area > 6 cm² associated with MR ≥ 3/4; **B)** Annular dilatation; **C)** Loss of the annular systolic contraction; **D)** ± Mitral papillary muscle dysfunction in the presence of concomitant ischemia

> **Ischemic papillary muscle dysfunction**: posteromedial muscle (perfusion by PDA)  +
  >> anterolateral muscle (double perfusion by diagonal and marginal arteries)

# CARPENTIER'S CLASSIFICATION

According to movement of the leaflets

| TYPE I | TYPE II | TYPE IIIa | TYPE IIIb |
|--------|---------|-----------|-----------|

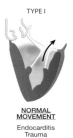 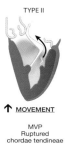 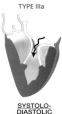 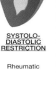 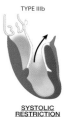

| **NORMAL MOVEMENT** | ↑ **MOVEMENT** | **SYSTOLO-DIASTOLIC RESTRICTION** | **SYSTOLIC RESTRICTION** |
|---|---|---|---|
| Endocarditis<br>Trauma<br>Annular dilatation | MVP<br>Ruptured<br>chordae tendineae | Rheumatic | Papillary muscle dysfunction<br><br>Displaced papillary muscle secondary to RWMA / LV dilatation |

# SEVERITY

|  | MILD MR (1/4) | MODERATE MR (2 to 3/4) | SEVERE MR (4/4) |
|---|---|---|---|
| **Veina contracta (mm)** | < 3 | 3 - 6.9 | ≥ 7 |
| **Regurgitant volume (mL/b)** | < 30 | 2/4: 30 - 44<br>3/4: 45 - 59 | ≥ 60 |
| **Regurgitant fraction (%)** | < 30 | 30 - 49 | ≥ 50 |
| **Regurgitant orifice (cm²) (prognostic value)** | < 0.20 | 2/4: 0.2 - 0.29<br>3/4: 0.3 - 0.39 | ≥ 0.40 |
| **Jet area** | Small central jet < 4 cm² or < 20% of LA area | Intermediate | Large central jet > 10 cm² (or > 40% of LA area) or eccentric jet along the LA wall (Coanda) |
| **Pulmonary vein flow rate** | Systolic dominance | Systolic attenuation | Systolic reversal |
| **Jet envelope on continuous Doppler** | Faint; parabolic | Intermediate | Dense; Early, triangular peak |
| **LA dimensions** | Normal |  | Dilatation |
| **LV dimensions** | Normal |  | Dilatation |
| **Angiography** | 1+ | 2+ | 3-4+ |

**FUNCTIONAL MR**: severe regurgitation when regurgitant orifice ≥ 0.20 cm² or regurgitant volume ≥ 30 mL/b or regurgitant fraction ≥ 50%

# HEMODYNAMIC CONSEQUENCES

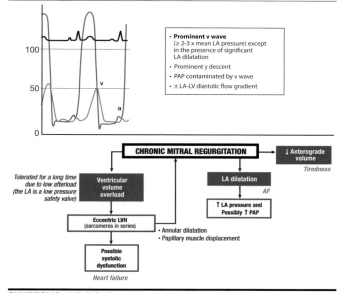

- **Prominent v wave**
  (≥ 2-3 x mean LA pressure) except
  in the presence of significant
  LA dilatation
- Prominent y descent
- PAP contaminated by v wave
- ± LA-LV diastolic flow gradient

## SYMPTOMS AND SIGNS

**SYMPTOMS**: Dyspnea; OTP; PND; symptoms of low output state; Palpitations (AF); Right heart failure

**APEX** : hyperdynamic; **dilated; lateralized**; ± palpable S3; palpable wave in left parasternal region (dilated LA kick)

**AUSCULTATION** : **Decreased S1** in the presence of a leaflet abnormality; early A2 and split S2; P2 > A2 in the presence of PHT; S3; diastolic rumble (↗ inflow)

**SYSTOLIC MURMUR**: spreads as far as (and invades) A2; **often holosystolic**; ± thrill; high-pitched; maximum at the apex; radiation to the axilla or left scapula (posteriorly directed murmur) or sternum and base (anteriorly directed murmur as in posterior leaflet MVP); not amplified post-PVC; decreased by standing up (increased by squatting); decreased during Valsalva; increased by clenching the fists (in contrast with aortic stenosis)

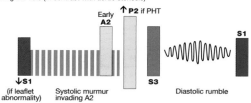

A Practical Handbook / **153**

**DDx: A)** VSD: murmur maximal in left parasternal region; thrill in left parasternal region; **B)** TR: murmur ↗ on inspiration; murmur maximal in left parasternal region; prominent jugular v wave

**ISCHEMIC PAPILLARY MUSCLE DYSFUNCTION**: mid-systolic or end-systolic murmur

## ECHOCARDIOGRAPHIC FOLLOW-UP

| MILD MR | MODERATE MR | SEVERE MR |
|---------|-------------|-----------|
| TTE every 3 to 5 years | TTE every 1 to 2 years | TTE 6 to 12 months |

TEE to clarify the anatomy, mechanism, severity and possibility of repair

Stress echocardiography PRN to detect ischemic MR and to measure PAP on exertion

## MANAGEMENT

**MEDICAL**: **little benefit of vasoactive agents in the presence of normal LVEF** (afterload is rarely increased except in HTN); anticoagulation in the presence of AF; aggressive treatment of LV dysfunction in the presence of functional MR (+ resynchronization)

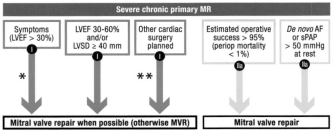

IIb: Consider Mitraclip when surgery is contraindicated in NYHA III or IV with favorable anatomy

\*IIb: Symptoms and LVEF < 30%    \*\* IIa: Moderate chronic primary MR (mitral valve repair)

**MITRAL VALVE REPAIR / ANNULOPLASTY**: Best candidates (in the absence of calcification)
→ **A)** Degenerative MR - MVP (posterior leaflet easier to repair); **B)** Annular dilatation; **C)** Papillary muscle dysfunction; **D)** Ruptured chordae tendineae; **E)** Leaflet perforation (endocarditis)

> Possible via a minimally invasive approach
> Warfarin for 3 months post-repair; ASA 80 indefinitely

**MVR**: opt for preservation of the subvalvular apparatus whenever possible (LVEF ↘ by 10% if loss of the subvalvular apparatus due to modification of LV geometry)

**MITRACLIP**: percutaneous transseptal repair; creation of a double orifice valve using a clip (equivalent to Alfieri procedure)

> ★ **EVEREST**: Mitraclip less effective than conventional surgery to reduce the degree of regurgitation
> **Candidates**: inoperable patient; mitral regurgitation with **regurgitant jet due to malcoaptation of segments A2 and P2**; functional or degenerative regurgitation (MVP or leaflet eversion); depth of coaptation < 11 mm; vertical length of coaptation > 2 mm

**FUNCTIONAL MR: ▶▶|** Chapter 3

# MITRAL VALVE PROLAPSE

2.4% of the population; female predominance

**DIAGNOSIS: A)** Mid-systolic click then murmur; **B) Displacement of one or both leaflets > 2 mm behind the plane of the mitral annulus (PLAX); C) ± Thickening of the leaflets by > 5 mm**

## ETIOLOGIES

a) **MVP syndrome**: young woman; benign; associated with OH - palpitations - anxiety; thin leaflets

b) **MVP with myxomatous thickening**: often males aged 40-70 years; thickening / redundancy of the leaflets; significant risk of progression; risk of ruptured chordae tendineae

c) **MVP associated with another disease**: Marfan; HCM; Ehlers-Danlos; osteogenesis imperfecta; *pseudoxanthoma elasticum;* Holt-Oram syndrome; *ostium secundum* ASD; Ebstein's anomaly

**CLINICAL FEATURES: mid-systolic click** then mid- or end-systolic murmur (often crescendo); normal S1; dynamic auscultation

> Mid-systolic click different from the aortic ejection click, as it occurs after the onset of the carotid upstroke

| DECREASED LEFT INTRAVENTRICULAR VOLUME | INCREASED LEFT INTRAVENTRICULAR VOLUME |
|---|---|
| Effect: ↗ duration of MVP murmur | Effect: ↘ duration of MVP murmur |
| **Maneuvers:**<br>• Tachycardia<br>• ↘ Afterload<br>• ↗ Contractility<br>• ↘ Venous return (standing; Valsalva) | **Maneuvers:**<br>• Bradycardia<br>• ↗ Afterload (clenched fists)<br>• ↘ Contractility<br>• ↗ Venous return (squatting; raising legs) |

**COMPLICATIONS**: Heart failure; Ruptured chordae tendineae; Thromboembolism; Endocarditis; AF; serious complications (including surgery) in 1/100 patient-years

> **TIA**: ASA 80 mg qd
> **AF**: anticoagulation if > 65 years or HTN or MR or history of heart failure
> **Stroke**: anticoagulation if MR or AF or LA thrombus or leaflets > 5 mm

# 4.6/ ACUTE MITRAL REGURGITATION

**ETIOLOGIES: A)** Endocarditis; **B)** Trauma - Iatrogenic; **C)** Ruptured chordae tendineae (idiopathic-spontaneous; myxomatous degeneration / MVP; Marfan; Ehlers-Danlos; endocarditis; acute rheumatic fever; trauma); **D)** Papillary muscle dysfunction or rupture (ischemia - MI); **E)** Prosthetic valve dysfunction

**HEMODYNAMIC CONSEQUENCES**: Acute MR → poorly compliant LA (significant v wave) → pulmonary congestion / PHT

> Acute MR → low anterograde flow

**PHYSICAL EXAMINATION**: **Decrescendo early systolic murmur** due to rapid equalization of pressures on both sides of the valve; **S3 and S4**; signs of PHT; early closure of pulmonary valve (early P2); pulmonary overload; hypotension; tachycardia

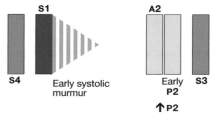

**MANAGEMENT**: Urgent surgery in the presence of heart failure

> **Medical treatment**: Nitroprusside (± Dobutamine) while waiting for surgery; IABP

## 4.7/ TRICUSPID STENOSIS

**ETIOLOGIES**: **Rheumatic** (majority); usually associated with MS

> **Other causes (rare)**: Congenital atresia; RA tumor; Carcinoid syndrome (TR >> TS); PPM lead; Extracardiac tumor; Thrombus; Endomyocardial fibrosis; Endocarditis; SLE

**SEVERITY**: Significant TS when valve area ≤ 1 cm² or mean gradient ≥ 5 mmHg or pressure halftime > 190 ms

**JUGULAR**: Prominent a wave; Loss of y descent

**AUSCULTATION: diastolic rumble in lower left parasternal region with ↗ on inspiration** (± thrill); murmur ↗ on **Mueller maneuver** (inspiration against closed glottis) or during exercise

> Opening snap following that of MS in lower left parasternal region
> Diastolic rumble of the MS; Opening snap

**SIGNS OF RIGHT HEART FAILURE** (ascites; HSM; peripheral edema; JVD)

**MANAGEMENT**: operation if **severe symptomatic TS or severe TS with concomitant mitral surgery**

> Open commissurotomy vs TVR (bioprosthesis) vs Balloon valvuloplasty

## 4.8/ TRICUSPID REGURGITATION

**ETIOLOGIES**: **Secondary / Functional** (majority); secondary to dilatation of the tricuspid annulus following dilatation of the RV (sPAP > 55 mmHg; RV infarction; PS; DCM; left heart failure...)

> **Primary causes**: Rheumatic; Endocarditis; Ebstein's anomaly; Prolapse (associated with MVP); Carcinoid; Papillary muscle dysfunction / Ruptured chordae tendineae; Trauma; Marfan; RA; Radiotherapy; AV canal defect; Endomyocardial fibrosis; Myxoma; PPM lead; Repeated biopsy (heart transplant); anorectics; SLE

| | MILD TR (1/4) | MODERATE TR (2 – 3/4) | SEVERE TR (4/4) |
|---|---|---|---|
| Jet area (central) cm² | < 5 | 5 - 10 | > 10 |
| Vena contracta (mm) | | | ≥ 7 |
| PISA radius (mm) | ≤ 5 | 6 - 9 | > 9 |
| Tricuspid E (m/sec) | | | > 1 |
| Jet envelope on continuous Doppler | Faint; parabolic | Intermediate | Dense; Early, triangular peak |
| Hepatic vein flow | Systolic dominance | Systolic attenuation | Systolic reversal |

> **Other criteria**: tricuspid annulus ≥ 40 mm (or > 21 mm/m²); D-shaped septal curvature; RV - RA dilatation; EROA ≥ 0.4 cm²; regurgitant volume ≥ 45 mL/b

**INSPECTION**: Cachexia; Jaundice; Pulsatile orbits

**JUGULAR**: Prominent c-v wave; loss of x descent; prominent y descent; ± venous thrill; Kussmaul

**PALPATION**: left parasternal heave; RV lift

**AUSCULTATION**: Right S3 (↗ on inspiration); ↗ P2 if PHT; holosystolic murmur in lower left parasternal region (early systolic if primary TR); murmur ↗ on inspiration (Carvallo's sign); **murmur ↗ on Mueller's maneuver**

**SIGNS OF RIGHT HEART FAILURE** (ascites; pulsatile liver; HSM; peripheral edema; JVD)

**MANAGEMENT - SECONDARY TR**: Tricuspid annuloplasty during mitral surgery in the presence of: **A)** Severe TR or **B)** Mild-to-moderate TR with dilatation of the tricuspid annulus (≥ 40 mm) or in the presence of PHT or right heart failure

**MANAGEMENT - PRIMARY TR**: Bioprosthesis TVR or Annuloplasty if severe symptomatic TR or severe TR with progressive RV dilatation / dysfunction or severe TR with concomitant mitral surgery

> **TR secondary to endocarditis in IDU**: total excision of the valve is possible
> **Carcinoid syndrome**: ▶▶| Chapter 5 - RCM

# 4.9/ PULMONARY STENOSIS

▶▶| Chapter 7 - Congenital heart disease

**ETIOLOGIES: Congenital** (majority)

> **Fusion of commissures**: thin, dome-shaped valve; treatment by balloon valvuloplasty
> **Dysplastic valve**: thickened leaflets; Noonan syndrome; surgical treatment

**OTHER ETIOLOGIES (RARE)**: Carcinoid; extrinsic compression (tumor; aortic sinus aneurysm); Rheumatic; Supravalvular or subvalvular obstruction (congenital)

**SEVERITY**: Severe PS if peak gradient > 64 mmHg

# 4.10/ PULMONARY REGURGITATION

**ETIOLOGIES: A)** Annular dilatation or dilatation of PA (PHT); **B)** Endocarditis; **C)** Following correction of congenital PS - TOF; **D)** Congenital; **E)** Trauma; **F)** Carcinoid; **G)** Rheumatic; **H)** Syphilis

| | MILD PR (1/4) | MODERATE PR (2 TO 3/4) | SEVERE PR (4/4) |
|---|---|---|---|
| **Jet envelope on continuous Doppler** | Faint; Slow deceleration | Intermediate | Dense; Marked deceleration; early end of diastolic flow (± anterograde diastolic flow) |

> **Other criteria**: D-shaped septal curvature; RV dilatation; PHT < 100 ms

**PALPATION**: left parasternal heave; systolic beat in the 2nd intercostal space (PA dilatation)

**AUSCULTATION**: Delayed P2; systolic click (PA dilatation); mid-systolic ejection murmur ( ↗ flow); right S3 and S4 (increased on inspiration)

> **Diastolic murmur:** soft, low-pitched (in the absence of PHT); ↗ on inspiration
> **Graham Steell murmur:** decrescendo high-pitched diastolic murmur in the presence of dilatation of the pulmonary annulus secondary to PHT; accentuated P2; starts after A2; ↗ on inspiration; signs of PHT; TR murmur

# 4.11/ MULTIVALVULAR HEART DISEASE

**AS & MS:** Aortic transvalvular gradient underestimated (low flow)

**AS & MR:** MR increased due to high left intraventricular pressure; the aortic transvalvular gradient can be underestimated (low flow); operate on the mitral valve when MR is severe or in the presence of significant mitral structural disease

**AR & MR:** MR accentuates AR causing more severe pulmonary congestion; severe LV dilatation (accentuating MR)

# 4.12/ VALVE PROSTHESES

| MECHANICAL PROSTHESES | BIOPROSTHESES |
|---|---|
| • High thrombo-embolic risk<br>• Excellent durability<br>• **Prefer in patients < 60 years** | • Risk of structural deterioration (Mitral >> Aortic)<br> - Decreased risk in patients > 65 years<br>• **Prefer in the presence of: A) Bleeding risk; B) Difficult anticoagulation; C) > 70 years; D) Small LVOT (stentless bioprosthesis); E) Woman of childbearing potential; F) Patient preference** |
| • Double-leaflet (St-Jude; Carbo-Medics; ATS Medical)<br>• Tilting-disk (Medtronic-Hall; Omnicarbon) | • Stented porcine bioprosthesis (Mosaic)<br>• Stented bovine pericardium bioprosthesis (Carpentier-Edwards; Mitroflow)<br>• Stentless bioprosthesis<br> - Less obstructive; prefer in patients with small LVOT<br>• Homograft: cadaveric valve<br> - Used for complex aortic valve endocarditis<br>• Ross procedure: autologous transplant of the patient's P valve to the Ao valve; use a cadaveric valve for the P valve<br> - Use in young patients / women of childbearing potential<br>• Percutaneous bioprosthesis (TAVI):<br> - Deployed by balloon (Edwards-Sapien; Sapien XT)<br> - Self-expanding bioprosthesis (Corevalve) |

**COMPLICATIONS**: **A)** Structural deterioration; **B)** Pannus; **C)** Patient-prosthesis mismatch (▸▸| Chapter 1 - Echocardiography); **D)** Thrombosis; **E)** Embolism; **F)** Endocarditis (vegetation; abscess; fistula; dehiscence; destruction); **G)** Periprosthetic leak; **H)** Hemolysis related to periprosthetic regurgitation (↗ LDH; ↗ Bilirubin; ↘ Haptoglobin; Schistocytes); **I)** Dehiscence (rule out endocarditis); **J)** Bleeding secondary to anticoagulants; **K)** Pseudoaneurysm

> **Structural deterioration**: TAVI is possible (valve-in-valve)
> **Periprosthetic regurgitation**: Percutaneous closure with Amplatzer prosthesis (with 3D TEE guidance); indicated if the patient is not a candidate for surgery with significant periprosthetic regurgitation and secondary heart failure or hemolysis (transfusion-dependent); transseptal or transapical approach (M valve); retrograde arterial approach (Ao valve)

**MECHANICAL VALVE**: thromboembolic risk → 1-2 per 100 patient-years (aortic) and 2-3 per 100 patient-years (mitral)

**PORCINE BIOPROSTHESIS**: **structural deterioration** in 30% of patients at 10 years
> 10% at 10 years in patients > 65 years

**PROSTHETIC THROMBOSIS**: dyspnea; ↘ closing sound; *de novo* murmur
> **Diagnosis**: TTE - TEE - Fluoroscopy
> **Risk**: 0.1%/ year for aortic valve; 0.35%/year for mitral valve (with adequate treatment)

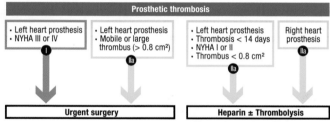

**Prosthetic thrombosis**

| · Left heart prosthesis<br>· NYHA III or IV<br>**I** | · Left heart prosthesis<br>· Mobile or large thrombus (> 0.8 cm²)<br>**IIa** | · Left heart prosthesis<br>· Thrombosis < 14 days<br>· NYHA I or II<br>· Thrombus < 0.8 cm²<br>**IIa** | Right heart prosthesis<br>**IIa** |

**Urgent surgery** ← → **Heparin ± Thrombolysis**

rtPA 10 mg bolus then 90 mg IV over 120 min
Mortality: 4-12% / Embolism: 15%

## ANTITHROMBOTIC THERAPY

| MITRAL VALVE REPAIR / ANNULOPLASTY |
| --- |
| · Warfarin for 3 months (INR 2-3)  · ASA 80 mg qd indefinitely |

| BIOPROSTHESIS |
| --- |
| · ASA 80 mg qd indefinitely<br>· ± Warfarin 3 months postoperatively (INR 2-3); Class IIa recommendation for bioprosthesis MVR;<br>· Class IIb recommendation for bioprosthesis AVR |

| MECHANICAL PROSTHESIS (MODERN) | |
| --- | --- |
| **Low risk**<br>**AVR with no risk factors***<br>· Warfarin indefinitely (INR 2-3)<br>· ASA 80 mg qd indefinitely | **High risk**<br>**AVR with risk factors* or MVR**<br>· Warfarin indefinitely (INR 2.5-3.5)<br>· ASA 80 mg qd indefinitely |

**\* Risk factors: AF / LV dysfunction / History of thromboembolic disease / Hypercoagulability**

**EMBOLISM DESPITE WARFARIN THERAPY**: **A)** If INR 2-3 → target INR 2.5-3.5; **B)** If INR 2.5-3.5 → target INR 3.0-4.0; **C)** If patient not taking ASA → add ASA

**EXCESSIVE ANTICOAGULATION**: **A)** Life-threatening bleeding → Prothrombin complex concentrate (or FFP) + vitamin K 5-10 mg IV (max: 1 mg/min); **B)** INR > 10 without bleeding → suspend Warfarin; vitamin K 2.5 mg PO

## FOLLOW-UP

| BIOPROSTHESIS | MECHANICAL VALVE |
|---|---|
| • Baseline TTE to 2-4 weeks after discharge<br>• Annual follow-up (± TTE if new symptoms and signs)<br>• After 10 years: annual TTE | • Baseline TTE to 2-4 weeks after discharge<br>• Annual follow-up (± TTE if new symptoms and signs) |

**AT FOLLOW-UP**: Physical examination; ECG; CXR; ± Laboratory tests (CBC; BUN / Creatinine; Clotting assessment; INR; Blood cultures); Prophylactic antibiotics

# 4.13/ INFECTIVE ENDOCARDITIS

## MICROBIOLOGY

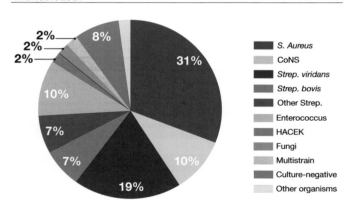

Pie chart legend:
- S. Aureus — 31%
- CoNS — 10%
- Strep. viridans — 19%
- Strep. bovis — 7%
- Other Strep. — 7%
- Enterococcus — 10%
- HACEK — 2%
- Fungi — 2%
- Multistrain — 2%
- Culture-negative — 8%
- Other organisms

**Culture-negative:**

Previous antibiotic; *Coxiella burnetii; Bartonella sp.; Aspergillus sp.; Mycoplasma pneumonia; Brucella sp.; Legionella pneumophila; Tropheryma whipplei; Bartonella sp.;* Fungi (*Candida sp.; Aspergillus sp.*); Antiphospholipid syndrome; Marantic endocarditis; Porcine bioprosthesis allergic response; Rheumatic carditis; Polyarteritis nodosa...

| | |
|---|---|
| **S.aureus (including MRSA)** | • Aggressive acute endocarditis; marked toxicity<br>• Metastatic infection; valve destruction<br>• Mortality 25-40% (left heart) |
| **Coagulase-negative Staphylococcus - CoNS (S. epidermidis; S. lugdunensis)** | • Foreign body infection / prostheses<br>• Nosocomial infection |
| **Streptococcus viridans (sanguis; mutans; mitis; salivarius...)** | • Oropharyngeal flora; alpha-hemolytic<br>• **Subacute endocarditis**<br>• Highly sensitive to penicillin |
| **Streptococcus bovis (gallolyticus)** | • GI flora; associated with polyps and colon cancer<br>• **Subacute endocarditis**<br>• Highly sensitive to penicillin |
| **Beta-hemolytic Streptococci (groups A - B - C - G)** | • Frequent intracardiac and extracardiac complications; abscess |
| **Enterococci (faecalis and faecium)** | • GI flora<br>• Associated with urinary tract infection/nosocomial infection<br>• Treatment requires bactericidal activity **(synergism with gentamicin)** |
| **HACEK**<br>• **Haemophilus sp.**<br>• **Aggregatibacter sp. (previously Actinobacillus)**<br>• **Cardiobacterium hominis**<br>• **Eikenella corrodens**<br>• **Kingella sp.** | • Fastidious Gram-negative bacilli<br>• Upper respiratory tract infections - Oropharyngeal flora<br>• Positive blood culture after 5 days of incubation (sometimes longer)<br>• Large vegetation |
| **Other micro-organisms (can cause culture-negative endocarditis)** | • **Coxiella burnetii (Q fever)**: subacute endocarditis; elevated IgG titer<br>• **Bartonella sp.**: Culture-negative endocarditis (perform serology or specific culture technique); cat scratch disease<br>• **Fungi (Candida)**: Risk factors: immunodepression - prosthesis - central line - IDU; invasive endocarditis<br>• **Others**: Brucella sp.; Tropheryma whipplei; Mycoplasma sp.; Legionella sp. |

## RISK FACTORS

**RISK FACTORS**: MVP; congenital heart disease (bicuspid aortic valve; VSD; patent ductus arteriosus); rheumatic disease; degenerative valvular heart disease; prosthesis or intracardiac device; hospitalization - nursing home; central line; hemodialysis; history of endocarditis

**IDU (INJECTION DRUG USERS)**: S.aureus (most frequent organism); mostly involving the tricuspid valve (look for septic pulmonary emboli)

**PROSTHETIC VALVE ENDOCARDITIS (PVE)**

> **Early (< 12 months post-op): CoNS; S. aureus; Gram-negative bacilli; Fungi (Candida); Corynebacterium sp; Legionella sp**
> **Late (> 12 months post-op): similar microbiology to community-acquired native valve endocarditis**
> Mortality due to S. aureus PVE: > 45%

# MODIFIED DUKE CRITERIA

| DEFINITE ENDOCARDITIS | POSSIBLE ENDOCARDITIS |
|---|---|
| • 2 major criteria or<br>• 1 major + 3 minor criteria or<br>• 5 minor criteria | • 1 major + 1 minor or<br>• 3 minor criteria |

**MAJOR CRITERIA**

**1. Positive blood culture**

   **A)** Typical microorganism on ≥ 2 separate blood cultures
- Strep. viridans; Strep. bovis; HACEK; S.areus or
- Community-acquired Enterococcus with no primary site

   **B)** Sustained bacteremia
- **Slow method**: ≥ 2 positive blood cultures taken at an interval of ≥ 12 h or
- **Rapid method**: 3/3 positive blood cultures or the majority of ≥ 4 blood cultures are positive (taken by different venipunctures); the first and last cultures were taken at an interval of > 1 h

   **C)** Coxiella burnetii (Q fever): ≥ 1 positive culture bottle or IgG titer > 1:800

**2. Endocardial involvement**

   **A)** Positive echocardiography
- Oscillating intracardiac mass (on valve or supporting structures, or in the path of regurgitant jets, or on foreign body) in the absence of an alternative explanation or
- Abscess or
- De novo prosthetic dehiscence

   **B)** De novo valvular regurgitation

**Minor criteria**

   **1. Predisposition** (heart disease or IDU)

   **2. Fever** ≥ 38°C

   **3. Vascular phenomenon**: arterial embolism; septic pulmonary infarction; mycotic aneurysm; intracranial hemorrhage; conjunctival hemorrhage; Janeway lesion

   **4. Immunological phenomenon** (subacute endocarditis): glomerulonephritis; Osler's nodes; Roth's spot; positive rheumatoid factor; vasculitis

   **5. Microbiological evidence**: positive blood culture but not meeting the major criterion or serological evidence of active infection (with organism consistent with infective endocarditis)

*Li JS, Sexton DJ, Mick N, et al. Clin Infect Dis 2000;30:633*

# SYMPTOMS AND SIGNS

**SYMPTOMS**: fever; chills; night sweats; weight loss; dyspnea; cough; stroke; headache; nausea / vomiting; myalgia; arthralgia; retrosternal chest pain; back pain; abdominal pain; confusion

**SIGNS**: fever; neurological signs; signs of peripheral embolism; clubbing

> **Cardiac murmur**: in 85% of cases (uncommon in subacute endocarditis)
> **Splinter hemorrhages**: proximal nail fold; red lines
> **Petechiae**: conjunctiva; oral mucosa and palate; extremities
> **Osler's nodes**: small, painful subcutaneous nodule on fingertips (sometimes more proximal)
> **Janeway lesion**: painless, erythematous or hemorrhagic macular lesion on palms and soles
> **Roth's spot**: oval retinal hemorrhage (with central pallor)
> **Splenomegaly**: more frequent in subacute endocarditis

## PERIPHERAL EMBOLISM

> **Risk factors**: vegetation > 10 mm / mobile; mitral valve (anterior leaflet); *S.aureus*; *Candida*
> **Uncommon after 2 weeks of effective treatment**
> Stroke; digital infarction; septic arthritis; discitis; splenic or renal infarction; splenic abscess; coronary embolism; mesenteric embolism; pulmonary embolism

**STROKE: A) Cardioembolic; B) Intracranial hemorrhage**: ruptured mycotic aneurysm or arteritis with rupture or hemorrhagic transformation of a stroke

> **Dx: A) MRI angiography or CT angiography; B) Conventional angiography** to exclude small aneurysms (< 2 mm) not seen on non-invasive imaging
> **Indication for intervention:** progressing or ruptured aneurysm or > 7 mm
>    - **Small aneurysm without rupture**: monitor (possible improvement with antibiotics)
> **When valve surgery is indicated: A) Stroke without bleeding** → surgery **without delay** (except with extensive brain damage / coma); **B) Intracranial bleeding** → wait **> 4 weeks**
> **Management of anticoagulation:** stop anticoagulation in patients with mechanical valve > 2 weeks in the presence of stroke (class IIa recommendation)

**HEART FAILURE: A)** Valve destruction; **B)** Ruptured chordae tendineae; **C)** Fistula; **D)** Purulent myocarditis; **E)** Coronary embolism; **F)** Valve obstruction

**ARF: A)** Immune complex glomerulonephritis (↘ complement); **B)** Renal embolism (renal infarction); **C)** Prerenal ARF; **D)** Gentamicin toxicity; **E)** Interstitial nephritis (secondary to antibiotics)

**AV BLOCK / CONDUCTION DISORDERS**: perivalvular abscess

## ECHOCARDIOGRAPHY

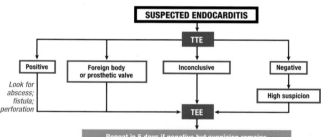

**SENSITIVITY: TTE** → 70% (50% for prosthesis); **TEE** → 96% (92% for prosthesis)

**VEGETATION**: Oscillating mass with independent movement; atrial aspect for M and T valves; ventricular aspect for Ao and P valves; on the surface of implanted intracardiac material

> **DDx**: Old vegetation; Non-bacterial thrombotic endocarditis (marantic); Antiphospholipid syndrome / SLE (Libman-Sacks); degenerative changes / myxomatous valve; Lambl's excrescences; ruptured chordae tendineae; $Ca^{2+}$; nodule - RA; thrombus; fibroelastoma

**LOOK FOR: vegetation; abscess** (not communicating with the lumen) **/ pseudoaneurysm** (pulsatile; colour-Doppler flow detected); **prosthetic dehiscence** (± rocking motion); valvular aneurysm (saccular bulging); intracardiac fistula; valve perforation - channel; purulent pericarditis; obstruction; early mitral valve closure in acute AR (with restrictive diastolic pattern)

## MANAGEMENT

**ANTIBIOTIC TREATMENT**: Target → eradication of microorganisms; bactericidal antibiotic action; sufficient serum concentrations (to penetrate the vegetation by diffusion); minimal toxicity

> **MIC**: Minimum inhibitory concentration (to inhibit growth)
> **MBC**: Minimum bactericidal concentration (to reduce the inoculum)

**DURATION:** from the first day on which blood cultures ar negatives

> **Positive operative tissue cultures**: entire antimicrobial course after valve surgery

| PNC-SENSITIVE *STREP. VIRIDANS* OR *STREP. BOVIS* - MIC < 0.12 µG/ML | | |
|---|---|---|
| PNC G | 12-18 million U / day IV (4-6 doses) | 4 weeks |
| Ceftriaxone | 2 g / day IV or IM (1 dose) | 4 weeks |
| PNC G (or Ceftriaxone) + Gentamicin | 12-18 million U / day IV (4-6 doses) 3 mg/kg / day IV or IM (1 dose) | 2 weeks 2 weeks |
| Vancomycin | 30 mg/kg / day IV (2 doses) | 4 weeks |

- **Prosthesis: A)** 6 weeks therapy of PNC G (24 million U / day) or Ceftriaxone (with or without gentamicin for the first 2 weeks); **B)** 6 weeks therapy of Vancomycin
- Serum Vancomycin levels: trough 10-15 µg/mL
- Serum Gentamicin levels (3 divided doses): peak serum 3-4 µg/mL; trough < 1 µg/mL

| *STREP. VIRIDANS* OR *STREP. BOVIS* RELATIVELY RESISTANT - MIC 0.12 – 0.50 µG/ML | | |
|---|---|---|
| PNC G + Gentamicin | 24 million U / day IV (4-6 doses) 3 mg/kg / day IV or IM (1 dose) | 4 weeks 2 weeks |
| Vancomycin | 30 mg/kg / day IV (2 doses) | 4 weeks |

- **Prosthesis**: 6 weeks therapy
- Ceftriaxone: consider as an alternative if the isolate is susceptible

| METHICILLIN-SENSITIVE STAPHYLOCOCCUS - NO FOREIGN BODY | | |
|---|---|---|
| Cloxacillin | 12 g / day IV (4-6 doses) | 6 weeks |
| Cefazolin | 6 g / day IV (3 doses) | 6 weeks |
| Vancomycin (ß-lactam allergy evaluation) | 30 mg/kg / day IV (2 doses) | 6 weeks |

- Uncomplicated right heart endocarditis: 2 weeks

| METHICILLIN-RESISTANT STAPHYLOCOCCUS - NO FOREIGN BODY | | |
|---|---|---|
| Vancomycin | 30 mg/kg / day IV (2 doses) | 6 weeks |
| Daptomycin | ≥ 8 mg/kg / day IV (1 dose) | 6 weeks |

| METHICILLIN-SENSITIVE STAPHYLOCOCCUS - PROSTHESIS | | |
|---|---|---|
| Cloxacillin + Rifampicin + Gentamicin | 12 g / day IV (4-6 doses) 900 mg / day IV or PO (3 doses) 3 mg/kg / day IV or IM (2-3 doses) | ≥ 6 weeks ≥ 6 weeks 2 weeks |

| METHICILLIN-RESISTANT STAPHYLOCOCCUS - PROSTHESIS | | |
|---|---|---|
| Vancomycin + Rifampicin + Gentamicin | 30 mg/kg / day IV (2 doses) 900 mg / day IV or PO (3 doses) 3 mg/kg / day IV or IM (2-3 doses) | ≥ 6 weeks ≥ 6 weeks 2 weeks |

- Rifampin: caution in relation to multiple drug interactions

| ENTEROCOCCUS SPP. | | |
|---|---|---|
| Ampicillin + Gentamicin | 2 g IV every 4 h 3 mg/kg / day IV or IM (2-3 doses) | 4-6* weeks 2-6 weeks (6 weeks with prosthetic valve) |
| Ampicillin + Ceftriaxone *(E. faecalis)* | 2 g IV every 4 h 4 g / day IV or IM (2 doses) | 6 weeks 6 weeks |
| Vancomycin + Gentamicin | 30 mg/kg / day IV (2 doses) 3 mg/kg / day IV or IM (3 doses) | 6 weeks 6 weeks |

\* 4 weeks with < 3 months duration of symptoms (6 weeks with ≥ 3 months)

| HACEK | | |
|---|---|---|
| Ceftriaxone | 2 g / day IV or IM  (1 dose) | 4 weeks (6 weeks if prosthesis) |

| EMPIRICAL TREATMENT (BEFORE PATHOGEN IDENTIFICATION) – COMMUNITY–ACQUIRED NATIVE VALVE OR LATE PROSTHETIC VALVE (> 12 MONTHS) | |
|---|---|
| Ampicillin + Cloxacillin + Gentamicin | 2 g IV every 4 h 12 g / day IV (4-6 doses) 3 mg/kg / day IV or IM |

| EMPIRICAL TREATMENT (BEFORE PATHOGEN IDENTIFICATION) – EARLY PROSTHETIC VALVE (< 12 MONTHS) OR NOSOCOMIAL ENDOCARDITIS | |
|---|---|
| Vancomycin + Gentamicin + Rifampin | 30 mg/kg / day IV (2 doses) 3 mg/kg / day IV or IM 900 mg / day IV or PO (3 doses) |

## PROPHYLACTIC ANTIBIOTICS

**Candidates**
  **a)** Prosthetic valve (or prosthetic valve material)
  **b)** History of infective endocarditis
  **c)** Congenital heart disease
    1. Unrepaired cyanotic heart disease
      (including palliative conduits and shunts)
    2. Complete repair with prosthetic material
      < 6 months
    3. Repair with residual defect close to
      prosthesis / patch (preventing
      endothelialization)
  **d)** Transplant recipient with regurgitation on
    a structurally abnormal valve

**Procedure**
  • Dental procedure involving the gums
    or periapical region of the tooth or
    perforation of the oral mucosa

• **Amoxicillin 2 g PO** (60 min before the operation) or
• Cephalexin 2 g PO or Azithromycin 500 mg PO or Clindamycin 600 mg PO or
• Cefazolin or Ceftriaxone 1 g IM or IV

## SURGICAL INDICATIONS

- Coronary CT angiography can provide coronary artery evaluation before cardiac surgery

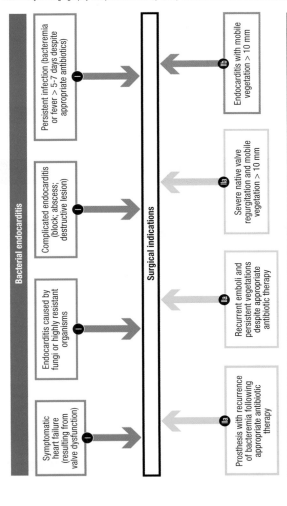

**Bacterial endocarditis**

Symptomatic heart failure (resulting from valve dysfunction) — I

Endocarditis caused by fungi or highly resistant organisms — I

Complicated endocarditis (block; abscess; destructive lesion) — I

Persistent infection (bacteremia or fever > 5-7 days despite appropriate antibiotics) — I

**Surgical indications**

Prosthesis with recurrence of bacteremia following appropriate antibiotic therapy — IIa

Recurrent emboli and persistent vegetations despite appropriate antibiotic therapy — IIa

Severe native valve regurgitation and mobile vegetation > 10 mm — IIa

Endocarditis with mobile vegetation > 10 mm — IIb

I: Removal of implantable cardiac device (pacemaker or ICD) if documented infection of the system

IIa: Removal of implantable cardiac device (pacemaker or ICD) if endocarditis due to *S.aureus* or fungi

# 4.14/ CARDIAC IMPLANTABLE ELECTRONIC DEVICE INFECTION

**MICROBIOLOGY**: CoNS (42%); Sensitive *S. aureus* (25%); MRSA (4%); Gram-negative bacilli (9%); Multistrain (7%); Culture-negative (7%)

**PATHOGENESIS**

**A)** Pocket infection (during procedure or secondary to skin erosion) → ± propagation of infection to intravascular leads → ± intracardiac propagation of infection

**B)** Bacteremia *(S. aureus)* → hematogenous pocket and/or lead infection

**ASSESSMENT**: blood cultures x 2; TEE if blood cultures positive (rule out vegetation adherent to the lead and/or the valve); culture of the pocket after explantation of the system; FDG PET-CT (rule out increased FDG uptake)

**MANAGEMENT**

**A) Superficial skin infection** without involvement of the pocket and system → oral antibiotics against Staphylococcus for 7 to 10 days

**B) Pocket infection and/or skin erosion**: complete removal of the system (even in absence of systemic infection) + ATB

**C) Documented system infection** (lead endocarditis and/or valve endocarditis and/or bacteremia with pocket involvement): complete removal of the system + ATB (risk of clinically significant pulmonary embolism during percutaneous lead removal if vegetation on electrode > 2 cm)

**D) Valve endocarditis** (without documented system infection): complete removal of the system (± implantation of a new epicardial system) + ATB

**E) Occult Staphylococcus bacteremia**: complete removal of the system + ATB

**EMPIRICAL ANTIBIOTICS**: Vancomycin (then according to the organism / sensitivity)

**DURATION OF ANTIBIOTICS**: **A)** 7-10 days if skin erosion with no inflammatory changes; **B)** 10-14 days if pocket infection; **C)** > 2-4 weeks IV if bacteremia (repeat TEE in 2 weeks in the case of lead vegetation); **D)** > 4-6 weeks if complication (valve endocarditis; septic thrombophlebitis; osteomyelitis)

**OPTIMAL TIMING FOR PLACEMENT OF A NEW DEVICE (CONTRALATERAL): A)** Skin erosion / Pocket infection: in the absence of bacteremia; **B)** Positive blood cultures: absence of bacteremia x > 72 h post-explantation; **C)** Valve endocarditis: wait > 14 days before reimplanting an endovenous system

**TEMPORARY PACEMAKER**: Use active fixation lead

# 4.15/ RHEUMATIC FEVER

Autoimmune reaction 2 to 4 weeks after group A beta-hemolytic Streptococcus sore throat (*S. pyogenes*)

## JONES' CRITERIA

| **Major criteria** | **Minor criteria** |
|---|---|
| 1) Carditis and valvulitis | • Arthralgia |
| 2) Migratory arthritis (swollen joints) | • Fever |
| 3) Sydenham's chorea (CNS inflammation; late manifestation) | • Elevation of inflammatory markers (ESR - CRP) |
| 4) Erythema marginatum (trunk; proximal limbs) | • Prolonged PR |
| 5) Subcutaneous nodules | |

**Diagnosis: group A Streptococcal sore throat followed by:**
• 2 major criteria or
• 1 major criterion + 2 minor criteria

## CARDITIS

**PANCARDITIS**: **Valvulitis (MR >> AR)**; LV dysfunction; pericarditis

**PHYSICAL EXAMINATION (IN A CONTEXT OF ACUTE RHEUMATIC FEVER)**:
Tachycardia; ↘ S1; ↗ P2 in the case of severe MR; S3; holosystolic murmur; **Carey Coombs murmur** (mid-diastolic murmur secondary to turbulence and increased mitral diastolic flow); early diastolic decrescendo murmur in the case of AR; pericardial friction rub; TR murmur

**LONG-TERM SEQUELAE: Progressive mitral valve disease (MS >> MR)** which becomes symptomatic after several decades; Ao or T valve involvement is possible

## PRIMARY PREVENTION

Start antibiotics < 10 days after onset of sore throat

PNC V 500 mg PO bid for 10 days

## SECONDARY PREVENTION

| **Candidate** | **Agent** | **Duration** |
|---|---|---|
| All patients with history of rheumatic fever (with or without carditis) due to the high risk of recurrence (class I recommendation) | • PNC G 1.2 million U IM every 4 weeks (or every 3 weeks if residual cardiac lesion) or<br>• PNC V 200 mg PO bid or<br>• Sulfadiazine 1 g PO daily | • Persistent valvular heart disease: > 10 years since last episode (until age of 40 years minimum; long term if in contact with children)<br>• History of carditis but no sequelae: > 10 years since episode (until age of 21 years minimum)<br>• Absence of carditis: > 5 years since episode (until age of 21 years minimum) |

- Bonow RO, Mann DL, Zipes DP, Libby P. *Braunwald's Heart Disease. A textbook of cardiovascular medicine.* Elsevier. 2012. 1961 p.
- Nishimura RA, Otto CM, Bonow RO. 2014 AHA/ACC Guideline for the Management of Patients With Valvular Heart Disease. *JACC;* 2014; *63*; e57-e185.
- 2008 Focused Update Incorporated Into the ACC/AHA 2006 Guidelines for the Management of Patients With Valvular Heart Disease: A Report of the American College of Cardiology/American Heart Association Task Force on Practice Guidelines (Writing Committee to Revise the 1998 Guidelines for the Management of Patients With Valvular Heart Disease) Endorsed by the Society of Cardiovascular Anesthesiologists, Society for Cardiovascular Angiography and Interventions, and Society of Thoracic Surgeons. *JACC;* 2008; *52;* e1-e142.
- Echocardiographic Assessment of Valve Stenosis: EAE/ASE Recommendations for Clinical Practice. *JASE* 2009; *22;* 1-23.
- Recommendations for Evaluation of the Severity of Native Valvular Regurgitation with Two-dimensional and Doppler Echocardiography. *JASE* 2003; *16;* 777-802.
- Nietlispach F, Johnson M, Moss RR et al. Transcatheter closure of paravalvular defects using a purpose-specific occlude. *JACC interventions.* 2010; *3;* 759-765.
- Webb J, Rodès-Cabau J, Fremes S et al. Transcatheter aortic valve implantation: a canadian cardiovascular society position statement. *CJC;* 2012; *28;* 520-528.
- Jayasuriya C, Moss RR, Munt B. Transcatheter aortic valve implantation in aortic stenosis: the role of echocardiography. *JASE;* 2011; *24;* 15-27.
- 2012 ACCF/AATS/SCAI/STS Expert consensus document on transcatheter aortic valve replacement. *JACC;* 2012; *59;* 1200-1254.
- Feldman T, Foster E, Glower DG et al. Percutaneous repair or surgery for mitral regurgitation. *NEJM* 2011; *364;* 1396-1406.
- Mauri L, Garg P, Massaro JM, et al. The EVEREST II Trial: design and rationale for a randomized study of the Evalve MitraClip system compared with mitral valve surgery for mitral regurgitation. *Am Heart J* 2010; *160;* 23-9.
- 2015 ESC Guidelines for the management of infective endocarditis: The Task Force for the Management of Infective Endocarditis of the ESC. *EHJ* 2015; *36;* 3075-3128.
- Infective Endocarditis in Adults: Diagnosis, antimicrobial therapy, and management of complications: A scientific statement for healthcare professionals from the AHA. *Circulation* 2015; *132;* 1435-1486.
- Murdoch DR, Corey CR, Hoen B, et al. Clinical presentation, etiology, and outcome of infective endocarditis in the 21st century. *Arch Intern Med* 2009; *169;* 463.
- Gordon SV, Pettersson GB. Native-valve Infective Endocarditis - When does it require surgery? *NEJM* 2012; *366;* 2519-2521.
- Update on Cardiovascular Implantable Electronic Device Infections and Their Management: A Scientific Statement From the American Heart Association. *Circulation.* 2010; *121;* 458-477
- Baddour LM, Cha Y-M, Wilson WR. Infections of Cardiovascular Implantable Electronic Devices. *NEJM* 2012; *367;* 842-849.
- Marijon E, Mirabel M, Celermajer DS, at al. Rheumatic heart disease. *Lancet* 2012; *379;* 953-64.
- Guidelines for the diagnosis of rheumatic fever. Jones Criteria, 1992 update. Special Writing Group of the Committee on Rheumatic Fever, Endocarditis, and Kawasaki Disease of the Council on Cardiovascular Disease in the Young of the American Heart Association. *JAMA.* 1992; *268;* 2069.
- UpToDate 2015

# Diseases of the Pericardium & Myocardium

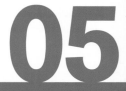

## 05

| 5.1/ | Diseases of the pericardium: etiologies | 172 |
|------|------|------|
| 5.2/ | Acute pericarditis | 173 |
| 5.3/ | Incessant and recurrent pericarditis | 174 |
| 5.4/ | Cardiac tamponade | 174 |
| 5.5/ | Constrictive pericarditis | 177 |
| 5.6/ | Congenital anomalies of the pericardium | 179 |
| 5.7/ | Cardiomyopathies - Classification | 179 |
| 5.8/ | Hypertrophic cardiomyopathy | 181 |
| 5.9/ | Dilated cardiomyopathy | 184 |
| 5.10/ | Restrictive cardiomyopathy | 184 |
| 5.11/ | Cardiac amyloidosis | 187 |
| 5.12/ | Arrhythmogenic right ventricular dysplasia (ARVD) | 188 |
| 5.13/ | Isolated left ventricular noncompaction | 190 |
| 5.14/ | Takotsubo (stress) cardiomyopathy | 191 |
| 5.15/ | Myocarditis | 191 |
| 5.16/ | Indications for endomyocardial biopsy | 193 |
| 5.17/ | Cardiac tumors | 194 |
| 5.18/ | Cardiac complications of cancer | 196 |

# 5.1/ DISEASES OF THE PERICARDIUM: ETIOLOGIES

## IDIOPATHIC (MOST COMMON)

## INFECTIOUS

> **Viral:** echovirus; coxsackievirus; adenovirus; EBV; CMV; HCV; HIV; influenza; parvovirus B19
> **Bacterial:** Pneumococcus; Staphylococcus; Streptococcus; Mycoplasma; Lyme; *Haemophilus influenzae;* Meningococcus; Gonococcus; *Coxiella burnetii; Legionella* spp*; Listeria* spp
> **Mycobacteria:** *M. tuberculosis; M. avium*
> **Fungi:** histoplasmosis; coccidioidomycosis
> **Parasites:** toxoplasmosis; echinococcosis
> **Infective endocarditis** (extension)

## INFLAMMATORY - IMMUNE

> **Collagen diseases:** SLE; RA; Scleroderma; Sjögren
> **Vasculitis:** PAN; Giant cell arteritis; Churg-Strauss; Takayasu; Behçet
> Sarcoidosis
> Still disease
> **Dressler's syndrome:** late post MI or late post-cardiac surgery or late post-trauma
> Myopericarditis
> Inflammatory bowel disease
> Acute rheumatic fever (pancarditis)
> **Medications:** Procainamide; Hydralazine; Cyclosporine; Doxorubicin; Cyclophosphamide...

## NEOPLASTIC

> **Primary:** mesothelioma; angiosarcoma; lipoma; paraganglioma
> **Secondary:** Lung; Breast; Lymphoma; Kaposi sarcoma; GI carcinoma; melanoma; sarcoma...

## RADIOTHERAPY

## EARLY POST-MYOCARDIAL INFARCTION (2-4 DAYS)

## EARLY POST-CARDIAC SURGERY

## HEMOPERICARDIUM

> Trauma
> Free wall rupture (infarction)
> Aortic dissection
> **Iatrogenic:** PCI; pacemaker; ablation of arrhythmia; ASD closure; valve repair / replacement; endomyocardial biopsy

## TRAUMA

> Contusion; Penetrating injury; Post-CPR

## CONGENITAL

> Cyst
> Congenital absence of pericardium

## OTHER

> Renal failure - Uremia
> Dialysis
> Anorexia nervosa
> Chylopericardium
> Hypothyroidism or Hyperthyroidism
> Amyloidosis
> Heart failure (transudate)
> Severe PHT (transudate)
> Familial Mediterranean fever; TRAPS syndrome

**EARLY POST-MI PERICARDITIS (< 1 WEEK):** extension of transmural necrosis to the pericardium (with localized pericarditis); **localized ST elevation; look for ventricular rupture** if effusion associated; treatment with ASA 650 mg PO qid at tapered doses (avoid other NSAIDs) + Colchicine

**DRESSLER'S SYNDROME: Late** post-MI or post-cardiac surgery or post-trauma pericarditis; **autoimmune phenomenon;** polyserositis; fever; treatment with NSAID + Colchicine

**RADIATION-INDUCED PERICARDITIS: A) Acute; B) Late:** several months to several years; pericarditis - effusion - constriction - effusion / constriction

**METASTATIC PERICARDIAL EFFUSION:** Management → pericardiocentesis with drainage; intrapericardial chemotherapy or sclerosing agent; radiotherapy; pericardial window (surgical via left minithoracotomy or percutaneous approach)

**CHRONIC PERICARDIAL EFFUSION: Look for and treat an underlying cause**; look for systemic inflammation (CRP); **when idiopathic →** monitor by regular TTE **vs.** trial of NSAID / colchicine **vs.** pericardiocentesis (if chronic and > 20 mm; if symptomatic; if suspicion of bacterial or neoplastic aetiology)

**DIALYSIS-ASSOCIATED PERICARDITIS:** Now more frequent than uremic pericarditis; occurs even with normal plasma urea; consider intensifying dialysis

**BACTERIAL PERICARDITIS:** Direct extension of pneumonia or endocarditis or hematogenous spread or iatrogenic; **toxic patient;** urgent pericardiocentesis / urgent surgical drainage (± pericardiotomy; ± pericardiectomy)

# 5.2/ ACUTE PERICARDITIS

Inflammation of the pericardium

**Dry vs serous vs fibrinous pericarditis (fibrin; granulation; adhesions; scarring) vs suppurative (bacterial) vs hemorrhagic**

**PRESENTATION:** Retrosternal chest pain **(pleuritic; radiation to trapezius; worse in supine position; relieved by sitting foward)**; dyspnea

**CLINICAL FEATURES:** ± fever; ± tachycardia; ± signs of tamponade

> **Pericardial friction rub: 1 or 2 or 3 components (systole; rapid ventricular filling; atrial kick);** evanescent; left parasternal region; patient seated, leaning forward in forced expiration

**ECG: 4 phases**
1. **Diffuse ST elevation (concave); PR segment depression; mirror changes in aVR**
2. Normalization of ST segment with depression of the J point
3. T wave inversion
4. T wave normalization

**ASSESSMENT:** ECG; TTE; Creatinine - BUN; CBC; liver tests; CXR; ESR - CRP; Troponin (if ↗: consider myopericarditis or MI)

> ± ANA; ANCA; RF; PPD; HIV; HCV; TSH; BNP; tumor work-up; chest CT scan and/or cardiac MRI; Ferritin (Still disease); ACE (Sarcoidosis); Serology for *Coxiella burnetii* or for Lyme disease
> ± Pericardial aspiration (looking for cancer cells - cytology; cultures / mycobacterium culture; PCR for TB; Adenosine deaminase); Biopsy (cancer; TB)

**DIAGNOSIS: Clinical diagnosis: ≥ 2 out of 4 criteria**

| Pleuritic and positional retrosternal chest pain | Pericardial friction rub (pathognomonic) | Typical ECG changes | Pericardial effusion |
| --- | --- | --- | --- |

**MANAGEMENT**

**IBUPROFEN 600 to 800 mg every 6 to 8 h** > 10 to 14 days (with tapering based on clinical response)

/or
**ASA 650 mg PO qid**

**+**

**PPI** daily

**+**

**COLCHICINE 0.5 mg bid for 3 months if > 70 kg (0.5 mg daily if < 70 kg)**
(★ COPE and ★ ICAP studies)

> Look for and treat any specific cause
> Analgesia - Narcotics PRN
> Rest / avoid exercise until complete resolution of symptoms (athletes: 3 months)
> **Corticosteroids: not recommended as first-line therapy**, as risk factor for recurrence
> **Hospitalization: A)** Fever; **B)** Subacute course; **C)** Failure to respond within 7 d to NSAID; **D)** Large pericardial effusion (> 20 mm) and/or tamponade; **E)** Myopericarditis; **F)** Trauma; **G)** Underlying cause; **H)** Immunosuppression; **I)** Receiving anticoagulant

**COMPLICATIONS:** pericardial effusion; tamponade; constriction

## 5.3/ INCESSANT AND RECURRENT PERICARDITIS

**INCESSANT PERICARDITIS:** recurrence of symptoms on withdrawal of treatment

**RECURRENT PERICARDITIS:** new episode after a symptom-free interval of > 4-6 weeks
> "Self-reactivity" sometimes develops following the first episode

**MANAGEMENT**

1. **Rule out a specific cause**
2. Resume NSAID with tapering over > 12 weeks; assess the response to therapy with CRP
3. Colchicine (★ CORP; ★ CORP-2) for ≥ 6 months
4. Avoid corticosteroids (in case of contraindications to ASA / NSAID / Colchicine → Prednisone 0.2-0.5 mg/kg daily for several weeks then gradual tapering)
5. **Last resort:** Azathioprine; IV immunoglobulins; anti-IL-1 (e.g. Anakira); Pericardiectomy

## 5.4/ CARDIAC TAMPONADE

**THE PERICARDIUM** is a closed sac with a low volume reserve; accumulation of fluid induces increased intrapericardial pressure and **compression of the heart chambers** (R > L)

> **Normal volume of pericardial fluid:** < 50 mL

**Increase then equalization of diastolic pressures in heart chambers ≈ INTRAPERICARDIAL PRESSURE ≈ 15-20 mmHg**

**CLINICAL FEATURES:** tachypnea; tachycardia; diaphoresis; signs of hypoperfusion
> **Beck's triad:** hypotension; muffled heart sounds; JVD
> **Jugular:** attenuated y descent

## PULSUS PARADOXUS: ↘ > 10 mmHg of SBP on inspiration

> Difference between the two pressures on sphygmomanometry when:
>    **1.** Onset of Korotkoff sounds (expiration only)
>    **2.** Korotkoff sounds are audible throughout the respiratory cycle

> **Pathophysiology:** cardiac transmission of respiratory variations of intrathoracic pressure is maintained

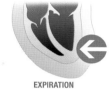

### Inspiration

**INSPIRATION**
↗ Venous return to R heart
↓
Displacement of septum towards the L
↓
↘ Filling and
↘ LV stroke volume

### Expiration

**EXPIRATION**
Septum towards the R

Pulsus paradoxus

> **Tamponade and absence of pulsus paradoxus:** AR; ASD; severe LV dysfunction; LVH; RVH; severe hypotension; pericardial adhesions; localized effusion

> **DDx of pulsus paradoxus:** constrictive pericarditis (effusion-constriction); pulmonary embolism; RV infarction; pulmonary disease with marked variations of intrathoracic pressure (asthma; COPD; OSAHS); obesity; ascites; severe hypotension / hemorrhage; pectus excavatum

**ECG:** low voltage; electrical alternans

**CXR:** rounded and enlarged heart shadow

**FLUOROSCOPY:** abolition of cardiac pulsation

**TTE:** pericardial effusion (anterior to aorta on PLAX); **RA collapse during its relaxation** after the peak of the R wave (very sensitive and specific if > 1/3 of cardiac cycle); **early diastolic RV collapse after T wave** (absent if RVH); abnormal respiratory movement of the septum; plethoric IVC

> **Exaggerated respiratory variations of transvalvular flow**
>    · Measure the first E wave following the start of inspiration and expiration
>    · **Mitral valve**: ↘ E on inspiration; variation > 30% (Eexp - Einsp / Eexp)
>    · **Tricuspid valve**: ↘ E on expiration; variation > 60% (Eexp - Einsp / Eexp)

> **Pulmonary veins:** predominance of **systolic** flow (↘ Y wave)
> **Hepatic veins**: expiration → ↘ anterograde flow and ↗ diastolic reversal (A wave)

|  | TAMPONADE | CONSTRICTION |
|---|---|---|
| **Pulsus paradoxus** | Present | Possible (1/3) |
| **Jugular** | Attenuation of Y wave | Prominent Y wave "M or W" Pattern |
| **Effect of inspiration on CVP** | Reduction (normal effect) | Kussmaul (increase or absence of reduction) |

|  | TAMPONADE | CONSTRICTION |
|---|---|---|
| **Equalization of diastolic pressures** | + | + |
| **Square root sign (ventricular curve)** | Absent | + |
| **Ventricular interdependence (discordance of RV and LV systolic pressures during breathing)** | Present | Present |
| **Valve flow variations** | • M valve: ↘ E on inspiration; **variation > 30 %**<br>• T valve: ↘ E on expiration; **variation > 60 %** | • M valve: ↘ E on inspiration; **variation > 25 %**<br>• T valve: ↘ E on expiration; **variation > 40 %** |
| **Pulmonary vein flow** | Systolic | Diastolic |
| **Hepatic vein flow** | ↗ Diastolic reversal on expiration | ↗ Diastolic reversal on expiration |

## PERICARDIOCENTESIS

1. Patient in 45° supine; subxiphoid approach (1 cm below the xyphoid process and 1 cm to the patient's left); local anesthesia
2. Needle introduced at an angle of 30-45° to the skin aiming for the left scapula while applying negative pressure on the syringe (± echocardiographic guidance)
3. Confirm the correct position of the needle: contrast in the case of echocardiographic guidance; insertion of a guide into the pericardial sac in the case of fluoroscopic guidance
4. Insertion of a dilator followed by a Pigtail catheter
   > Remove the drain when it drains **< 50 mL/day**

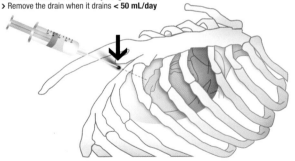

> **Indications: A)** Tamponade; **B)** Diagnosis of pericardial effusion (metastases; bacterial pericarditis; TB)
> **Contraindication**: Aortic dissection with hemopericardium; ventricular rupture; coagulopathy; inaccessible effusion
> **Complications (1-2%)**: Perforation of right heart chambers; coronary laceration; pneumothorax; hepatic puncture; arrhythmia; arterial bleeding
> **Surgical drainage**: Following trauma or ventricular rupture or loculated / organized effusion or when biopsy is required or bacterial pericarditis
> **Pericardial window (pericardiotomy)**: During reaccumulation / frequent recurrence; surgical or balloon

# 5.5/ CONSTRICTIVE PERICARDITIS

Pericardial fibrosis / calcification / adhesions

**ETIOLOGIES: Idiopathic; Postoperative; Viral pericarditis; Recurrent pericarditis; Post-radiotherapy; TB;** Other (infectious; neoplastic; collagen disease; uremia; post-trauma; sarcoidosis)

**CONSEQUENCE: limited filling of heart chambers**

> Rapid early diastolic ventricular filling (prominent Y wave), which then ceases abruptly at mid-diastole (rigid pericardium)

**PRESENTATION: systemic venous congestion mimicking right heart failure**

**CLINICAL FEATURES:** JVD; **prominent Y wave** (normal X descent; "M or W" pattern); **Kussmaul's sign** (increase or absence of decrease of CVP on inspiration); ± pulsus paradoxus (especially in the case of effusion - constriction); anasarca; hepatomegaly; pulsatile liver; signs of liver disease; jaundice; cardiac cachexia; low output state

> **Pericardial knock:** high-pitched early diastolic sound at the apex or left parasternal region corresponding to the abrupt cessation of ventricular filling (± palpable)

> **DDx of Kussmaul's sign: RV infarction; pulmonary embolism; RCM; TS; RA tumor; severe right heart failure**

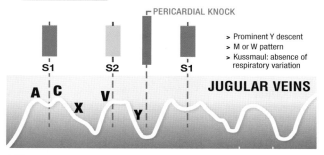

┌ PERICARDIAL KNOCK

S1      S2      S1

A  C      V

X        Y

**JUGULAR VEINS**

> Prominent Y descent
> M or W pattern
> Kussmaul: absence of respiratory variation

**CXR:** Pericardial calcifications

**CT SCAN AND MRI:** pericardial thickening **> 4 mm** (20% of patients have normal thickness); calcifications (CT scan); pericardial adhesions to the myocardium (MRI)

**TTE:** abrupt cessation of ventricular filling at early diastole; abnormal respiratory movement of the septum (septal bounce); restrictive ventricular filling pattern; plethoric IVC

> **Exaggerated respiratory variations of transvalvular flow**
> • Measure the first E wave following the start of inspiration and expiration
> • **Mitral valve**: ↘ E on inspiration; variation > 25% (Eexp - Einsp / Eexp)
> • **Tricuspid valve**: ↘ E on expiration; variation > 40% (Eexp - Einsp / Eexp)

  - Variations masked if ↗ LA pressure (unmasked by asking the patient to sit up)
  - **DDx:** RV infarction; pulmonary embolism; pleural effusion; COPD (COPD: ↗ SVC anterograde systolic flow velocity > 20 cm/s on inspiration)

> **Pulmonary veins**: predominance of **diastolic flow** (↗ Y wave)
> **Hepatic veins: expiration** → decreased anterograde flow and increased diastolic reversal (A wave)
> **Tissue Doppler imaging of septal mitral annulus: E' > 8 cm/s** (*annulus paradoxus*)

## CARDIAC CATHETERIZATION

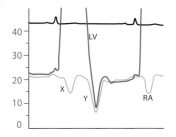

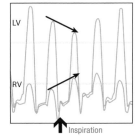

**ATRIAL CURVE:**
• Prominent Y descent
• W or M pattern
• Kussmaul

**VENTRICULAR CURVE:**
• Square root sign

**VENTRICULAR CURVES:**
• Equalization of end-diastolic pressures
• Respiratory discordance of ventricular systolic pressures

> **Ventricular curve: square root sign**: rapid initial ventricular filling, then increase and **equalization of end-diastolic pressures** of the chambers (≈ 20 mmHg)
> • LVEDP - RVEDP < 5 mmHg
>   - Can be detected with a bolus in the presence of dehydration
> **Interdependence**: RV and LV systolic pressure discordance during respiration

## INSPIRATION

↓ Intrathoracic pressure
↓ Pulmonary venous pressure

(no change of intrapericardial pressure and LA pressure)

↓↓ PV - LA PRESSURE GRADIENT
=
↓ venous return to LV
(septum shifted to the left)

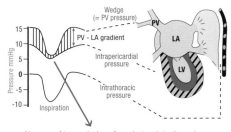

Absence of transmission of respiratory intrathoracic pressure variations to the intrapericardial compartment (isolated by the thickened pericardium)

**Adapted from**: *Bunnell IL, Holand JF, Griffith GT, Greene DG. Hemodynamics during induced cardiac tamponade in man. Am J Med 1960;25:640-6*

## MANAGEMENT

1. Diuretics (beware of decreased preload)
2. Avoid BB-CCB (compensatory tachycardia to maintain cardiac output)
3. **Pericardiectomy**: the only definitive treatment (perioperative mortality: 5-15%)
4. NSAID in acute effusive / constrictive pericarditis

# 5.6/ CONGENITAL ANOMALIES OF THE PERICARDIUM

## PERICARDIAL CYST

Often adjacent to right chambers

Cardiac MRI PRN; Conservative management (except when compressive)

## CONGENITAL ABSENCE OF THE PERICARDIUM

Most often partial absence of the left pericardium

**COMPLICATIONS:** hernia / strangulation of part of the heart; retrosternal chest pain - syncope - sudden death

**ECG:** Incomplete RBBB; poor precordial progression of R wave

**CXR:** Marked levoposition; loss of right heart contour; interposition of lung between Ao and main PA

**TTE:** Unusual imaging window (PLAX); RV appears dilated; exaggerated heart movements; abnormal movement of interventricular septum

**CARDIAC MRI:** Marked levoposition; presence of lung parenchyma between Ao and main PA and between inferior heart surface and diaphragm; ± hernia of part of the heart

**TREATMENT:** Pericardioplasty (in the presence of symptoms or hernia)

# 5.7/ CARDIOMYOPATHIES - CLASSIFICATION

Myocardial disease (abnormal structure and function) in the absence of CAD - HTN - valvular heart disease - congenital heart disease

▶▶| Classification (following page)

# CARDIOMYOPATHIES

Branches: **HCM** → **DCM** → **RCM** → **ARVD** → **UNCLASSIFIED**

## HCM

**NON-FAMILIAL**
- **OBESITY**
- **ATHLETIC TRAINING**
- **AMYLOIDOSIS** (AL / senile)
- **ACROMEGALY**

**FAMILIAL**

**SARCOMERIC PROTEIN MUTATIONS**
- β myosin-binding protein C
- β myosin heavy chain
- Troponin I
- Troponin T
- α-tropomyosin
- Myosin light chain
- Actin
- α-myosin
- Titin
- Troponin C
- LIM protein

**SYNDROMIC HCM**
- Noonan's syndrome
- LEOPARD syndrome
- Friedreich's ataxia
- Beckwith–Wiedemann syndrome
- Swyer's syndrome

**GLYCOGEN STORAGE DISEASES**
- Pompe
- PRKAG2
- Forbes
- Danon (LAMP2)

**LYSOSOMAL STORAGE DISEASES**
- Anderson–Fabry
- Hurler's

**DISORDERS OF FATTY ACID METABOLISM**

**CARNITINE DEFICIENCY**

**PHOSPHORYLASE B KINASE DEFICIENCY**

**MITOCHONDRIAL CYTOPATHIES**

**FAMILIAL AMYLOIDOSIS (TTR)**

**FAMILIAL, UNKNOWN GENE**

## DCM

**NON-FAMILIAL**
- **IDIOPATHIC**
- **MYOCARDITIS** (infectious / toxic / auto-immune; see Etiologies)
- **EOSINOPHILIC** (Churg–Strauss syndrome)
- **DRUG-INDUCED CARDIOTOXICITY**
- **CARDIOTOXINS** (alcohol, cocaine, amphetamines; anabolic steroids)

**PREGNANCY**

**ENDOCRINE**
- Thyroid disease
- Pheochromocytoma
- Acromegaly

**NUTRITIONAL**
- Thiamine (Berber)
- Carnitine
- Selenium
- Hypophosphatemia
- Hypocalcemia

**KAWASAKI**

**TACHYCARDIOMYOPATHY**

**VIRAL PERSISTENCE**

**PERIPARTUM CM**

**HIV**

**METALS** (phosphorus, mercury; cobalt)

**SARCOIDOSIS**

**FAMILIAL**

**SARCOMERIC PROTEIN MUTATIONS** (see HCM)

**Z-BAND**
- LIM protein
- TCAP

**CYTOSKELETAL GENES**
- Dystrophin
- Desmin
- Metavinculin
- Sarcoglycan complex
- CRYAB
- Epicardin

**MUSCULAR DYSTROPHY**
- Becker (dystrophin)
- Duchenne (dystrophin)
- Emery–Dreifuss

**NUCLEAR MEMBRANE**
- Lamin A/C (LMNA)
- Emerin

**MILDLY DILATED CM**

**INTERCALATED DISC PROTEIN MUTATIONS** (see ARVD)

**SCN5A MUTATION**

**MITOCHONDRIAL CYTOPATHIES**

**HAEMOCHROMATOSIS**

**FAMILIAL, UNKNOWN GENE**

## RCM

**NON-FAMILIAL**
- **IDIOPATHIC**
- **AMYLOIDOSIS** (AL / senile)
- **SARCOIDOSIS**
- **SCLERODERMA**

**ENDOMYOCARDIAL DISEASES**
- Endomyocardial fibrosis
- Hypereosinophilic syndrome (Loeffler)
- Idiopathic
- Drugs (serotonin, methysergide, ergotamine, mercurial agents, busulfan)

**CARCINOID HEART DISEASE**

**METASTATIC CANCERS**

**RADIOTHERAPY**

**DRUGS (ANTHRACYCLINES)**

**DIABETES**

**FAMILIAL**

**FAMILIAL AMYLOIDOSIS**
- Transthyretin (neuropathy)
- Apolipoprotein (nephropathy)

**SARCOMERIC PROTEIN MUTATIONS**
- Troponin I
- Myosin light chain

**HAEMOCHROMATOSIS**

**DESMINOPATHY**

**PSEUDOXANTHOMA ELASTICUM**

**ANDERSON–FABRY**

**GLYCOGEN STORAGE DISEASE**

**HURLER'S SYNDROME**

**GAUCHER'S DISEASE**

**FAMILIAL, UNKNOWN GENE**

## ARVD

**NON-FAMILIAL**

**FAMILIAL**

**INTERCALATED DISC PROTEIN MUTATIONS (DESMOSOME)**
- Plakoglobin 2 (PKP2)
- Desmoglein 2
- Desmoplakin 2
- Plakoglobin

**CARDIAC RYANODINE RECEPTOR (RYR2)**

**TRANSFORMING GROWTH FACTOR-B3 (TGFB3)**

**FAMILIAL, UNKNOWN GENE**

## UNCLASSIFIED

**NON-FAMILIAL**
- **TAKOTSUBO**

**FAMILIAL**

**LV NON-COMPACTION**
- Barth syndrome (Tafazzin)
- Lamin A/C
- ZASP
- α-dystrobrevin

**Adapted from**: Elliott P, Andersson B, Arbustini E, et al. Classification of the cardiomyopathies: a position statement from the european society of cardiology working group on myocardial and pericardial diseases. EHJ 2008, 29; 270-276.

# 5.8/ HYPERTROPHIC CARDIOMYOPATHY

LV hypertrophy without dilatation and with no identifiable cause (see DDx)

**Obstructive HCM (intraventricular gradient at rest or on exercise) versus non-obstructive HCM (gradient < 30 mmHg)**    +

Autosomal dominant; sarcomere protein gene

PATHOPHYSIOLOGY

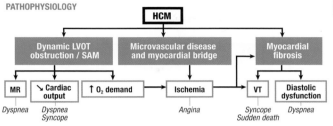

DIFFERENTIAL DIAGNOSIS

> Valvular heart disease; subaortic membrane; HTN (regression of LVH with tight blood pressure control); amyloidosis (TTR; AL); CRF; isolated basal septal hypertrophy in the elderly; acromegaly; phaeochromocytoma
> Syndromic: Noonan; LEOPARD; Friedreich's ataxia
> Glycogen storage disease; Lysosomal storage disease (Anderson-Fabry); Mitochondrial cytopathy
  • Symmetrical LVH; WPW (Danon and PRKAG2)
> High-level athlete

|  | ATHLETE | HCM |
|---|---|---|
| **Genetic test or family history** | Negative | Positive |
| **Diastolic dysfunction** | Absent | Present |
| **LV end-diastolic diameter** | > 55 mm | < 45 mm |
| **SAM** | Absent | Present |
| **Asymmetrical LVH** | Absent | Present |
| **Severe LVH (> 17 mm)** | Absent | Present |
| **Regression of LVH after stopping training** | Present | Absent |
| **VO₂ max > 110% predicted** | Present | Absent |
| **Scar / fibrosis on MRI** | Absent | Present |

PRESENTATION: dyspnea; retrosternal chest pain; syncope; AF; malignant arrhythmia; sudden death
> Progression to DCM with systolic dysfunction ("burn-out" HCM): < 5%

CLINICAL FEATURES: rapid carotid upstroke with **pulsus bisferiens** ("*spike and dome*");    +
**3 components at apex** (early systolic wave; late systolic wave; S4); paradoxical split S2; **left parasternal systolic ejection murmur (↗ on Valsalva or on standing)**; MR murmur (radiation to axilla)

ECG: LVH; LAH; T - ST abnormalities (diffuse T wave inversion in apical HCM); Q waves; arrhythmias

**TTE (± CONTRAST): A)** LV wall **≥ 15 mm** (that is not explained solely by loading conditions); asymmetrical septal hypertrophy (septum / posterior wall **> 1.5 : 1**) and/or apical hypertrophy and/or anterolateral hypertrophy or concentric; ↗ LV mass; **B) SAM** (mid-to-late systolic MR with posterior jet); **C)** Dynamic intraventricular gradient **≥ 30 mmHg** amplified by Valsalva maneuver (continuous Doppler shows **a late-peaking dagger-shaped appearance**); **D)** Diastolic dysfunction; **E)** Structural abnormality of the mitral valve (elongated leaflets; abnormal insertion of anterolateral papillary muscle); **F)** LA dilatation; **G)** Apical aneurysm    +

> **Exercice echocardiography**: in symptomatic patients to detect a significant dynamic intraventricular gradient (≥ 50 mmHg) when absent at rest

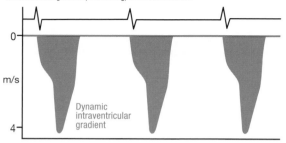

> **DDx of Dynamic intraventricular gradient**: Takotsubo; cardiac amyloidosis; anterior myocardial infarction (basal hyperdynamism); post-AVR (AS with LVH); sigmoid septum in eldery people; hypertensive heart disease; small hyperdynamic LV

**CARDIAC CATHETERIZATION**

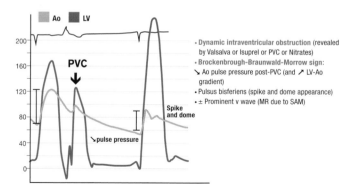

- **Dynamic intraventricular obstruction** (revealed by Valsalva or Isuprel or PVC or Nitrates)
- **Brockenbrough-Braunwald-Morrow sign**: ↘ Ao pulse pressure post-PVC (and ↗ LV-Ao gradient)
- Pulsus bisferiens (spike and dome appearance)
- ± Prominent v wave (MR due to SAM)

**STRESS TEST:** evaluate functional capacity; look for abnormal BP response (↘ **BP > 20 mmHg**  + **or absence of increase of BP > 20 mmHg**); combine with echocardiography to demonstrate dynamic obstruction; repeat stress test every 2-3 years in clinically stable patients

**CARDIAC MRI:** LVH; Rule out apical HCM; late gadolinium enhancement (interventricular septum; free wall; RV insertion sites) with **≥ 10% of LV mass associated with increase SCD risk**    +

**BIOPSY**: disorganized myocyte architecture; interstitial fibrosis

**GENETIC TEST**: indicated routinely (Class I); enables cascade genetic screening of the relatives; positive in 60-70% of cases

## MANAGEMENT

> Avoid strenuous exertion / competitive sports
> **Hypotension due to LVOT obstruction**: volume; BB; Phenylephrine
> **Anticoagulation** for AF irrespective of CHADSVASc score
> **Family screening**: 1st degree relatives; clinical and/or genetic screening

| 12 - 18 YEARS OR COMPETITIVE SPORTSMAN | > 18 YEARS |
|---|---|
| ANNUAL ECG / TTE | ECG / TTE EVERY 5 YEARS |

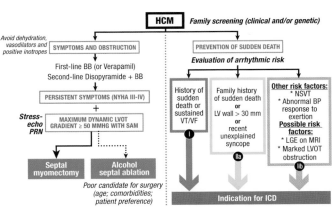

**HCM** — *Family screening (clinical and/or genetic)*

*Avoid dehydration, vasodilators and positive inotropes*

**SYMPTOMS AND OBSTRUCTION**

First-line BB (or Verapamil)
Second-line Disopyramide + BB

**PERSISTENT SYMPTOMS (NYHA III-IV)**
+
*Stress-echo PRN* — **MAXIMUM DYNAMIC LVOT GRADIENT ≥ 50 MMHG WITH SAM**

**Septal myomectomy**   **Alcohol septal ablation**

*Poor candidate for surgery (age; comorbidities; patient preference)*

**PREVENTION OF SUDDEN DEATH**

*Evaluation of arrhythmic risk*

History of sudden death or sustained VT/VF **I**

Family history of sudden death or LV wall > 30 mm or recent unexplained syncope **IIa**

**Other risk factors:**
* NSVT
* Abnormal BP response to exertion
**Possible risk factors:**
* LGE on MRI
* Marked LVOT obstruction **IIb**

**Indication for ICD**

> **Septal myomectomy**: preferable in most cases (especially young patients; septum > 30 mm; other concomitant surgical indication; structural abnormality of mitral valve)
  • **Complications**: mortality (1%); complete AV block (2%); LBBB; iatrogenic VSD (< 1%); Ao valve lesion (AR)
> **Alcohol septal ablation:** selective injection of alcohol into perforating septal coronary branches; under ultrasound guidance (with intracoronary contrast); "controlled" infarction targeting the basal ventricular septum at the site of SAM
  • **Complications**: mortality (2%); complete AV block (10-20%); RBBB; in-hospital VT (5%); repeat procedures (12%); possible long-term arrhythmic risk

**PROGNOSIS**: cardiovascular death 1-2 % / year; the majority of patients have a **similar life expectancy to that of the general population**; identify patients with increased risk of sudden death

**HCM RISK-SCD (5 years):** $= 1 - 0.998^{\text{Prognostic index}}$; **consider ICD if 5-year risk ≥ 6%**

> **Prognostic index:** $= [0.15939858 \times \text{maximal wall thickness (mm)}] - [0.00294271 \times \text{maximal wall thickness}^2 \text{ (mm}^2)] + [0.0259082 \times \text{LA diameter (mm)}] + [0.00446131 \times \text{maximal LVOT gradient (mmHg)}] + [0.4583082 \times \text{familial history SCD}] + [0.82639195 \times \text{NSVT}] + [0.71650361 \times \text{unexplained syncope}] - [0.01799934 \times \text{age (years)}]$

## 5.9/ DILATED CARDIOMYOPATHY

Ventricular dilatation and systolic dysfunction

**Idiopathic in 50% of cases**

CLINICAL FEATURES: JVD; lateralized and enlarged apex; S3; S4; AV valve regurgitation

COMPLICATIONS: Heart failure; arrhythmias; conduction disorders; thromboembolism; sudden death

ECG: Sinus tachycardia; arrhythmias; T - ST abnormalities; LVH; poor precordial progression of R wave; conduction disorders

TTE: Spherical LV; thinned walls; dilated chambers; MR (Carpentier I and IIIb); limited aortic valve opening; LVOT VTI < 18 cm; ↘ dP/dT; thrombus; diastolic dysfunction; pericardial effusion; PHT

ASSESSMENT: CXR; CBC; Electrolytes; Phosphorus; Calcium; Renal function; LFTs; TSH; CK; ANA; ESR; CRP; Iron assessment; HIV; Urinalysis; Blood glucose; Lipid profile; ± Lyme antibody titer; ± Urine metanephrines; ± BNP

> **Family screening / Genetic Test**: consider when: **A)** DCM is possibly familial; **B)** DCM with AV block and/or sudden death in the family (LMNA; SCN5A)

## SPECIFIC ENTITIES

TACHYCARDIOMYOPATHY: secondary to sustained supraventricular or ventricular tachycardia; recovery of LV function by aggressive rhythm control or rate control within 4 weeks

> **AF**: BB; Amiodarone x 1 month then cardioversion; Digoxin; RF ablation

ALCOHOLIC CARDIOMYOPATHY: improvement of LVEF with abstinence

> **Harmful effects of alcohol (heavy drinking)**: systolic and/or diastolic dysfunction; HTN; CAD **(decreased risk with low consumption / 1 to 2 standard drinks per day)**; stroke; arrhythmia - AF; sudden death; hypertriglyceridemia

OBESITY-RELATED CARDIOMYOPATHY: Secondary to ↗ cardiac output and myocardial fat infiltration; LV dilatation then LV dysfunction

> Suspect when BMI > 40 kg/m² (for more than 10 years); Diagnosis of exclusion

CHAGAS DISEASE (TRYPANOSOMIASIS): *Trypanosoma cruzi*; transmission of the parasite by *Triatominae* bugs

> **Early infection**: Acute myocarditis; ± meningoencephalitis / skeletal muscle involvement / nerve involvement
> • **Treatment**: Nifurtimox or Benznidazole
> • **Reactivation**: Immunosuppression / HIV / heart transplant
> **Latent infection**: Mild lymphocytic myocarditis
> **Chagas cardiomyopathy:** 30% of patients; several years after infection; autoimmune myocarditis (little or no residual parasites); dilatation of chambers; ventricular dysfunction (RV then LV); apical and inferolateral aneurysm; thrombus (apex; RAA); embolism; ventricular arrhythmia; blocks; cardiac dysautonomia

## 5.10/ RESTRICTIVE CARDIOMYOPATHY

High filling pressure secondary to **rigid myocardium** due to **myocardial or endomyocardial fibrosis or following infiltration of the myocardium by a substance**

PRESENTATION: dyspnea; weakness; edema / anasarca; AF

CLINICAL FEATURES: JVD; Kussmaul's sign; S3; S4; palpable apex (contrary to constriction); AV valve regurgitation; hepatomegaly; ascites; peripheral edema

ECG: **low voltage**; conduction disorders; poor precordial progression of R wave; AF +

TTE: **bi-atrial dilatation; normal or decreased ventricular volume**; normal or slightly +
increased wall thickness; sparkling myocardium; thickening of valves / interatrial septum;
diastolic dysfunction with restrictive pattern; effusion

| | CONSTRICTION | RESTRICTION |
|---|---|---|
| **Y descent** | Prominent | Prominent |
| **Pulsus paradoxus** | Sometimes present (1/3) | Absent |
| **Palpable apex** | No | Yes |
| **Pericardial knock** | Present | Absent |
| **LV filling pressure > 25 mmHg** | Rare | Frequent |
| **Square root sign** | Present | Present |
| **LVEDP - RVEDP (equalization of diastolic pressures)** | < 5 mmHg | > 5 mmHg |
| **RVEDP / RVSP (pulse pressure)** | > 0.33 | < 0.33 |
| **sPAP** | < 50 mmHg | > 50 mmHg |
| **Ventricular interdependence (discordant respiratory variations of RV and LV pressures)** | Present (pressure discordance) | Absent (pressure concordance) |
| **Diastolic pattern** | Restrictive | Restrictive |
| **Respiratory variations of transvalvular flow** | Exaggerated • **M valve**: > 25 % variation • **T valve**: > 40 % variation | Normal • **M valve**: about 5% variation |
| **Mitral septal annulus E`** | > 8 cm/s | < 8 cm/s |
| **Hepatic veins: ↗ diastolic reversal** | Expiratory | Inspiratoire |
| **Ventricular wall thickness** | Normal | ± Increased |
| **Pericardial thickness** | ± Increased | Normal |
| **Atrial dimensions** | ± LA dilatation | Bi-atrial dilatation ++ |
| **Abnormal respiratory movement of the septum** | Present | Absent |
| **BNP** | Often normal | Increased |

BIOPSY: Rule out infiltration (amyloidosis; sarcoidosis; Gaucher; Hurler's)

MANAGEMENT

> Treatment of underlying cause
> Control of blood volume is difficult (hypotension if ↘ preload)
> Caution with BB and CCB: cardiac output depends on HR (**fixed stroke volume** due to poor filling)

## SPECIFIC ENTITIES

SCLERODERMA: microvascular spasm with ischemia and necrosis / fibrosis

**HEMOCHROMATOSIS:** tissue iron deposits (heart; liver; gonads; pancreas; skin)

> Autosomal recessive; HFE gene mutation
>   - **Secondary iron overload:** repeated transfusions; ineffective erythropoiesis
> **Pentad:** heart failure; cirrhosis; impotence; DM; arthritis
> **Cardiac involvement: diastolic dysfunction - RCM (possibly followed by systolic dysfunction); LV dilatation - DCM;** conduction disorders
> **Assessment:** ↗ ferritin (> 200 µg/L in premenopausal women; > 300 µg/L in men or postmenopausal women); ↗ transferrin saturation (> 50% in women and > 60% in men)
> **MRI:** ↘ relaxation time on T2* (< 20 ms)
> **TREATMENT:** Phlebotomies; Chelator (Deferoxamine)

**FABRY DISEASE:** X-linked; α-galactosidase A deficiency; accumulation of glycosphingolipids in lysosomes

> **Diagnosis:** ↗ urinary globotriaosylceramide; skin biopsy
> Variable degree of enzyme deficiency: **A) Total deficiency:** neuropathies; renal / skin / cardiac involvement; stroke; **B) Partial deficiency:** isolated cardiac involvement is possible
> **Cardiac involvement:** LVH mimicking HCM; Diastolic dysfunction - RCM; angina / myocardial infarction (endothelial infiltration); HTN; MVP
> **Management:** enzyme replacement therapy

**SARCOIDOSIS:** multisystem noncaseating granulomas (particularly in lungs / reticulo-endothelial system / skin)

> **Cardiac involvement:** infiltration of cardiac conduction tissue and myocardium (IV septum; LV free wall); blocks; ventricular arrhythmias; RCM; systolic LV dysfunction; LV dilatation; LV aneurysm; RWMA not corresponding to coronary anatomy; pericarditis; valvular heart disease; cor pulmonale (pulmonary fibrosis)
> **Biopsy:** often falsely negative
> **MRI:** late gadolinium enhancement reflecting intramural or subepicardial fibrosis (often anteroseptal or inferolateral)
> **PET-FDG:** demonstrates patchy zones of fibrosis and/or inflammation
> **Management:** Corticosteroids; Plaquenil; Methotrexate; Cyclophosphamide; ICD; Transplant (risk of recurrence)

**ENDOMYOCARDIAL FIBROSIS (DAVIES DISEASE):** Tropical regions; ± eosinophilia; fibrosis / thrombus / endocardial obliteration (obliteration of apex; papillary muscle fibrosis; AV valve regurgitation); bi-atrial dilatation; diastolic dysfunction with restrictive pattern

**LOEFFLER ENDOCARDITIS (HYPEREOSINOPHILIC SYNDROME):** Eosinophilia > 1 500 cells/µL with multisystem involvement (lung; CNS; GI; skin)

> **Cardiac involvement:** myocarditis followed by replacement of the myocardium by thrombus then formation of endomyocardial fibrosis; fibrosis / thrombus / endocardial obliteration (apex; posterior mitral leaflet; posterobasal wall); RCM; AV valve regurgitation; embolism
> **Management:** anticoagulation; Corticosteroids; Hydroxyurea; Interferon; endocardiectomy; valve replacement / repair

**CARCINOID SYNDROME:** Gastrointestinal tract (small bowel) or bronchial tumor; release of serotonin by the tumor and liver metastases; ↗ urinary 5-HIAA

> **Symptoms:** skin flushing; diarrhea; bronchospasm; hypotension
> **Cardiac involvement:** Fibrous endomyocardial plaques in right heart chambers; tricuspid and pulmonary valve disease with thickening / retraction / rigidity of leaflets (TR and PR due to malcoaptation; ± TS; ± PS); right ventricular dilatation and dysfunction
>   - Involvement of left chambers in the presence of R→L shunt or lung metastases
> **Management:** Somatostatin analogs; embolization of liver metastases; TVR if severe symptoms and/or dilatation – progressive RV dysfunction (despite adequate control of the cancer)

# 5.11/ CARDIAC AMYLOIDOSIS

Interstitial infiltration of a protein demonstrating apple-green birefringence when stained with Congo Red

## PRIMARY AMYLOIDOSIS (AMYLOIDOSIS AL)

**Plasma cell dyscrasia** (plasma cell clone); tissue deposits of a portion of **immunoglobulin light chains**

**CARDIAC INVOLVEMENT (50% OF PATIENTS):** median survival = 15 months; LVH; RCM; progressive LV dysfunction; ischemia (microvascular infiltration); conduction disorders; atrial disease; sudden death (pulseless electrical activity)

**SYSTEMIC INVOLVEMENT:** OH; peripheral / autonomic neuropathy; carpal tunnel; periorbital purpura; ecchymoses; macroglossia; RUQ pain; onychodystrophy; renal failure / nephrotic syndrome

**CLINICAL FEATURES:** hypotension / OH; JVD; Prominent X and Y waves; Kussmaul; S4 rarely present (atrial disease); pleural effusions; hepatomegaly; anasarca

**ECG: microvoltage (despite LVH on TTE)** ; AF; pseudo-infarction; blocks $+$

**TTE:** thickened walls; small ventricular chamber; dynamic LVOT obstruction; valvular / interatrial septum infiltration; sparkling myocardium; diastolic dysfunction; possible systolic dysfunction; pericardial effusion; bi-atrial dilatation

**CARDIAC MRI:** rapid accumulation of contrast in myocardium (**rapid wash-out from blood**); circumferential subendocardial or patchy transmural late gadolinium enhancement; atrial left gadolinium enhancement

**DIAGNOSIS:** biopsy of abdominal adipose tissue (positive in > 70% of cases) or gums or salivary glands or kidney or rectum or endomyocardial tissue

> If Congo Red positive → **Distinguish primary (AL) from familial (TTR) amyloidosis**
>  • Serum and urinary immunofixation (± SPEP and UPEP)
>  • Electron microscopy immunohistochemistry techniques
>  • Abnormal kappa / lambda light chain ratio
> Bone marrow biopsy: % plasma cells; rule out MM and Waldenström

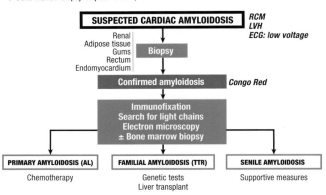

## MANAGEMENT

> Cautious use of Lasix; **particular caution with vasodilators and Digoxin**
> Anticoagulation in the presence of AF or atrial disease (A wave < 20 cm/s)
> **Anti-plasma cell chemotherapy**: Melphalan / Dexamethasone or Cyclophosphamide / Thalidomide / Dexamethasone; High-dose chemotherapy combined with autologous bone marrow transplantation as required

## FAMILIAL AMYLOIDOSIS

**Mutant transthyretin protein (TTR) (in the majority of cases)**

Autosomal dominant; most patients develop clinical features after the age of 40 years

**PRESENTATION:** various degrees of cardiac / conduction tissue / peripheral nerve / renal involvement

**TREATMENT: liver transplant** (mutant TTR produced by the liver)

## SENILE CARDIAC AMYLOIDOSIS

Non-mutant transthyretin protein (TTR)

Rare extracardiac involvement

**SUSPECT:** in an elderly patient with heart failure + LV wall thickening + normal chamber dimensions; frequent blocks; AF

**DIAGNOSIS:** endomyocardial biopsy

Median survival: 7.5 years

# 5.12/ ARRHYTHMOGENIC RIGHT VENTRICULAR DYSPLASIA (ARVD)

RV dysfunction (regional or global) secondary to infiltration of the myocardium by fibrous / adipose tissue

> **Triangle of dysplasia**: lesion of the RV inflow tract, RV outflow tract and apex of the RV
> LV is sometimes involved; can mimic DCM

**AUTOSOMAL DOMINANT:** majority of cases; desmosome protein gene

> **Autosomal recessive: Naxos syndrome** (plakoglobin; woolly hair; palmoplantar keratoderma); **Carvajal syndrome** (desmoplakin; palmoplantar keratoderma; predominant LV involvement)

**4 PHASES**

1. Asymptomatic
2. Arrhythmic (palpitations; syncope; VT – sudden death)
3. Right heart failure
4. Biventricular failure / DCM

**DIAGNOSIS:** requires the presence of several criteria

| MAJOR CRITERIA | MINOR CRITERIA |
|---|---|

### 01. Structural lesion

**TTE**
a) RV: **regional akinesia or dyskinesia or aneurysm +**
b) **PLAX RVOT ≥ 32 mm or PSAX RVOT ≥ 36 mm** (end-diastole) or FAC ≤ 33%

**MRI**
a) RV: regional akinesia or dyskinesia or dyssynchrony +
b) RV end-diastolic volume ≥ 110 mL/m² (M) or ≥ 100 mL/m² (F) or RVEF ≤ 40%

**Angiography**
• RV: regional akinesia or dyskinesia or aneurysm

---

**TTE**
a) RV: regional akinesia or dyskinesia +
b) PLAX RVOT 29 to 32 mm or PSAX RVOT 32 to 36 mm (end-diastole) or FAC 33% to 40%

**MRI**
a) RV: regional akinesia or dyskinesia or dyssynchrony +
b) RV end-diastolic volume 100 to 110 mL/m² (M) or 90 to 100 mL/m2 (F) or RVEF 40 to 45%

### 02. Tissue characterization (biopsy)

**Residual myocytes < 60%** with fibrous **replacement** of RV free wall with or without fat replacement

---

Residual myocytes 60 - 75% with fibrous replacement of the RV free wall with or without fat replacement

### 03. Repolarization abnormalities

**T wave inversion in V1-V2-V3** (absence of cRBBB with QRS ≥ 120 ms)

---

• T wave inversion in V1-V2 (absence of RBBB with QRS ≥ 120 ms) or V4 or V5 or V6
• T wave inversion in V1-V2-V3-V4 with cRBBB

### 04. Depolarization / conduction abnormalities

**Epsilon wave in V1-V2-V3 (low amplitude signal between the end of the QRS and the start of the T wave)**

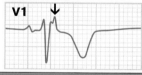

---

• Late potentials (SAECG): ≥ 1/3 positive parameters (absence of QRS ≥ 110 ms on basic ECG)
a) Filtered QRS ≥ 114 ms
b) Terminal QRS (< 40 µV) ≥ 38 ms
c) RMS (Root mean square) of terminal 40 ms ≤ 20 µV
• QRS: S nadir to the end of the QRS ≥ 55 ms in V1- V2-V3 (absence of cRBBB)

### 05. Arrhythmias

**NSVT or VT with LBBB morphology with superior axis** (negative QRS in II - III - aVF and positive QRS in aVL)

---

• NSVT or VT of RVOT, LBBB morphology with inferior axis (positive QRS in II - III - aVF and negative QRS in aVL) or unknown axis
• > 500 PVCs per 24 h

### 06. Family history

• **1st degree relative meeting the criteria**
• **1st degree relative with histologically confirmed diagnosis**
• **Pathogenic mutation**

---

• History of ARVD in 1st degree relative (but impossible to verify criteria)
• Sudden death < 35 years in a 1st degree relative with suspected ARVD
• Confirmed ARVD (histology or criteria) in a 2nd degree relative

---

• **Definitive diagnosis:** 2 major or 1 major + 2 minor or 4 minor (different categories)
• **Borderline diagnosis:** 1 major + 1 minor or 3 minor (different categories)
• **Possible diagnosis:** 1 major or 2 minor (different categories)

*Marcus FI, McKenna WJ, Sherrill D, et al. Diagnosis of Arrhythmogenic Right Ventricular Cardiomyopathy/Dysplasia. Proposed Modification of the Task Force Criteria. Circulation. 2010;121; 1533-1541.*

**OTHER ELEMENTS TO LOOK FOR: A)** ↗ QRS duration > 100 ms in V1 (delayed activation of RV; RBBB); **B)** Multiple RV scars on electrophysiological voltage mapping; **C)** Fat infiltration of RV on MRI (marked inter-observer variability)

**DDX: A)** DCM; **B)** Uhl's anomaly (zones in RV with absence of myocardium; endocardium and epicardium are continuous); **C)** Idiopathic RVOT VT (ECG / SAECG / TTE all normal); **D)** Myocarditis; **E)** Sarcoidosis

**MANAGEMENT**

> Avoid competitive sports or symptomatic exertion; Screening in 1st degree relatives
> Treatment of heart failure: ACE inhibitors; BB; Heart transplantation PRN
> ICD:
  a) **Secondary prevention**: documented sustained VF / VT
  b) **Primary prevention**: consider ICD → unexplained syncope; frequent NSVT; family history of premature sudden death; extensive disease (extensive RV involvement; LV involvement); marked QRS prolongation; VT induction during EPS
  c) **Frequent shocks**: Sotalol; Amiodarone; VT ablation

# 5.13/ ISOLATED LEFT VENTRICULAR NONCOMPACTION

Failure of endomyocardial compaction during embryogenesis

Prominent trabeculations with deep intertrabecular crypts

**Isolated** (autosomal dominant or sporadic) vs **associated with congenital heart disease** (Ebstein; RVOT or LVOT obstruction; complex heart disease)

**PRESENTATION:** heart failure; arrhythmia; sudden death; embolism

**TTE (± CONTRAST): thin epicardial layer with thick non-compacted endomyocardial layer** (predominantly apical and middle portions of inferior and lateral walls); **intertrabecular crypts continuous with the intraventricular cavity** (blood flow on color Doppler); RWMA; LV dysfunction; thrombus; abnormal papillary muscle

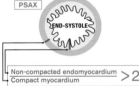

| Non-compacted endomyocardium | > 2 |
| Compact myocardium | |

| **LV NONCOMPACTION** | | |
|---|---|---|
| **HEART FAILURE** | **EMBOLIC RISK** | **RISK OF SUDDEN DEATH** |
| ↓ | ↓ | ↓ |
| STANDARD TREATMENT (NONISCHEMIC CM) | ANY CONDITION REQUIRING A/C OR THROMBOEMBOLIC HISTORY OR LEFT INTRAVENTRICULAR THROMBUS OR LVEF < 35-40% | **ASSESSMENT OF ARRHYTHMIC RISK** EVERY 1-2 YEARS (HOLTER) |
| ↓ | | ↓ |
| PERSISTENT SEVERE SYMPTOMS | | SECONDARY PREVENTION OR LVEF < 35% OR FAMILIAL HISTORY OF SUDDEN DEATH OR UNEXPLAINED SYNCOPE OR NSVT |
| ↓ | ↓ | ↓ |
| **TRANSPLANT** | **WARFARIN** | **CONSIDER ICD** |

**05**

MRI: non-compacted endomyocardium / compacted myocardium ratio > **2.3 in diastole**

MANAGEMENT: screening of 1st degree relatives (TTE); avoid competitive sports

## 5.14/ TAKOTSUBO CARDIOMYOPATHY (STRESS CARDIOMYOPATHY)

Transient systolic dysfunction involving the apex (± midventricular walls) in the absence of any significant CAD; often following an intense emotional or physical stress

> Secondary to catecholamine surge
> Postmenopausal women in > 90% of cases
> **Variants**: isolated midventricular lesion or reverse Takotsubo (basal akinesia)

PRESENTATION: Retrosternal chest pain; ST elevation on ECG or diffuse T wave inversion (with ↗ QT); ↗ troponin (limited); negative coronary angiography

> **Complications**: hemodynamic instability (LVOT obstruction ± SAM secondary to basal hyperdynamism in 15% of cases); heart failure; arrhythmias; thromboembolism; MR (SAM)
> **Complete recovery of LV function in 1 to 3 months; good prognosis**

CARDIAC MRI: myocardial edema; apical akinesia; absence of fibrosis - necrosis

DDX: Intracranial hemorrhage or SAH (often **basal and mid-ventricular akinesia**); major stroke; Pheochromocytoma (rule out if recurrence); Vasospasm; Cocaine; Amphetamines; Myocarditis

MANAGEMENT

> Carvedilol (alpha / beta blocker)
> ACE inhibitor (stop after recovery)
> TTE at 1 and 3 months (consider alternative diagnosis if LV dysfunction persists)
> **Anticoagulation: A)** Anticoagulant therapy if LV thrombi; **B)** Prophylactic anticoagulation may be considered to prevent LV thrombi (class IIb recommandation)
> **Hypotension / Shock**:
  • **Severe systolic dysfunction without LVOT obstruction**: Amines (cautiously); IABP as required
  • **LVOT obstruction**: BB (avoid amines); Volume (in absence of overload); Phenylephrine (cautiously)

## 5.15/ MYOCARDITIS

Inflammation of the myocardium

DALLAS CRITERIA: presence of **inflammatory cells** (lymphocytes) ± **myocyte necrosis** on biopsy; poor sensitivity (often falsely negative)

ETIOLOGIES

> **Virus:** Coxsackievirus; echovirus; adenovirus; parvovirus B19; CMV; HSV6; HIV; influenza; HCV; EBV
> **Bacteria / Spirochete:** TB; *Chlamydia pneumoniae; Streptococcus; Mycoplasma pneumoniae; Treponema pallidum; Clostridium*; Diphtheria; Whipple; Lyme
> **Fungi:** *Aspergillus; Candida; Coccidioides; Cryptococcus; Histoplasma*
> **Parasites:** Chagas; Schistosomiasis; Echinococcosis
> **Toxins:** Anthracyclines; Cocaine; 5-FU; phenytoin; cyclophosphamide; arsenic; iron; radiotherapy; alcohol; amphetamines; carbon monoxide; heatstroke; hypothermia; insect / snake bite
> **Hypersensitivity:** clozapine; sulfonamides; cephalosporins; tetracyclines; PNC; tricyclic antidepressants; allopurinol; dobutamine; diuretics
> **Autoimmune:** giant cell myocarditis; Churg-Strauss; Sjögren; inflammatory bowel disease; celiac disease; sarcoidosis; SLE; Takayasu arteritis; Wegener; dermatomyositis; Kawasaki; RA; scleroderma; thyrotoxicosis

## PATHOPHYSIOLOGY

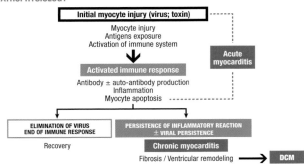

## PRESENTATION

**Compatible symptoms:** Acute retrosternal chest pain mimicking myocardial infarction or pericarditis; heart failure; palpitations; syncope; sudden death; cardiogenic shock; viral prodromes; fever

| + ≥ 1 DIAGNOSTIC CRITERION | | | |
|---|---|---|---|
| **ECG:** AV block (Lyme; giant cell; sarcoidosis); branch block; ST-T abnormalities; PVCs; VT - VF; AF; sinus arrest; low voltage; Q waves | **Myo-cardio-cytolysis:** elevated troponins | **Structural / functional abnormalities (TTE):** RWMA; systolic dysfunction; ventricular dilatation; wall thickening; effusion; thrombus | **MRI (Lake Louise criteria)** · Early gadolinium enhancement on T1 indicating inflammation (myocardium vs skeletal muscle enhancement ratio > 4.0) · Late gadolinium enhancement indicating fibrosis (intramural or subepicardial; often anteroseptal or inferolateral) · ↗ T2 signal intensity indicating edema (myocardium vs skeletal muscle signal ratio > 2.0) |

> **Fulminant lymphocytic myocarditis**: < 2 weeks after a viral infection; hemodynamic instability; diffuse LV dysfunction (rarely dilatation); wall thickening (edema); good prognosis with support

> **Giant cell myocarditis**: heart failure (evolving over several weeks to several months); blocks; ventricular arrhythmias; deterioration despite treatment; often underlying autoimmune disease (thymoma; Crohn); median survival < 6 months; Treatment: immunosuppression; transplant

> **Acute lymphocytic myocarditis**: may mimic acute MI (with negative coronary angiography) or may present with progressive LV dysfunction / dilatation or fulminant myocarditis; can progress to DCM

> **Eosinophilic myocarditis**: Hypersensitivity or Loeffler endocarditis or acute necrotizing eosinophilic myocarditis
> • **Hypersensitivity**: drug reaction; rash; fever; multiple organ dysfunction; eosinophilia; Myocarditis; Treatment with corticosteroids
> • **Acute necrotizing eosinophilic myocarditis**: rare; poor prognosis

> **Chronic active myocarditis**: insidious; LV systolic dysfunction (sometimes diastolic with restrictive pattern); ± viral persistence

**DEFINITIVE DIAGNOSIS:** myocarditis with **histological and/or immunohistological proof** ✛ on biopsy

**CONSEQUENCES:** viral persistence and/or persistent activation of immune system; chronic myocarditis; myocyte necrosis / fibrosis; remodeling; DCM; arrhythmia - sudden death

**MANAGEMENT**

> Avoid strenuous exertion / competitive sports for ≥ 6 months

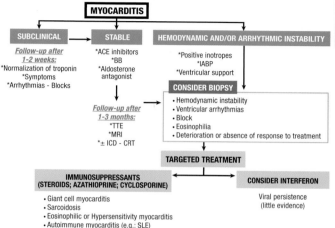

# 5.16/ INDICATIONS FOR ENDOMYOCARDIAL BIOPSY

1. Heart failure for **< 2 weeks** with hemodynamic compromise **(fulminant lymphocytic myocarditis; necrotizing eosinophilic myocarditis; giant cell myocarditis)** (I;B)

2. Heart failure for **2 weeks to 3 months** with LV dilatation and ventricular arrhythmias or AV block (2nd or 3rd degree) or absence of response to treatment (1-2 weeks) **(giant cell myocarditis or eosinophilic myocarditis)** (I;B)

3. Heart failure for > 3 months with LV dilatation and ventricular arrhythmias or AV block (2nd or 3rd degree) or absence of response to treatment (1-2 weeks) **(sarcoidosis or Chagas)** (IIa;C)

4. Heart failure with dilated cardiomyopathy and suspicion of allergic reaction and/or eosinophilia (eosinophilic myocarditis) (IIa; C)

5. Heart failure with suspicion of anthracycline cardiomyopathy (detect at an early stage of cardiotoxicity) (IIa; C)

6. Heart failure with unexplained RCM (IIa; C)

7. Suspected cardiac tumor (with the exception of myxoma), when noninvasive method is inconclusive (IIa; C)

**COMPLICATIONS OF BIOPSY:** 3%; venous access (arterial puncture; pneumothorax; bleeding); arrhythmia; blocks - RBBB; valve injury; cardiac perforation; tamponade; death; stroke (LV biopsy)

# 5.17/ CARDIAC TUMORS

## METASTASIS

Direct extension; hematogenous; extension via IVC (Hypernephroma; intravenous leiomyomatosis)

Lung; Breast; Lymphoma; Leukemia; Kaposi; Esophagus; Melanoma; Stomach; Mesothelioma; Thyroid; Renal; Extracardiac sarcoma

## PRIMARY TUMORS

**75 % benign**                                                                    +

**SYSTEMIC FEATURES:** fever; malaise; weight loss; anemia

**EMBOLIC PHENOMENA:** tumor embolism or thromboembolism

**CARDIAC SIGNS: depending on the site of the tumor**; blocks - arrhythmia; valve obstruction or regurgitation; SVC syndrome; coronary artery compression; hemorrhagic pericardial effusion (angiosarcoma; lymphoma); heart failure

**DIAGNOSIS:** TTE; TEE; CT scan or MRI (**mass visible if > 1 cm**); biopsy; metastatic work-up of malignant tumors; PET scan
> **MRI:** distinction between tumor and thrombus (according to gadolinium enhancement); tissue characterization

## MYXOMA

Pedunculated mass with stalk attached to the endocardium (often interatrial septum)

**LA (80%); RA (10%); > 90% are solitary**

**PRESENTATION:** Constitutional symptoms; embolisms (tumor fragment or thrombus); valve obstruction (can vary according to the position; look for tumor "plop"); extracardiac metastases

**Recurrence in 3% of cases**; TTE follow-up for life

Family screening (5 to 10% are familial)
> **Carney complex:** autosomal dominant; multiple intracardiac and extracardiac myxomas; high recurrence rate; cutaneous lentigines; other tumors (testicular; pituitary; thyroid)

**TREATMENT:** surgical resection

## PAPILLARY FIBROELASTOMA

On **valvular endocardium** (80-90%); aortic valve (40%; aortic side); mitral valve (30%; ventricular side); rarely endocardium of LA or LV; solitary (90%)

Friable lesion measuring about 1 cm; resembles a sea anemone; adherent thrombus; 45% have a stalk (1-3 mm)

**COMPLICATIONS:** thromboembolism

**TREATMENT:** surgical resection (especially if embolism or mobile or > 1 cm)

## LIPOMA

Especially subendocardial (also subepicardial or myocardial)

Predominantly solitary (multiple in the case of tuberous sclerosis)

**MRI:** fatty mass

**COMPLICATIONS:** obstruction; pericardial effusion; block; arrhythmias

**TREATMENT:** surgical resection when symptomatic

## LIPOMATOUS HYPERTROPHY OF INTERATRIAL SEPTUM

Excessive fat accumulation in the interatrial septum

**Thickening spares the fossa ovale; dumbbell appearance**

Associated with obesity and age > 70 years

**COMPLICATIONS:** Blocks; arrhythmias; SVC obstruction (rare)

## RHABDOMYOMA

Children; **associated with tuberous sclerosis** (autosomal dominant; epilepsy; skin lesions; hamartomas)

Ventricles > atria; **multiple lesions; spontaneous regression**

## FIBROMA

Children (sometimes adults)

Solitary intramural mass; interventricular septum or LV free wall

**TREATMENT:** Surgical resection when symptomatic (arrhythmia; blocks; obstruction)

## HEMANGIOMA / LYMPHANGIOMA

Intrachamber (ventricle > atrium) / intramural / epicardium / pericardium

Coronary angiography sometimes demonstrates the tumor blood supply

**PRESENTATION:** asymptomatic; palpitations; heart failure; pericardial effusion; obstruction; embolism; AV block

**TREATMENT:** echocardiographic follow-up (may increase in size or disappear); surgical resection when symptomatic

## MALIGNANT TUMORS

**ANGIOSARCOMA**
> - **RA in 90% of cases** (intramural mass protruding into the chamber)
> - Frequent pericardial involvement
> - Metastasis at presentation in 70-80% of cases (lung; liver; CNS; bone)
> - Mean survival: 10 months
> - **Treatment:** Surgery; Radiotherapy; Chemotherapy (Doxorubicin); Neoadjuvant chemotherapy (reduce tumor size prior to surgery); IL-12; autologous transplant (with ex vivo resection); transplant; palliative care

**RHABDOMYOSARCOMA**
> - Children - young adults
> - Multiple lesions (60%); no predilection for a particular chamber
> - Aggressive, invasive tumor; metastases (lungs; lymph nodes)
> - Survival < 1 year

#### LEIOMYOSARCOMA

> **LA (70-80 %)**; solitary (70%)
> Rapid growth; metastases; mean survival: 6 months

#### CARDIAC LYMPHOMA

> Right heart (70%); solitary (66%)
> Pericardial effusion (50%)
> Frequent extracardiac disease at the time of presentation
> **Treatment:** Anthracycline; Radiotherapy; Rituximab

## 5.18/ CARDIAC COMPLICATIONS OF CANCER

**COMPLICATIONS: A)** Metastases; **B)** Pericardial effusion; **C)** Tamponade; **D)** Constriction (radiotherapy); **E)** SVC obstruction; **F)** Valvular heart disease (metastases: infective endocarditis or non-bacterial thrombotic endocarditis; radiotherapy; obstruction; carcinoid); **G)** CAD (common risk factors; cancer chemotherapy; radiotherapy); **H)** Hyperviscosity (erythrocytosis or thrombocytosis or leukocytosis; ↗ Ig); **I)** Cardiotoxicity of chemotherapy and radiotherapy

**ANTHRACYCLINE TOXICITY:** (Doxorubicin; Daunorubicin; Epirubicin; Idarubicin)

> **Acute toxicity:** myocarditis; pericarditis; pericardial effusion; arrhythmia; ventricular dysfunction
> **Chronic toxicity: type I cardiotoxicity (irreversible, dose-dependant damage)** leading to ↘ LVEF / DCM
> **Risk factors for toxicity: cumulative dose > 350 mg/m²**; bolus; females; young; > 65 ans; risk factors for heart disease; history of heart disease; mediastinal radiotherapy; **Trastuzumab (TTE every 3 months during treatment) or Cyclophosphamide or Paclitaxel;** baseline LVEF < 55 %

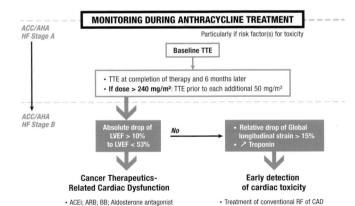

**MONITORING DURING ANTHRACYCLINE TREATMENT**

*ACC/AHA HF Stage A*

Particularly if risk factor(s) for toxicity

Baseline TTE

• TTE at completion of therapy and 6 months later
• If dose > 240 mg/m²: TTE prior to each additional 50 mg/m²

*ACC/AHA HF Stage B*

Absolute drop of LVEF > 10% to LVEF < 53%  —*No*→  • Relative drop of Global longitudinal strain > 15%
• ↗ Troponin

**Cancer Therapeutics-Related Cardiac Dysfunction**

• ACEi; ARB; BB; Aldosterone antagonist
• Hold or discontinue chemotherapy (± Cardiac MRI to confirm LV dysfonction)

**Early detection of cardiac toxicity**

• Treatment of conventional RF of CAD
• Limit the cumulative dose
• Continuous infusion instead of bolus
• Epirubicin (less cardiotoxic)
• Dexrazoxane
• Cardioprotective agents (ACEi; ARB; BB)

**MEDIASTINAL RADIOTHERAPY:** **fibrosis and calcification of cardiac structures;** complications often occur 10-20 years post-exposure; **higher risk with cumulative dose > 30 Gy**

> **Complications:** **A)** Accelerated CAD; **B)** Blocks / Conduction system disease; **C)** Valvular heart disease (thickening / fibrosis / calcification; predominant on left-sided valves; regurgitation > stenosis); **D)** Constrictive pericarditis; Pericardial effusion; **E)** Diffuse myocardial fibrosis with diastolic dysfunction / RCM; **F)** Carotid artery disease (Stroke – TIA); **G)** Aortic calcification / Porcelain aorta; **H)** Recurrent pleural effusions
> **Prevention:** minimize dose to the heart; cardiac shielding; reduction of dose-volume; decreased field; breath-holding; treatment of conventional risk factors of CAD
> **Monitoring after chest radiation exposure:** TTE 5-10 years after exposure then re-assess every 5 years; consider stress-test for CAD detection

## SPECIFIC CARDIAC COMPLICATIONS OF CHEMOTHERAPY

**LV DYSFUNCTION:** Anthracyclines (type I cardiotoxicity; permanent dose-dependant damage); Trastuzumab (type II cardiotoxicity; reversible damage; TTE every 3 months during therapy); Cyclophosphamide; Ifosfamide; Clofarabine; Docetaxel; Paclitaxel (in combination with Doxorubicin); Bevacizumab; Bortezomib; Dasatinib; Imatinib; Sunitinib

**ISCHEMIA / VASOSPASM:** Capecitabine; 5-Fluorouracil; Paclitaxel; Docetaxel; Bevacizumab (arterial thromboses); Rituximab; Dasatinib; Erlotinib; Sorafenib; Cisplatin; Carboplatin; Interferon

**BRADYCARDIA:** Thalidomide; Paclitaxel; Docetaxel

**HTN:** Cisplatin; Docetaxel; Bevacizumab; Rituximab; Trastuzumab; Dasatinib; Sunitinib; Sorafenib; Cyclophosphamide; Tacrolimus; MMF; Sirolimus

**DEEP VEIN THROMBOSIS:** Cisplatin; Thalidomide; Bevacizumab; Rituximab; Lenalidomide; Erlotinib; Sorafenib

↗ **QT:** Anthracyclines; Vorinostat; Arsenic tiroxide; Dasatinib; Lapatinib; Nilotinib; Sunitinib; Lenalidomide; 5-fluorouracil; Cyclophosphamide; Trastuzumab

# /SOURCES

- Bonow RO, Mann DL, Zipes DP, Libby P. *Braunwald's Heart Disease. A textbook of cardiovascular medicine.* Elsevier. 2012. 1961 p.
- LeWinter MM. Acute pericarditis. *NEJM* 2014; *371*; 2410-2416.
- 2015 ESC Guidelines for the diagnosis and management of pericardial diseases: the Task Force on the Diagnosis and Management of Pericardial Diseases of the ESC. *EHJ* 2015; *42*; 2921-2964.
- Otto, CM. *Textbook of clinical echocardiography.* Saunders Elsevier. 2009. 519 p.
- Fitch MT, Nicks BA, Pariyadath M et al. Emergency pericardiocentesis. *NEJM* 2012; *366:* e17
- Spodick DH. Acute cardiac tamponade. *NEJM* 2003; *349:* 684-690
- American Society of Echocardiography Clinical Recommendations for Multimodality Cardiovascular Imaging of Patients with Pericardial Disease. *JASE* 2013; *26:* 965-1012
- Scheuermann-Freestone M, Orchard E, Francis J. Partial Congenital Absence of the Pericardium. *Circulation.* 2007; *116:* e126-e129
- Classification of the cardiomyopathies: a position statement from the european society of cardiology working group on myocardial and pericardial diseases. *EHJ* 2008; *29:* 270–276
- Contemporary Definitions and Classification of the Cardiomyopathies; An American Heart Association Scientific Statement. *Circulation.* 2006; *113:* 1807-1881
- Watkins H, Ashrafian H, Redwood C. Inherited Cardiomyopathies. *NEJM* 2011; *364;* 1643-56
- 2014 ESC Guidelines on diagnosis and management of hypertrophic cardiomyopathy. *EHJ* 2014; *35;* 2733-2779.
- Maron BJ, Ommen SR, Semsarian C. Hypertrophic Cardiomyopathy. Present and Future, With Translation Into Contemporary Cardiovascular Medicine. *JACC* 2014; *64;* 83-99.
- 2011 ACCF/AHA Guideline for the Diagnosis and Treatment of Hypertrophic Cardiomyopathy. *JACC* 2011; *58:* 1-52
- Kushwaha SS, Fallon JT, Fuster V. Restrictive cardiomyopathy. *NEJM* 1997, *336:* 267-276
- Gujja P, Rosing DR, Tripodi DJ. Iron overload cardiomyopathy. *JACC* 2010; *56:* 1001-1012
- Falk RH. Diagnosis and Management of the Cardiac Amyloidoses. *Circulation* 2005; *112:* 2047-2060.
- Marchs FI, McKenna WJ, Sherrill D. Diagnosis of arrhythmogenic right ventricular cardiomyopathy/dysplasia. *EHJ* 2010; *31;* 806–814
- Jenni R, Oechslin E N, van der Loo B; Isolated ventricular non-compaction of the myocardium in adults. *Heart* 2007; *93:* 11–15.
- Bybee KA, Prasad A. Stress-related cardiomyopathy syndromes. *Circulation.* 2008; *118:* 397-409
- Canadian Cardiovascular Society Consensus Conference guidelines on heart failure, update 2009: Diagnosis and management of right-sided heart failure, myocarditis, device therapy and recent important clinical trials. *CJC* 2009; *25:* 85-106.
- Kindermann I, Barth C, Mahfoud F et al. Update on Myocarditis. *JACC* 2012; *59:* 779-792.
- Sagar S, Liu PP, Cooper LT Jr. Myocarditis. *Lancet* 2012; *379:* 738–747
- Cooper LT Jr. Myocarditis. *NEJM* 2009; *360:* 1526-1538.
- Friedrich MG, Sechtem U, Schulz-Menger J. Cardiovascular Magnetic Resonance in Myocarditis: A JACC White Paper. *JACC;* 2009; *53:* 1475-1487.
- The Role of Endomyocardial Biopsy in the Management of Cardiovascular Disease. A Scientific Statement From the American Heart Association, the American College of Cardiology, and the European Society of Cardiology. *JACC* 2007; *50:* 1915-1933.
- Bruce CJ. Cardiac tumours: diagnosis and management. *Heart* 2011; *97:* 151-160
- Truong J, Yan AT, Cramarossa G. Chemotherapy-Induced Cardiotoxicity: Detection, Prevention, and Management. *CJC* 2014; *30;* 869-878.
- Yeh ETH, Bickford CL. Cardiovascular Complications of Cancer Therapy. *JACC* 2009; *53:* 2231-2247
- Expert Consensus for Multimodality Imaging Evaluation of Adult Patients during and after Cancer Therapy: A Report from the ASE and the EACI. *JASE* 2014; *27;* 911-939.
- UpToDate 2015

# Arrhythmias

# 06

| 6.1/ | Physiology | 200 |
| 6.2/ | Bradyarrhythmias | 201 |
| 6.3/ | Supraventricular tachyarrhythmias | 204 |
| 6.4/ | Atrial fibrillation | 210 |
| 6.5/ | Ventricular tachyarrhythmias | 219 |
| 6.6/ | Channelopathies | 224 |
| 6.7/ | Syncope | 227 |
| 6.8/ | Antiarrhythmic drugs (AAD) | 229 |
| 6.9/ | Amiodarone | 232 |
| 6.10/ | Permanent pacemaker (PPM) | 233 |
| 6.11/ | Cardiac resynchronization therapy (CRT) | 239 |
| 6.12/ | Implantable cardioverter-defibrillator (ICD) | 241 |

# 6.1/ PHYSIOLOGY

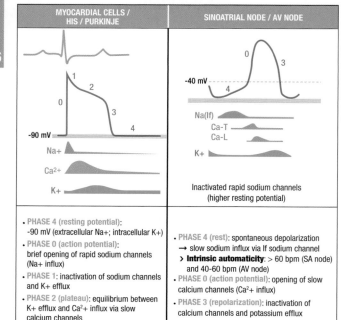

| MYOCARDIAL CELLS / HIS / PURKINJE | SINOATRIAL NODE / AV NODE |
|---|---|
| • PHASE 4 (resting potential): -90 mV (extracellular Na+; intracellular K+) <br> • PHASE 0 (action potential): brief opening of rapid sodium channels (Na+ influx) <br> • PHASE 1: inactivation of sodium channels and K+ efflux <br> • PHASE 2 (plateau): equilibrium between K+ efflux and Ca2+ influx via slow calcium channels <br> • PHASE 3 (rapid repolarization): K+ efflux | • PHASE 4 (rest): spontaneous depolarization → slow sodium influx via If sodium channel <br> > **Intrinsic automaticity**: > 60 bpm (SA node) and 40-60 bpm (AV node) <br> • PHASE 0 (action potential): opening of slow calcium channels (Ca2+ influx) <br> • PHASE 3 (repolarization): inactivation of calcium channels and potassium efflux |

## ARRHYTHMIC MECHANISMS

1) ABNORMAL AUTOMATICITY: ↗ phase 4 diastolic depolarization

2) REENTRY: two conduction pathways with different conduction velocities and refractory periods; requires one-directional conduction block in one of the pathways of the circuit

3) TRIGGERED ACTIVITY: abnormality during repolarization

> **Early afterdepolarization**: Torsade de pointes
> **Delayed afterdepolarization**: Digoxin poisoning; idiopathic VT; catecholaminergic polymorphic VT

| SINOATRIAL NODE | |
|---|---|
| **Sinus bradycardia** | • **HR < 60 bpm; normal morphology of P wave**<br>• **Etiologies**: benign; vagal hypertonia; athletes; sick sinus syndrome (SSS); drugs (BB; CCB; Digoxin; Ivabradine; Clonidine; Propafenone; Amiodarone); post-cardiac surgery; ischemia / myocardial infarction; myocarditis; infiltrative cardiomyopathy; Lyme disease; coronary angiography; meningitis; intracranial hypertension; stroke; hypoxia; hypothyroidism; hypothermia; Gram-negative bacillus sepsis; cervical / mediastinal tumor; OSAHS; familial SSS (SCN5A mutation); Chagas, ...<br>• **Management**: observation; Atropine 0.5 mg; PPM if symptomatic |
| **Sinus arrest / Sinus pause** | • **Sudden absence of sinus P wave; the duration of the pause is not a multiple of the intrinsic P–P interval**<br>   &gt; Ventricular asystole if absence of escape rhythm by latent pacemakers<br>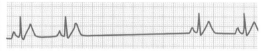<br>• **Etiologies**: ▶▶\| Sinus bradycardia<br>• **Tachy-bradycardia syndrome**: supraventricular tachyarrhythmia alternating with sinus bradycardia; ± sinus pause following conversion of the tachyarrhythmia; associated with sick sinus syndrome (SSS)<br>• **Management**: PPM if symptomatic |
| **Sinoatrial block (SA exit block)** | • **Sinoatrial block, 2nd degree - Mobitz I**: progressive reduction of P-P interval then absence of P wave; duration of the pause < twice the P-P interval; group beating<br>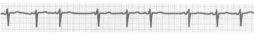<br>• **Sinoatrial block, 2nd degree - Mobitz II**: sudden absence of P wave; the duration of the pause is a **multiple of the intrinsic P–P interval**<br>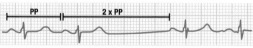 |
| **Wandering atrial pacemaker** | • Passive and gradual shift from a dominant pacemaker focus of the sinoatrial node to a latent atrial pacemaker; a single pacemaker controls rhythm at any one time; possible shift of control back to the sinoatrial node<br>• **Mechanism**: vigorous vagal tone (benign phenomenon) |
| **Chronotropic incompetence** | • **Inability to achieve > 80% HRmax predicted during a stress test (in the presence of sufficient exercise)**<br>   &gt; **Chronotropic index**: observed HR reserve (HRmax on stress test - resting HR) / (HRmax predicted for age - resting HR); chronotropic incompetence if **< 80 %**<br>• **Consequences**: exercise intolerance; factor of poor prognosis |

| AV CONDUCTION: AV NODE / HIS–PURKINJE SYSTEM | |
|---|---|
| **First degree AV block** | • **PR > 200 ms** in sinus rhythm<br>• **Narrow QRS**: delayed AV node conduction (↗ AH)<br>• **Wide QRS**: delayed AV node conduction (↗ AH) or His-Purkinje conduction (↗ HV)<br>   › **Bifascicular block (RBBB + LAHB or RBBB + LPHB or LBBB)**: consider a lesion of the third branch in the presence of prolonged PR |
| **2nd degree AV block, Mobitz I (Wenckebach)** | • **Progressive prolongation of the PR interval (with progressive shortening of the RR interval)** until a P wave is blocked; the RR interval including the non-conducted P wave is **less than twice the R–R interval of the previous cycle; group beating**<br>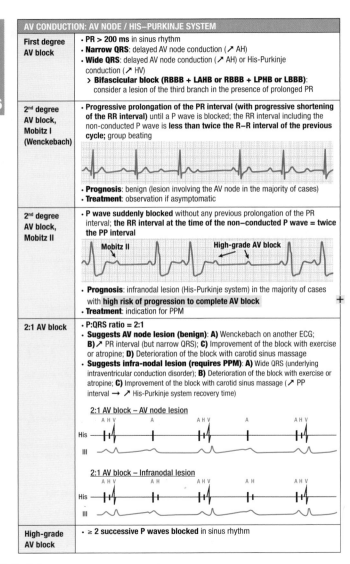<br>• **Prognosis**: benign (lesion involving the AV node in the majority of cases)<br>• **Treatment**: observation if asymptomatic |
| **2nd degree AV block, Mobitz II** | • **P wave suddenly blocked** without any previous prolongation of the PR interval; **the RR interval at the time of the non–conducted P wave = twice the PP interval**<br>Mobitz II    High-grade AV block<br>• **Prognosis**: infranodal lesion (His-Purkinje system) in the majority of cases with **high risk of progression to complete AV block**<br>• **Treatment**: indication for PPM |
| **2:1 AV block** | • **P:QRS ratio = 2:1**<br>• **Suggests AV node lesion (benign): A)** Wenckebach on another ECG; **B)** ↗ PR interval (but narrow QRS); **C)** Improvement of the block with exercise or atropine; **D)** Deterioration of the block with carotid sinus massage<br>• **Suggests infra-nodal lesion (requires PPM): A)** Wide QRS (underlying intraventricular conduction disorder); **B)** Deterioration of the block with exercise or atropine; **C)** Improvement of the block with carotid sinus massage (↗ PP interval → ↗ His-Purkinje system recovery time)<br>2:1 AV block – AV node lesion<br>A H V   A   A H V   A   A H V<br>His<br>III<br>2:1 AV block – Infranodal lesion<br>A H V   A H V   A H   A H V<br>His<br>III |
| **High-grade AV block** | • **≥ 2 successive P waves blocked** in sinus rhythm |

| **Complete AV block (3rd degree)** | • **Absence of AV conduction**<br>• **Intranodal block**: junctional escape rhythm; narrow QRS; **HR 40–60 bpm**<br>• **Infrahisian block**: ventricular escape rhythm (unreliable and unstable); wide QRS; **HR 15–40 bpm**<br><br>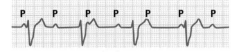<br><br>• **Etiologies**: degenerative; drugs; congenital; ischemia - MI; vagal hypertonia; surgery; calcified AS; progressive familial heart block (Lenègre's disease; SCN5A or TRPM4 mutation); electrolyte disorders; myocarditis; endocarditis; tumor; Chagas; Lyme disease; rheumatoid nodule; AVR; TAVI; hypothyroidism; polymyositis; dilated cardiomyopathy (lamin A/C); infiltrative cardiomyopathy (amyloidosis; sarcoidosis; scleroderma); muscular dystrophy...<br>• **Treatment**: Rule out a reversible cause; PPM |

## ELECTROPHYSIOLOGICAL STUDY OF CONDUCTION TISSUE

INDICATION: in the presence of a strong suspicion of significant and symptomatic bradyarrhythmia, but in the absence of a clearly documented abnormality

| **SNRT: Sinus node recovery time** | • Continuous rapid atrial stimulation (30 s) then stopped<br>• **SNRT**: interval between last paced beat and the first sinus return beat<br>• **CSNRT (corrected SNRT)**: = SNRT - CL in sinus rhythm<br>> **Normal CSNRT**: < 525 ms<br>• Low sensitivity (65%) but high specificity (95%) |
|---|---|
| **AV conduction** | 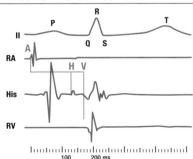<br><br><u>Intervals measured</u><br>• **AH**: AV node conduction; normal 55-125 ms<br>• **His conduction time**: normal < 25 ms<br>• **HV**: infra-His conduction time; normal: 35-55 ms<br>> **HV > 100 ms**: possible risk of complete AV block<br>> **Short HV**: **A)** Ventricular pre-excitation; **B)** PVC or idioventricular rhythm isorythmic with SR |

# 6.3/ SUPRAVENTRICULAR TACHYARRHYTHMIAS

## ATRIAL PREMATURE COMPLEXES

**ATRIAL PREMATURE COMPLEXES (APC)**: premature P wave in the cardiac cycle; arises from an atrial focus outside of the sinoatrial node; different morphology from that of the sinoatrial node; sometimes situated in the T wave (look for abnormal morphology of the T wave)

> **Modifiers**: Couplets; Bigeminy; Trigeminy; Salvo
> **Noncompensatory pause**: the APC depolarizes and resets the sinoatrial node; the interval between the two P waves before and after the APC < **twice the intrinsic PP interval**
> **Compensatory pause**: failure of the APC to depolarize the sinoatrial node; the interval between the two P waves before and after the APC = **twice the intrinsic PP interval**
> **Blocked atrial premature complex**: the P wave is not followed by a QRS complex (AV-His-Purkinje system in refractory period); the pause is usually noncompensatory

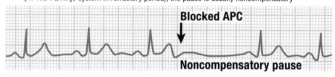

**Blocked APC**

**Noncompensatory pause**

## SUPRAVENTRICULAR TACHYARRHYTHMIAS

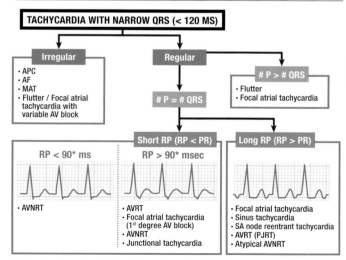

**TACHYCARDIA WITH NARROW QRS (< 120 MS)**

**Irregular**
- APC
- AF
- MAT
- Flutter / Focal atrial tachycardia with variable AV block

**Regular**

**# P > # QRS**
- Flutter
- Focal atrial tachycardia

**# P = # QRS**

**Short RP (RP < PR)**

RP < 90* ms
- AVNRT

RP > 90* msec
- AVRT
- Focal atrial tachycardia (1st degree AV block)
- AVNRT
- Junctional tachycardia

**Long RP (RP > PR)**
- Focal atrial tachycardia
- Sinus tachycardia
- SA node reentrant tachycardia
- AVRT (PJRT)
- Atypical AVNRT

*70 msec for intracardiac VA interval (90 msec for surface ECG VA interval)

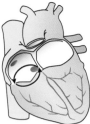

**Atrial Flutter**

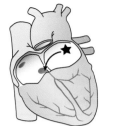

**Focal atrial tachycardia**

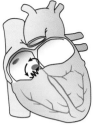

**AVNRT: nodal reentry**

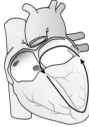

**Orthodromic AVRT**

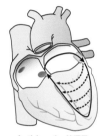

**Antidromic AVRT**

| RESPONSE TO ADENOSINE (OR VAGAL MANEUVER) | |
|---|---|
| **Sudden arrest** | **Slowing then re–acceleration** |
| • AVNRT<br>• AVRT<br>• SA node reentrant tachycardia<br>• (Focal atrial tachycardia) | • Sinus tachycardia<br>• Focal atrial tachycardia<br>• AF; Flutter<br>• Nonparoxysmal junctional tachycardia |

## SINUS TACHYCARDIA

**100-200 bpm (HRmax = 220 - age)**; nonparoxysmal (progressive onset and termination);  +
normal P waves; secondary to sympathetic stimulation

ETIOLOGIES: fever / sepsis; hypotension; hyperthyroidism; anemia; anxiety; pain; exercise;
hypovolemia; pulmonary embolism; ischemia; heart failure; shock; drugs (atropine; catecholamines;
adriamycin); alcohol; cocaine; high output state; pregnancy

INAPPROPRIATE SINUS TACHYCARDIA: increased automaticity / sinus dysautonomia

> **Diagnosis**: sinus HR > 100 bpm at rest; mean 24-h HR > 90 bpm; diagnosis of exclusion (rule
out physiological sinus tachycardia or focal AT from the high RA)

> **Management**: Rule out an underlying cause (anemia; hyperT4); Ivabradine; BB; radiofrenquency modification of sinoatrial node as last resort

POSTURAL ORTHOSTATIC TACHYCARDIA SYNDROME (POTS): orthostatic intolerance with significant increase of HR during the first 10 min after standing (HR > 120 bpm or HR increased by > 30 bpm)

> **Management**: fluids; NaCl; raise the head of the bed; training; elastic stockings; BB; Fludrocortisone; Midodrine; SSRI

SINOATRIAL NODAL REENTRANT TACHYCARDIA (SANRT): paroxysmal tachycardia; abrupt onset; P wave identical to P wave in SR

> **Management**: vagal maneuver; Adenosine; BB; CCB; RF ablation

## ATRIAL FLUTTER

ATRIAL FREQUENCY: **300 bpm** (slowed by class IC AA with risk of 1:1 conduction)

VENTRICULAR FREQUENCY: **150 or 100 or 75 bpm** (2:1 or 3:1 or 4:1 conduction)

| TYPICAL ATRIAL FLUTTER | ATYPICAL ATRIAL FLUTTER |
|---|---|
| • **Cavotricuspid isthmus-dependent macroreentrant flutter:** atrial flutter counterclockwise around the tricuspid valve annulus (most common) versus clockwise flutter<br>• **ECG:** sawtooth flutter waves (regular and identical); **negative waves in II-III-aVF and positive waves in V1 in counterclockwise flutter** (and vice versa in clockwise flutter); 2:1 or 3:1 or 4:1 AV conduction<br><br>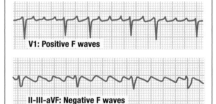<br>**V1: Positive F waves**<br><br>**II-III-aVF: Negative F waves**<br><br>MANAGEMENT<br>• ECV (50 J biphasic) or atrial overdrive or CCV (IV Ibutilide)<br>• AV node blocking agents (rate control more difficult than in AF)<br>• Class IC AAD (combined with AV node blocking agent) or class III AAD<br>• Thromboembolic prevention (▶▶| AF)<br>• **RF ablation of cavotricuspid isthmus**: success rate: 90-95%; **first-line long-term treatment;** target bidirectional block; 22-50% will have AF within 30 months | • **Cavotricuspid isthmus non-dependent macroreentrant flutter**<br><br>1) **IART (intra-atrial reentrant tachycardia):** macroreentrant circuit arising around a surgical scar following cardiac surgery<br><br>2) **Left atrial flutter post-AF ablation**<br><br>• **ECG**: variable morphology of flutter waves (depending on the circuit involved) and different from that of typical flutter<br><br>• **Management**: ECV; AV node blocking agents; AAD; RF ablation |

## FOCAL ATRIAL TACHYCARDIA

ATRIAL FREQUENCY: 150-250 bpm

THREE MECHANISMS: **A)** Automatic (incessant); **B)** Triggered activity; **C)** Microreentrant

ORIGIN: precise focus (pulmonary vein; atrial appendage; *crista terminalis;* SVC or IVC; coronary sinus; mitral annulus; fossa ovale)

ECG: **morphology of P wave different from that in SR**; isoelectric segment between P waves on all leads (unlike flutter); **long RP interval** +

> V1 - **Positive P wave**: = LA focus (negative P wave in aVL and I)
> V1 - **Negative or biphasic P wave**: = RA focus (positive or biphasic P wave in aVL)

MANAGEMENT: AV node blocking agent; Class IC or III AAD; ablation of arrhythmogenic focus with 3D electroanatomic mapping (85% success)

## MULTIFOCAL ATRIAL TACHYCARDIA (MAT)

ATRIAL FREQUENCY: **100-150 bpm**

IRREGULARLY IRREGULAR RHYTHM: absence of dominant pacemaker; variable morphology of P waves (**≥ 3 different morphologies**); variable PR interval; abnormal automaticity +

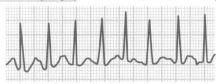

RISK FACTORS: COPD; age; Digoxin; Theophylline; hypomagnesemia

MANAGEMENT: correct underlying disease; nondihydropyridine CCB; Amiodarone; $Mg^{2+}$

## ATRIOVENTRICULAR NODAL REENTRANT TACHYCARDIA (AVNRT)

AVNRT: **150-250 bpm**; very regular rhythm (except at onset and termination) +

ONSET: **sudden; APC with long PR interval (anterograde conduction via the slow pathway)** +

SYMPTOMS: palpitations; anxiety; angina; syncope (↘ cardiac output; postconversion sinus pause; vasodepressive response)

| TYPICAL AVNRT | ATYPICAL AVNRT |
|---|---|
| • **Anterograde conduction via the slow pathway; retrograde conduction via the fast pathway (with retrograde atrial activation)**<br>• **ECG: Short RP < 90 ms; retrograde P wave hidden in the QRS or just after the QRS (pseudo-r' in V1; pseudo-S in II-III-aVF; absent on baseline ECG in sinus rhythm);** QRS *alternans* if very rapid | • 5-10 %<br>• Anterograde conduction via the rapid pathway; retrograde conduction via the slow pathway; **long RP** |

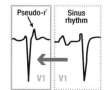 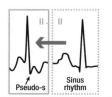

**MANAGEMENT**: vagal maneuver (Valsalva; carotid sinus massage); Adenosine; CCB; BB; ECV (50 J biphasic); class IC AAD (combined with AV node blocking agent); RF ablation

**RF ABLATION**: success rate > 95%; **first-line long-term treatment**                    +
> **Ablation of slow pathway**: inferoposterior to AV node (between the septal aspect of the tricuspid valve annulus and the ostium of the coronary sinus)
> **Complications**: AV block (1%); recurrence (5%); tamponade

---

## ATRIOVENTRICULAR REENTRANT TACHYCARDIA (AVRT) & ACCESSORY PATHWAY

**AVRT**: 150-250 bpm; very regular rhythm (except at onset)

**ACCESSORY PATHWAY (BUNDLE OF KENT)**: connection between atrium and ventricle (at the level of the AV sulcus) short-circuiting the AV node - His-Purkinje system; **retrograde    +
conduction only or anterograde (and retrograde) conduction**

**1) Accessory pathway with retrograde conduction only (30%)**: hidden pathway; absence of preexcitation
- **Associated arrhythmia**: orthodromic AVRT

**2) Accessory pathway with anterograde conduction (70%)**: ventricular pre-excitation; fusion of ventricular activations by the accessory pathway and by the AV - His-Purkinje system
- **Short or negative HV interval**                                                  +
- **Associated arrhythmias: A)** Orthodromic AVRT (retrograde conduction); **B)** Antidromic AVRT; **C)** Anterograde conduction of supraventricular arrhythmia (pre-excited AF)
- **ECG**: PR < 120 ms; wide QRS (> 120 ms) with delta wave; ST-T abnormalities (opposite direction to the QRS); maximized pre-excitation when AV node in refractory period

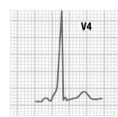

V4

| SITE OF PATHWAY | DELTA WAVE | | |
|---|---|---|---|
| | V1 | AVF | AVL |
| **Left lateral** | + | + | - |
| **Left septal or posterior** | + | - | + |
| **Right septal or posterior** | - | - | + |
| **Anterior or right lateral** | - | + | + |

**WOLFF-PARKINSON-WHITE SYNDROME**: symptoms compatible with tachyarrhythmia + ventricular pre-excitation

> **Benign pathway**: inefficient pathway with long refractory period; abrupt disappearance of pre-excitation on stress test (or intermittent loss during ECG or ambulatory monitoring)
> **Malignant pathway**: **refractory period < 250 ms**; able to maintain effective anterograde    +
conduction of possible AF (with risk of VF and sudden death)

**DEMONSTRATION OF AN ACCESSORY PATHWAY: A)** Eccentric retrograde atrial activation during ventricular stimulation or during orthodromic AVRT; **B)** Ventricular stimulation during AVRT induces atrial activation even when the His bundle is refractory; **C)** Ventricular stimulation induces atrial activation before activation of the His bundle; **D)** Ventricular stimulation at various frequencies associated with a stable VA interval (non-decremental VA conduction)

| ORTHODROMIC ATRIOVENTRICULAR REENTRANT TACHYCARDIA (AVRT) | ANTIDROMIC ATRIOVENTRICULAR REENTRANT TACHYCARDIA (AVRT) (5–10%) |
|---|---|
| • **Macro-reentrant tachycardia with anterograde conduction via the AV / His–Purkinje system and retrograde conduction via the accessory pathway**<br>• **ECG**: Narrow QRS; retrograde P wave following QRS **(short RP but > 70 ms intra-cardiac)**; negative retrograde P wave in lead I if left lateral bundle | • **Macro-reentrant tachycardia with anterograde conduction via the accessory pathway and retrograde conduction via the AV / His-Purkinje system; wide QRS tachycardia** |

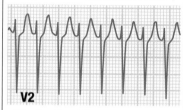

**V2**

| • If functional branch block ipsilateral to the accessory pathway: ↗ VA interval and ↗ tachycardia cycle length | |

**MANAGEMENT OF AVRT**: vagal maneuver; Adenosine (can precipitate AF); AV node blocking agent (can precipitate prexcited AF); ECV (50 J); AAD (IC; III); RF ablation of accessory pathway

**ABLATION OF THE ACCESSORY PATHWAY**: **first-line long-term treatment**; success rate: 95%
> **Complications**: 5% recurrence rate; vascular access; microembolism / stroke (left pathway); tamponade; AV block; coronary lesion
> **Asymptomatic pathway**: **EP study or observation is reasonable (IIa recommendation)**; ablation if high risk findings during EP study (**R-R < 250 ms** during induced AF; multiple accessory pathways; AVRT precipitating pre-excited AF; pathway with refractory period < 240 ms) or in patients with specific employment (e.g. pilot)

**PERMANENT FORM OF JUNCTIONAL RECIPROCATING TACHYCARDIA (PJRT)**:
incessant supraventricular tachycardia; posteroseptal accessory pathway (R > L); pathway with **slow retrograde one-directional** conduction; **long RP**; negative P wave in **II-III-aVF**

**MAHAIM PATHWAY**: accessory pathway in lateral wall of RV; distal connection to RV (atrioventricular connection) or to the right branch (atriofascicular connection); **similar conduction properties to those of the AV node (decremental conduction at higher HR)**; anterograde conduction only
> **Baseline ECG**: normal (minimal pre-excitation)
> **Associated arrhythmia**: antidromic AVRT (with **LBBB** morphology); QRS axis 0° and -75°; QRS < 150 ms; late precordial transition; HR 130-270 bpm

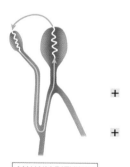

MAHAIM PATHWAY

| NONPAROXYSMAL JUNCTIONAL TACHYCARDIA | PAROXYSMAL JUNCTIONAL ECTOPIC TACHYCARDIA (JET) |
|---|---|
| • 70-130 bpm; nonparoxysmal = progressive onset ("warm-up")<br>• **Origin**: origin of AV node or His bundle; narrow QRS; abnormal automaticity<br>• **Etiologies**: Digoxin poisoning; post-cardiac surgery; electrolyte disorder; ischemia; MI; COPD; hypoxia; myocarditis<br>• **Management**: Treatment of underlying cause; BB; CCB | • 110-250 bpm; paroxysmal = sudden onset; more frequent in children; triggered by exercise or stress<br>• **Origin**: AV node or His bundle; narrow QRS; AV dissociation versus VA association<br>• **Management**: BB; AAD (IC; III); RF ablation |

# 6.4/ ATRIAL FIBRILLATION

**ATRIAL FREQUENCY**: **400-600 bpm**; absence of organized P wave with chaotic atrial fibrillation-rhythm; irregularly irregular ventricular rhythm

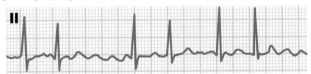

> **Lead V1**: sometimes prominent fibrillatory waves (mimicking atrial flutter), but absence of organized waves elsewhere

## CLASSIFICATION

| Paroxysmal AF | Terminates spontaneously or with intervention within < 7 days of onset |
|---|---|
| Persistent AF | Continuous AF, sustained > 7 days |
| Longstanding persistant AF | Continuous AF, sustained > 12 months |
| Permanent AF | No other attempt to restore and/or maintain SR |
| Nonvalvular AF | Absence of rheumatic MS, prosthetic heart valve or mitral valve repair |

**SYMPTOMS**: palpitations; tiredness; dyspnea; exercise intolerance; faintness; syncope (conversion pause or rapid AF in the presence of structural heart disease); systemic embolism; heart failure (tachycardiomyopathy)

| CCS SAF SCALE | |
|---|---|
| Class 0 | Asymptomatic |
| Class I | Minimal effect on quality of life |
| Class II | Minor effect on quality of life |
| Class III | Moderate effect on quality of life |
| Class IV | Severe effect on quality of life |

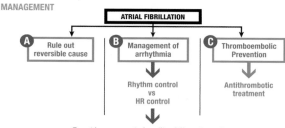

**ATRIAL FIBRILLATION**

**A** Rule out reversible cause

**B** Management of arrhythmia

Rhythm control vs HR control

**C** Thromboembolic Prevention

Antithrombotic treatment

· Target improvement of quality of life and symptoms
· Reduce hospitalizations

**RULE OUT REVERSIBLE CAUSE AND RISK FACTORS:** Alcohol ("holiday heart syndrome"); ischemia; myocarditis - pericarditis; structural heart disease / heart failure / cardiomyopathy / valvular heart disease / LVH / congenital heart disease / diastolic dysfunction; supraventricular tachycardia (tachycardia-induced AF); SSS; WPW; HTN; pulmonary embolism; hyperthyroidism; frequent V-Pace; OSAHS; vagal hypertonia (athlete; sleep); hyperadrenergism (exercise); postoperative; pneumonia; PHT

> **AF in young patient with structurally normal heart**: consider electrophysiological study to eliminate other supraventricular arrhythmia degenerating to AF (tachycardia-induced AF)

## MANAGEMENT OF ARRHYTHMIA

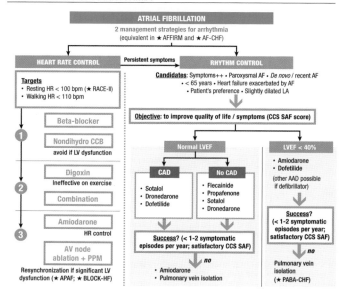

**ATRIAL FIBRILLATION**

2 management strategies for arrhythmia (equivalent in ★ AFFIRM and ★ AF-CHF)

**HEART RATE CONTROL** — Persistent symptoms → **RHYTHM CONTROL**

**Targets**
· Resting HR < 100 bpm (★ RACE-II)
· Walking HR < 110 bpm

**1** Beta-blocker

Nondihydro CCB
avoid if LV dysfunction

**2** Digoxin
Ineffective on exercise

Combination

**3** Amiodarone
HR control

AV node ablation + PPM

Resynchronization if significant LV dysfunction (★ APAF; ★ BLOCK-HF)

**Candidates:** Symptoms++ · Paroxysmal AF · *De novo* / recent AF
· < 65 years · Heart failure exacerbated by AF
· Patient's preference · Slightly dilated LA

**Objective:** to improve quality of life / symptoms (CCS SAF score)

**Normal LVEF**

**CAD**
· Sotalol
· Dronedarone
· Dofetilide

**No CAD**
· Flecainide
· Propafenone
· Sotalol
· Dronedarone

**Success?** (< 1-2 symptomatic episodes per year; satisfactory CCS SAF)

↓ *no*

· Amiodarone
· Pulmonary vein isolation

**LVEF < 40%**
· Amiodarone
· Dofetilide

(other AAD possible if defibrillator)

**Success?**
(< 1-2 symptomatic episodes per year; satisfactory CCS SAF?)

↓ *no*

Pulmonary vein isolation
(★ PABA-CHF)

| HEART RATE CONTROL STRATEGY | | | |
|---|---|---|---|
| **Diltiazem** | 0.25 mg/kg IV x 10 min (repeat 0.35 mg/kg PRN) | 120 - 480 mg PO qd | Hypotension; bradycardia; edema; negative inotrope; avoid if ↘ LVEF or pre-excited AF |
| **Verapamil** | 0.075 - 0.15 mg/kg IV x 2 min | 120 - 240 mg PO bid | |
| **Metoprolol** | 2.5 - 5 mg/kg IV x 2 min (3 doses every 5 min PRN) | 25 - 200 mg PO bid | Hypotension; bradycardia; tiredness; depression; asthma; negative inotrope; avoid if preexcited AF |
| **Nadolol** | 10 - 320 mg qd | | |
| **Esmolol** | **IV bolus**: 500 µg/kg; **Infusion**: 50-300 µg/kg/min (dilution: 2500 mg / 250 mL) | | |
| **Digoxin** | 0.25 mg IV (or PO) every 6 h (4 doses over 24 h; adjustment according to creatinine clearance) | 0.0625 to 0.25 mg qd | Digoxin toxicity; Nausea; Vomiting; Visual abnormalities; avoid in the presence of pre-excited AF |

| HEART RHYTHM CONTROL STRATEGY | | |
|---|---|---|
| **CLASS IC** | | |
| **Flecainide** | 50 - 150 mg PO bid   * Combine with AV node blocking agent | • **Efficacy at 1 year**: 30-50 % <br> • **Adverse effects**: ↗ QRS (caution if > 25%); VT; bradycardia; 1:1 flutter <br> • **Contraindications**: CAD or LV dysfunction (★ CAST) <br> • Pre-treatment stress test if > 50 years or high Framingham score |
| **Propafenone** | 50 - 300 mg PO tid   * Combine with AV node blocking agent | |
| **CLASSE III** | | |
| **Amiodarone** | Loading dose of 10 g over several weeks then 100 - 200 mg PO qd | • **Efficacy at 1 year**: 60-70 % (★ CTAF) <br> • **Avantage:** controls HR (BB effect) <br> • **Adverse effects**: ►►I Amiodarone |
| **Dronedarone** | 400 mg PO bid | • **Efficacy at 1 year**: 40 % <br> • ★ **ATHENA**: Paroxysmal AF; ↘ cardiac mortality with Dronedarone <br> • **Contraindications**: heart failure / LVEF < 40% (★ ANDROMEDA) or permanent AF (★ PALLAS) or Digoxin <br> • Monitor LFTs at 6 months |
| **Sotalol** | 40 - 160 mg PO bid | • **Efficacy at 1 year**: 30-50 % (★ CTAF) <br> • **Adverse effects**: ↗ QT; torsade de pointes; bradycardia; asthma (BB effect) <br> • **Avoid**: women > 65 years / CRF / LVEF < 40% / significant LVH / electrolyte disorders / ↗ QTc <br> • Monitoring of QT for 72 h; stop if QTc > 500 ms |
| **Dofetilide** | 0.125 to 0.5 mg PO bid (according to CrCl) | • **Complication**: torsade de pointes <br> • **Contraindications**: CrCl < 20 mL/min; hypokalemia; baseline QTc > 440 ms |

**"PILL IN THE POCKET" APPROACH**: AAD as needed (Flecainide 200 to 300 mg or Propafenone 450 to 600 mg) combined with Metoprolol 50 to 100 mg; indicated in the presence of occasional episodes in subjects with a healthy heart; initiate under cardiac monitoring to demonstrate safety of the approach

# CARDIOVERSION

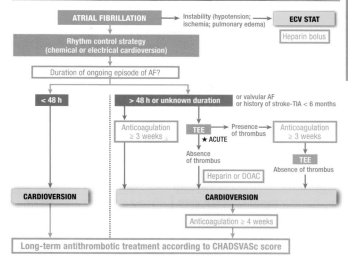

**ELECTRICAL CARDIOVERSION**: 200 J biphasic

> **Failure (5 %)**: Add AAD followed by another attempt of ECV (Amiodarone; Flecainide; Propafenone; Ibutilide; Sotalol)
> **Conversion then early recurrence of AF (ERAF) post-ECV**: Add AAD followed by another attempt of ECV

**CHEMICAL CARDIOVERSION**: only minimally effective when AF present for > 7 days

| CHEMICAL CARDIOVERSION | | |
|---|---|---|
| **Propafenone** | 450 to 600 mg PO | • Hypotension; 1:1 flutter; bradycardia; complete AV block |
| **Flecainide** | 200 to 300 mg PO | • Contraindicated in the presence of CAD or systolic dysfunction; administer with AV node blocking agent |
| **Procainamide** | 15-17 mg/kg IV x 60 min | • Hypotension<br>• **Efficacy**: 60 % |
| **Ibutilide** | 1 mg IV x 10 min; may repeat once if necessary | • Torsade de pointes (2-3%)<br>• Contraindicated if LVEF < 30% or significant LVH or ↗ QTc > 440 ms or SSS or hypokalemia<br>• Pretreat with $MgSO_4$ |
| **Vernakalant** | 3 mg/kg x 10 min then observation for 15 min then 2nd bolus of 2 mg/kg x 10 min PRN | • Blocks various atrial ionic channels (↗ refractory period)<br>• **Efficacy**: 50 % (★ ACT; ★ AVRO)<br>• **Adverse effects**: dysgeusia; Nausea; Hypotension; ↗ QT and QRS intervals<br>• **Contraindications**: hypotension; ACS during previous 30 days; NYHA III or IV; Severe AS; non-corrected QT > 440 ms; LVEF ≤ 35% |

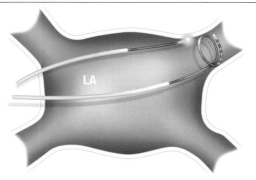

| PAROXYSMAL AF | PERSISTENT AF |
|---|---|
| • Triggered by **premature complexes arising in pulmonary veins** (90% of cases; ★ Haïssaguerre)<br>• **Ablation:** pulmonary vein isolation (electrical disconnection from the rest of the LA by radiofrequency ablation) | • Presence of a substrate **maintaining and perpetuating the arrhythmia**<br>• **Substrate**: structural and electrical remodeling of the atrium; fibrosis - inflammation - ↘ refractory period<br>• **Ablation**: pulmonary vein isolation combined with modification of the substrate (other radiofrequency lesions in the atria)<br> › Linear ablation (roof of LA and mitral annulus; ± cavotricuspid isthmus)<br> › Ablation of complex fractionated atrial electrograms sites (CFAE)<br> › No benefit in ★ STAR-AF |

OBJECTIVE: improve symptoms and quality of life

INDICATION: **AF with persistent and harmful symptoms (negative impact on quality of life) despite trial of drug treatment (class I or III AAD)**

SUCCESS RATE: **60-75% after 1 procedure and 75-90% after 2 procedures** (success rate 10-15% lower in the presence of persistent AF); improvement of quality of life; more effective than AAD for maintenance of SR

MAJOR COMPLICATIONS: **5 %;** vascular complication (1-2%); cardiac perforation / tamponade (1%); thromboembolism (1%); PV stenosis (0.5%); atrio-esophageal fistula; phrenic nerve palsy (diaphragmatic paralysis); atypical flutter; death (1/1,000)

CONTRAINDICATIONS: LA > 55 mm; significant structural heart disease; LA thrombus; long-term AF; mechanical MVR

PERIPROCEDURAL CONSIDERATIONS: TEE before the procedure; procedure performed under anticoagulation (continue warfarin; stop DOAC 12-24 h before the procedure); continue anticoagulation for 2 months post-op (then according to CHADSVASc score)

> **Early recurrence of AF post-PVI (< 3 months)**: secondary to acute inflammation; management by rhythm control then re-evaluate at 3 months

**PVI FOR PERSISTENT AF AND HEART FAILURE**: more effective than AV node ablation + resynchronization (★ PABA-CHF)

> ★ **AATAC-AF:** PVI superior to Amiodarone in relieving persistent AF in patients with congestive heart failure; PVI associated with ↘ all-cause mortality and ↘ hospitalization

**SURGICAL ABLATION OF AF**: indicated for symptomatic AF when concomitant cardiac surgery is planned

> **Paroxysmal AF:** pulmonary vein isolation (endocardial or epicardial) ± ablation line to mitral annulus

> **Persistent AF:** modified Cox-Maze procedure; requires bilateral atriotomy; ablation lines in LA to isolate pulmonary veins / isolate the posterior LA / create an ablation line between the pulmonary veins and mitral annulus; ablation lines at the cavotricuspid isthmus and between inferior and superior venae cavae; left atrial appendectomy; one-year success rate: 85% (63% in ★ CTSN AF)

# THROMBOEMBOLIC PREVENTION

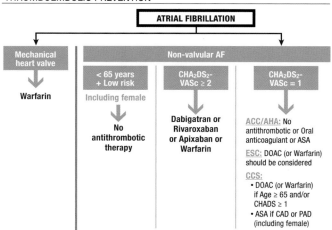

| CHADS₂ SCORE | | |
|---|---|---|
| Congestive heart failure and/or LVEF ≤ 40% | 1 point | **Stroke / year** |
| HTN | 1 point | 0 → 1.9 % |
| ≥ 75 years | 1 point | 1 → 2.8 % |
| | | 2 → 4.0 % |
| DM | 1 point | 3 → 5.9 % |
| | | 4 → 8.5 % |
| Stroke – TIA – Thromboembolism | 2 points | 5 → 12.5 % |
| | | 6 → 18.2 % |

*Gage BF, Waterman AD, Shannon W, et al. JAMA 2001;285:2864-70.*

| CHA₂DS₂-VASC SCORE | | |
|---|---|---|
| Recent decompensated HF and/or LVEF ≤ 40% | 1 point | **Stroke / year** |
| HTN | 1 point | 0 → 0 % |
| ≥ 75 years | 2 points | 1 → 1.3 % |
| DM | 1 point | 2 → 2.2 % 3 → 3.2 % |
| Stroke - TIA - Thromboembolism | 2 points | 4 → 4.0 % |
| Vascular disease (history of MI; PAD; Aortic plaque) | 1 point | 5 → 6.7 % 6 → 9.8 % 7 → 9.6 % |
| 65-74 years | 1 point | 8 → 6.7 % |
| Female | 1 point | 9 → 15.2 % |

*Lip GY, Nieuwlaat R, Pisters R, et al. Chest 2010;137:263–272.*

**BENEFIT OF WARFARIN IN PRIMARY PREVENTION**: ★ AFASAK-1 AND 2; ★ SPAF-1 and 2 and 3; ★ BAATAF; ★ CAFA; ★ SPINAF

> **Benefit of Warfarin**: relative risk of stroke ↘ by 64%                    +

> **Benefit of ASA**: relative risk of stroke ↘ by 19%

**WARFARIN ANTIDOTE**: vitamin K; prothrombin complex concentrate (Octaplex; Beriplex; Cofact; Proplex; factors II - VII - IX - X); FFP (8 units)

★ **ACTIVE-A**: Warfarin impossible; ASA + Plavix vs ASA; ↘ stroke but ↗ major bleeding

> **Indication for ASA-Clopidogrel**: when any form of oral anticoagulation is impossible but acceptable bleeding risk

---

## BLEEDING RISK ASSOCIATED WITH ANTICOAGULATION

**WARFARIN**: annual risk of major bleeding ≈ 3%                    +

| HAS-BLED SCORE | | |
|---|---|---|
| HTN (SBP > 160 mmHg) | 1 point | |
| Abnormal (liver or renal function)<br>· Creatinine ≥ 200 μmol/L or Dialysis<br>· AST - ALT > 3 x ULN or Bilirubin 2 x ULN or Cirrhosis | 1 point each | **Major bleeding/year** |
| Stroke | 1 point | 0 → 1.1 % 1 → 1.02 % |
| Bleeding (history; Anemia; Bleeding diathesis) | 1 point | 2 → 1.88 % |
| Labile INR | 1 point | **3 → 3.74 %** |
| Elderly (> 65 years) | 1 point | 4 → 8.7 % 5 → 12.5 % |
| Drugs (associated with a risk of bleeding) or Alcohol | 1 point each | |

*Pisters R, Lane DA, Nieuwlaat R, et al. Chest 2010;138:1093-100.*

**HAS-BLED ≥ 3**: **high bleeding risk**; try to correct reversible risk factors

**OTHER SCORES**: HEMORR₂HAGES; ATRIA

# DIRECT ORAL ANTICOAGULANTS (DOAC)

**CONTRAINDICATED: A)** Mechanical prosthetic valve; **B)** Moderate to severe mitral stenosis (usually of rheumatic origin)

| DABIGATRAN (PRADAXA) | RIVAROXABAN (XARELTO) | APIXABAN (ELIQUIS) | EDOXABAN (SAVAYSA; LIXIANA) |
|---|---|---|---|
| Direct thrombin inhibitor | Direct factor Xa inhibitor | Direct factor Xa inhibitor | Direct factor Xa inhibitor |
| Dose: 150 mg bid<br>• **110 mg bid**: ≥ 75 years; CrCl 30-49 mL/min with additional bleeding risk factor<br><br>Not studied in patients with CrCl < 30 mL/min | Dose: 20 mg qd<br>• **15 mg qd**: CrCl 30-49 mL/min<br><br>Not studied in patients with CrCl < 30 mL/min | Dose: 5 mg bid<br>• **2.5 mg bid**: ≥ 2 factors (≥ 80 years or ≤ 60 kg or creatinine ≥ 133 µmol/L)<br><br>Not studied in patients with CrCl < 25 mL/min | Dose: 60 mg qd<br>• **30 mg qd**: CrCl 30-49 mL/min<br><br>Not studied in patients with CrCl < 30 mL/min |
| ★ RELY<br>• **150 mg bid**: ↘ **stroke (superior to warfarin)**; comparable bleeding<br>• **110 mg bid**: non-inferior for stroke; ↘ **bleeding** | ★ ROCKET-AF<br>• 20 mg (15 mg if CrCl 30-49 mL/min): **non-inferior to warfarin for stroke**; comparable bleeding | ★ ARISTOTLE<br>• Apixaban 5 mg bid (2.5 mg bid not extensively studied): ↘ **stroke (superior to warfarin)**; ↘ **bleeding; ↘all-cause mortality** | ★ ENGAGE-AF<br>• **60 mg qd**: non-inferior for stroke (trend for superiority); ↘ **bleeding**<br>• **30 mg qd**: non-inferior for stroke (trend for inferiority); ↘ **bleeding; ↘ all-cause mortality** |
| Renal excretion: 80% | Renal excretion: 33% | Renal excretion: 25% | Renal excretion: 50% |

**FOLLOW-UP:** CrCl (Cockcroft-Gault) prior to initiation / when clinically indicated / ≥ 1 x / year

**CONSIDER REDUCED DOSE:** high bleeding risk (HAS-BLED ≥ 3); impaired renal function; drug interactions (P-gp and/or CYP3A4)

**★AVERROES:** AF with mean CHADS = 2; Warfarin impossible; Apixaban 5 mg bid versus ASA; early discontinuation (↘ stroke with Apixaban; similar bleeding)

**BLEEDING WITH DOAC:** Idarucizumab (Dabigatran; ★ RE-VERSE); Andexanet alpha (Rivaroxaban; Apixaban; Edoxaban); discontinue the anticoagulant; local compression; plasma expansion / transfusion; maintain diuresis to promote elimination; seek an opinion from a hematologist / pharmacist; consider prothrombin complex concentrates or activated factor VII or hemodialysis (Dabigatran)

| DOAC AND OTHER ANTICOAGULANTS | |
|---|---|
| **Switch from Warfarin → DOAC** | • INR < 2.0 → Start DOAC immediately<br>• INR 2.0 - 2.5 → Start DOAC on the following day |
| **Switch from IV Heparin → DOAC** | After stopping heparin |
| **Switch from LMWH → DOAC** | At the next scheduled dose of LMWH |
| **Switch from DOAC → LMWH or IV Heparin** | At the next scheduled dose of DOAC |
| **Switch from DOAC → Warfarin** | Stop DOAC when INR > 2.0 |

| PERIOPERATIVE USE OF DOAC | |
|---|---|
| **Surgery with low bleeding risk** (Dental extraction; cataract; endoscopy without biopsy; superficial skin surgery) | Continue DOAC (operate under DOAC) or skip the dose in the morning of the operation |
| **Surgery with intermediate bleeding risk** (Endoscopy with biopsy; prostate or bladder biopsy; angiography; electrophysiological intervention; pacemaker) | • **Apixaban – Rivaroxaban:** stop DOAC ≥ 24 h before the operation<br>• **Dabigatran:** stop DOAC ≥ 24 h (CrCl ≥ 80 mL/min) or ≥ 36 h (CrCl 50-80 mL/min) or ≥ 48 h (CrCl 30-50 mL/min) |
| **Surgery with high bleeding risk** (Lumbar puncture; spinal / epidural surgery; thoracic / abdominal / neurological / orthopedic surgery; liver or kidney biopsy; TURP) | • **Apixaban – Rivaroxaban:** stop DOAC ≥ 48 h before the operation<br>• **Dabigatran:** stop DOAC ≥ 48 h (CrCl ≥ 80 mL/min) or ≥ 72 h (CrCl 50-80 mL/min) or ≥ 96 h (CrCl 30-50 mL/min) |

## PERCUTANEOUS OCCLUSION OF LEFT ATRIAL APPENDAGE

★**PROTECT AF:** Watchman system non-inferior to warfarin for thromboembolic prevention; associated procedural complications; requires long-term antiplatelet therapy

INDICATION: high risk of stroke (CHADS ≥ 2) for whom anticoagulation is precluded

## ATRIAL FIBRILLATION AND CORONARY ARTERY DISEASE

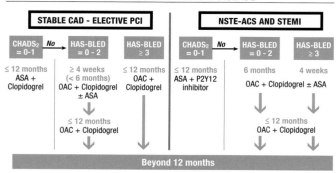

**OAC (Oral anticoagulation):**
Either Warfarin (INR 2.0 - 2.5) or DOAC (Dabigatran 110 mg bid; Rivaroxaban 15 mg qd; Apixaban 2.5 mg bid)

Proton pump inhibitor if risk of GI bleeding

★**WOEST:** 573 patients with an indication for anticoagulant therapy undergoing PCI (25-30% with ACS); Warfarin + Clopidogrel (versus Warfarin + Clopidogrel + ASA) associated with ↘ bleeding and ↘ mortality

## PRE-EXCITED ATRIAL FIBRILLATION

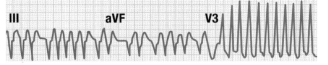

**III**  **aVF**  **V3**

**Irregularly irregular tachycardia with wide QRS**

COMPLICATIONS: **rapid AV conduction via an efficient accessory pathway (refractory period < 250 ms) → transformation to VF** +

MANAGEMENT: ECV stat; Procainamide or Ibutilide if hemodynamically stable; ablation of accessory pathway

> **Agents contraindicated**: AV node blocking agents predisposing to conduction via the accessory pathway (Digoxin; nondihydropyridine CCB; BB; Adenosine; IV Amiodarone)

## AF DETECTED BY PACEMAKER (SUBCLINICAL AF)

★ ASSERT: detection of subclinical atrial tachycardia (defined by HR > 190 bpm and duration > 6 min) associated with increased thromboembolic risk

> **Episode > 17.7 h (upper quartile of duration)**: significantly ↗ risk of stroke (fivefold)

★ TRENDS: atrial tachycardia (probable AF) ≥ 5.5 h associated with increased thromboembolic risk

CONSIDER ANTICOAGULATION: **A)** Episode lasting ≥ 24 h; **B)** Shorter episode in high-risk patient (cryptogenic stroke; TIA)

# 6.5/ VENTRICULAR TACHYARRHYTHMIAS

## PREMATURE VENTRICULAR COMPLEXES

**Premature ventricular depolarization during the cardiac cycle; wide QRS; T wave in opposite direction to the QRS**

MODIFIERS: couplet; bigeminy; trigeminy; monomorphic; polymorphic; associated with compensatory or noncompensatory pause; associated with retrograde atrial activation; interpolated complex; fusion complex; associated with echo (PVC → retrograde atrial activation → anterograde ventricular activation)

> **Compensatory pause**: interval between QRS before and after PVC = 2 x RR interval (failure of PVC to reset the sinoatrial node)

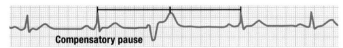

**Compensatory pause**

> **Interpolated PVC**: PVC between two beats of baseline rhythm with no modification of rhythm

PVC / MONOMORPHIC NSVT IN STRUCTURALLY NORMAL HEART: benign; risk of **tachycardiomyopathy** if frequent **(> 10,000 / 24 h)** and with a short coupling interval (< 300 ms) +

MANAGEMENT: Observation; intervention if symptoms or complications (tachycardiomyopathy); BB; AAD (IC; III); radiofrequency ablation

**PVC ASSOCIATED WITH AF**: elements in favor of PVCs rather than aberrant conduction →
fixed coupling interval / pause after wide QRS / bigeminy

## WIDE QRS TACHYCARDIA: DIFFERENTIAL DIAGNOSIS

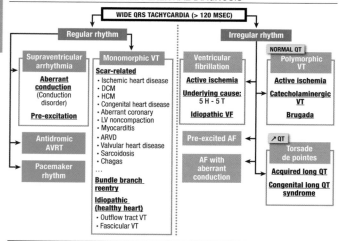

## WIDE QRS TACHYCARDIA: VT VERSUS ABERRANT CONDUCTION

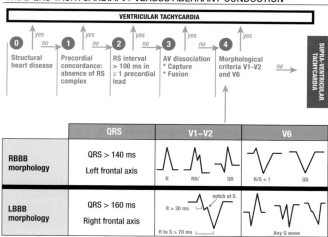

|  | QRS | V1–V2 | V6 |
|---|---|---|---|
| **RBBB morphology** | QRS > 140 ms<br>Left frontal axis | R    RSr´    QR | R/S < 1    QS |
| **LBBB morphology** | QRS > 160 ms<br>Right frontal axis | R > 30 ms    notch at S<br>R to S > 70 ms | Any Q wave |

**OTHER CRITERIA**

> **Supraventricular tachycardia with aberrant conduction: A)** Onset: Early P wave (APC); **B)** Change of PP interval precedes change of RR interval; **C)** QRS: identical to baseline rhythm; **D)** Stopped by vagal maneuver

> **Ventricular tachycardia: A)** Onset: Early QRS (PVC); **B)** Change of RR interval precedes change of PP interval; **C)** QRS: identical to PVC on baseline rhythm; **D)** Canon A wave; variable intensity of S1; variable SBP; **E)** -90° to 180° axis deviation

LOCALIZATION OF VT ON ECG

1) **V1 morphology**: LBBB (VT arises in RV and sometimes in LV septum); RBBB (VT arises in LV)

2) **Frontal axis**: Superior (VT arises in inferior wall); Inferior (VT arises in anterior wall)

3) **QRS V1 to V6: A)** Positive concordance → basal focus; **B)** Early QRS transition (V1-V2) → apical focus; **C)** Late QRS transition → midventricular focus

4) **QS complexes**: indicate the territory in which the arrhythmia arises (II-III-aVF = inferior; V4-V5-V6 = apical)

5) **Epicardial VT**: pseudo-Delta wave (initial portion of wide QRS)

# VENTRICULAR TACHYCARDIA (VT)

≥ 3 consecutive ventricular complexes; HR 110-250 bpm

> **Sustained**: > 30 s (or ECV necessary)                                          +

> AV dissociation or VA association (retrograde conduction)

MONOMORPHIC VENTRICULAR TACHYCARDIA: scar-related in the majority of cases;      +
look for structural heart disease

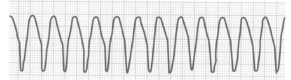

> **Acute management**: cardioversion (100 J biphasic) / defibrillation if absent pulse (200 J biphasic); Procainamide or Amiodarone (150 mg IV x 10 min then 1 mg/min x 6 h then 0.5 mg/min x 18 h) or Sotalol; ventricular overdrive; look for underlying cause

> **Secondary prevention**: First-line ICD; BB; Amiodarone (★ OPTIC); Sotalol; Mexiletine; RF ablation if repeated ICD shocks

VENTRICULAR TACHYCARDIA IN STRUCTURALLY NORMAL HEART

▶▶❙ Idiopathic ventricular tachycardia

BUNDLE BRANCH REENTRY TACHYCARDIA: in DCM; macro-reentry with anterograde conduction via the right bundle branch and retrograde conduction via the left bundle branch; Monomorphic VT with LBBB morphology

> **Management**: right bundle branch ablation

ACCELERATED IDIOVENTRICULAR RHYTHM (AIVR): 50-110 bpm; competition between sinoatrial node and a ventricular ectopic focus; increased automaticity; progressive onset and termination; associated with MI / reperfusion or Digoxin toxicity

> **Management**: observer; atropine PRN; « overdrive » auriculaire

POLYMORPHIC VENTRICULAR TACHYCARDIA WITH NORMAL QT: occurs during active myocardial ischemia or in genetic arrhythmia syndrome (▶▶❙ Channelopathies)

> **Acute management**: defibrillation; Rule out active ischemia; BB; Amiodarone; Lidocaine; correct electrolyte disorders

# IDIOPATHIC MONOMORPHIC VENTRICULAR TACHYCARDIA

Absence of structural heart disease; favorable prognosis

| | |
|---|---|
| **Outflow tract VT** | **MECHANISM**: myocyte calcium overload inducing triggered activity (delayed afterdepolarization); NSVT > sustained VT; 140-180 bpm; induced by exercise / stress / Isoproterenol<br>**RVOT VT**: LBBB morphology; inferior frontal axis; V3-V4 precordial transition<br>  › **DDx**: ARVD (abnormal SAECG / TTE / EPS)<br>  › **Management**: Adenosine; BB; Verapamil; class IC AAD; RF ablation (90% success rate)<br><br>V1       DIII<br><br>**LVOT VT**: 2 morphologies on ECG<br>  **1) RBBB - Inferior axis - S in V6**<br>  **2) LBBB - Inferior axis - early precordial R wave transition**<br>    **(V2 LVOT versus ≥ V3 RVOT)**<br>**VT ARISING IN SINUS OF VALSALVA**: LBBB; inferior axis<br>  › **Left sinus of Valsalva**: rS in I; V1 with "w" pattern or notch; early precordial transition<br>  › **Right sinus of Valsalva**: large R wave in V1; early precordial transition |
| **Fascicular VT** | **MECHANISM**: reentry in Purkinje system<br>**3 TYPES**:<br>  › **Left posterior hemibranch**: RBBB; Left superior frontal axis<br><br>V1      DI      DII<br><br>  › **Left anterior hemibranch**: RBBB; Right inferior frontal axis<br>  › **High septum**: Narrow QRS; normal axis<br>**MANAGEMENT**: Verapamil / Diltiazem; class III AAD; RF ablation |
| **Mitral annulus** | **ECG**: RBBB morphology; Dominant R in precordial leads |

# TORSADE DE POINTES

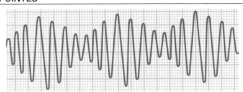

Polymorphic ventricular tachycardia; HR 200-250 bpm; twisting of QRS around the
isoelectric line (axis changes by 180° every 5-20 beats)

> **Associated with ↗ QT interval**: prolonged ventricular repolarization; QT > 500 ms; +
  ± prominent U wave
> **Mechanism**: triggered activity (early afterdepolarization)
> **Long RR - short RR sequence**

ETIOLOGIES - ACQUIRED LONG QT: Drugs (www.qtdrugs.org); AAD (IA; III); severe bradycardia;
electrolyte disorders (hypokalemia; hypomagnesemia); CNS lesion; ischemia; hypothermia;
anorexia; hypothyroidism; heart failure

> **Congenital long QT syndrome**: ►►| Channelopathies

MANAGEMENT: Mg$^{2+}$ (1-2 g IV); ventricular overdrive; Isoproterenol (pause-dependent TdP);
Lidocaine; BB with temporary pacemaker in place; correct underlying cause / correct electrolyte
disorders; PPM (in the case of pause-dependent TdP)

# VENTRICULAR FIBRILLATION (VF)

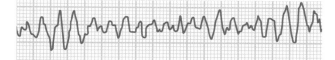

Chaotic ventricular rhythm; HR 400-600 bpm; absence of organized QRS - ST - T; fatal
within 3-5 min

ACUTE MANAGEMENT: immediate defibrillation (200 J biphasic) ± CPR (►►| Chapter 9); rule
out ischemia; look for underlying cause ("5 H and 5 T"); AAD to prevent recurrence (Amiodarone;
Lidocaine; Procainamide)

> **5 H - 5 T**: Hypovolemia; Hypoxia; Hydrogen (acidosis); Hypokalemia / Hyperkalemia; Hypothermia;
  Tension pneumothorax; Tamponade; Toxin; coronary Thrombosis; pulmonary Thrombosis

ELECTRICAL STORM: **≥ 3 episodes of VT/VF in 24 hours**                                    +

> **Management**: first-line BB; intubation / sedation; rule out ischemia or underlying cause;
  magnet over the ICD if inappropriate shocks; Amiodarone or Procainamide or Lidocaine
  (in the presence of ischemia); ventricular overdrive; reprogramming of ICD therapies;
  RF ablation; ventricular mechanical support

# IDIOPATHIC VENTRICULAR FIBRILLATION

DIAGNOSIS OF EXCLUSION: absence of structural heart disease and absence of an identifiable
channelopathy

EARLY REPOLARIZATION (HAÏSSAGUERRE PATTERN): association between VF and early
repolarization (J point elevation ≥ 1 mm on 2 contiguous inferior and/or lateral leads)

POSSIBLE MECHANISM: triggered by PVC with short coupling interval (arising in Purkinje system)

MANAGEMENT: ICD; Isoproterenol for electrical storm; Quinidine; catheter ablation of PVCs
triggering VF; assessment of first-degree relatives

## 6.6/ CHANNELOPATHIES

### CONGENITAL LONG QT SYNDROME (LQTS)

**ABNORMAL QT:** QTc ≥ 450 ms (male) or ≥ 460 ms (female)

> **50th percentile of LQTS cohorts**: QTc > 480 ms                                    +

**TRANSMISSION**: autosomal dominant form (Romano-Ward syndrome) or recessive form (deafness; Jervell & Lange-Nielsen syndrome)

| SCHWARTZ SCORE | | |
|---|---|---|
| **ECG** | **Clinical features** | **Family history** |
| • QTc ≥ 480 ms: 3 points<br>• QTc 460-479 ms: 2 points<br>• QTc > 450-459 ms (male): 1 point<br>• QTc after 4 min of recovery on stress test ≥ 480 ms: 1 point<br>• TdP: 2 points<br>• Alternating T wave: 1 point<br>• Notched T wave on 3 leads: 1 point | • Syncope on exercise / stress: 2 points<br>• Syncope without stress: 1 point | • Family member with LQTS: 1 point<br>• Sudden death in first degree relative before the age of 30 years: 0.5 point |

**≤ 1 point:** low probability
**1.5 to 3 points:** intermediate probability
**≥ 3.5 points:** high probability

*Schwartz PJ, Moss AM, Vincent GM, et al.*
*Circulation 1993; 88: 782-784.*

| LQT1 | LQT2 | LQT3 |
|---|---|---|
| KCNQ1 mutation | KCNH2 mutation | SCN5A mutation |
| **Trigger**: exercise; swimming; stress | **Trigger**: noise / alarms; postpartum | **Trigger**: rest / sleep |
| Wide-based T wave | Notched or biphasic T wave | Long isoelectric segment then narrow-based T wave |
| | | |
| **Management**: first-line BB (significant protection); ± ICD | **Management**: BB (moderate protection); ± ICD | **Management**: Mexiletine; Flecainide; Ranolazine; Low protection by BB; ± ICD |

**COMPLICATIONS**: syncope; TdP; sudden death

**MANAGEMENT**: avoid trigger; avoid drugs that ↗ QT; correct electrolyte; avoid strenuous exercise; BB (first-line); DDD or AAI pacemaker for pause-dependent TdP (especially associated with LQT3); sympathectomy

> **Risk factors for sudden death**: syncope; QTc > 500 ms; complex ventricular arrhythmia; Jervell and Lange-Nielsen
> **ICD**: A) Secondary prevention of sudden death; B) Syncope on BB therapy

### SHORT QT SYNDROME (SQTS)

**ECG**: **QTc interval ≤ 340 ms with HR < 100 bpm;** high amplitude T wave; short or absent    +
ST segment

COMPLICATIONS: AF; syncope; VF; sudden death

DIFFERENTIAL DIAGNOSIS: hyperkalemia; hypercalcemia; hyperthermia; acidosis; Digoxin

MANAGEMENT: Quinidine; Sotalol; ICD for secondary prevention

## BRUGADA SYNDROME

TRANSMISSION: autosomal dominant; sodium channel gene mutation (SCN5A; 20% of patients) or unidentified mutation

DIAGNOSTIC CRITERIA

| | |
|---|---|
| • Pattern 1 on ECG (≥ 2 leads: V1-V2-V3); spontaneous or with drug challenge (sodium channel blocking agent) **or** <br> • Pattern 2 or 3 (≥ 2 leads: V1-V2-V3) with conversion to Pattern 1 with drug challenge | **≥ 1 CLINICAL CRITERIA** <br> • Polymorphic VF or VT <br> • Family history of sudden death < 45 years <br> • Pattern 1 in the family <br> • VT during programmed stimulation <br> • Unexplained syncope <br> • Nocturnal agonal respiration |

*Wilde AA, Antzelevitch C, Borggrefe M et al. Circulation 2002; 106; 2514-2519.*

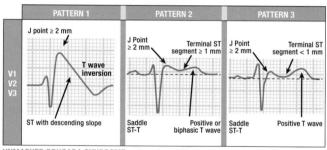

UNMASKED BRUGADA SYNDROME: sodium channel blocking agent (challenge with Procainamide 10 mg/kg IV x 10 min or Flecainide 400 mg PO); Drugs (www.brugadadrugs.org); fever; hypokalemia or hyperkalemia; leads V1-V2-V3 in 2nd or 3rd intercostal space; Cocaine; alcohol

COMPLICATIONS: Polymorphic VT (triggered by rest / sleep) / VF; sudden death (particularly in men in their forties); AF; SSS; conduction disorder

MANAGEMENT: Quinidine and/or Isoproterenol for electrical storm

> ICD: **A)** Secondary prevention of sudden death; **B)** Spontaneous pattern 1 with syncope

## CATECHOLAMINERGIC POLYMORPHIC VT

TRANSMISSION: autosomal dominant (ryanodine receptor gene mutation - RyR2) or autosomal recessive (calsequestrin gene mutation - CASQ2)

MYOCYTE CALCIUM OVERLOAD: triggered activity with delayed afterdepolarization

PRESENTATION: Polymorphic VT induced by exercise / stress; bidirectional VT

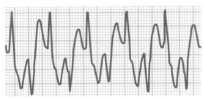

DIAGNOSIS: structurally normal heart; normal ECG

> **Exercise** → bidirectional VT and/or polymorphic PVCs and/or polymorphic VT

MANAGEMENT: BB (first-line treatment; Nadolol 1-2 mg/kg); CCB (Verapamil); Flecainide; Sympathectomy; avoid vigorous exercise

> **Titration of drug treatment**: guided by stress test and Holter
> **ICD**: **A)** Secondary prevention of sudden death; **B)** Syncope on BB therapy

## GENETIC TESTING FOR FAMILIAL ARRHYTHMIAS

OBJECTIVE: **A)** Family screening; **B)** Establish / confirm a diagnosis

| DISEASE | GENE | INDICATIONS FOR GENETIC TESTING |
|---|---|---|
| **Long QT syndrome** | Identification of a causal mutation: 75% (KCNQ1; KCNH2; SCN5A; KCNE1; KCNE2) | a) Cardiac arrest + long QT (family screening)<br>b) Syncope + long QT (family screening / diagnosis / treatment)<br>c) Asymptomatic long QT (family screening / diagnosis / treatment) |
| **Brugada syndrome** | Identification of a causal mutation: 20% (SCN5A) | a) Cardiac arrest + Brugada syndrome (family screening)<br>b) Syncope + Brugada syndrome (family screening)<br>c) Asymptomatic + Pattern 1 (family screening) |
| **ARVD – Arrhythmogenic RV dysplasia** | Identification of a causal mutation: 50% (PKP2; DSP; ± DSG2 - DSC2) | a) ARVD satisfying diagnostic criteria (family screening)<br>b) Suspected ARVD (diagnostic criterion) |
| **Catecholaminergic polymorphic VT** | Identification of a causal mutation: 50% (RYR2; ± CASQ2) | Suspected catecholaminergic polymorphic VT (family screening) |
| **Hypertrophic cardiomyopathy** | Identification of a causal mutation: 50% (MYH7; MYBPC3; ± TNNT2 - TNNI3 - TMP1) | a) HCM with clinical diagnosis (family screening)<br>b) HCM with pre-excitation (PRKAG2; LAMP2; GLA) |
| **Familial dilated cardiomyopathy** | Identification of a causal mutation: 20 % (MYBPC3; MYH7; TNNT2; LMNA; SCN5A) | a) Probable familial DCM (family screening)<br>b) Familial DCM + high-grade conduction disorder / atrial arrhythmia: LMNA and SCN5A |
| **Sudden death** | **Indication for targeted genetic testing**: negative autopsy in the presence of familial clinical signs of a particular phenotype (for family screening) | |

# 6.7/ SYNCOPE

**Brief loss of consciousness secondary to transient global cerebral hypoperfusion; resolves spontaneously; rapid recovery**

**DDX OF LOSS OF CONSCIOUSNESS:** Syncope; Aborted cardiac arrest; Epilepsy; Conversion / Psychogenic; Ischemic (vertebrobasilar TIA); Migraine; Metabolic disorder (Hypoglycemia; Poisoning; Hypoxemia; Hyperventilation); Traumatic (cerebral commotion)

**DDX OF SYNCOPE: A)** Neurocardiogenic (vasovagal); **B)** OH (dysautonomia; drugs; dehydration; alcohol); **C)** Cardiogenic syncope; **D)** Carotid sinus hypersensitivity; **E)** Situational syncope (cough; defecation; laughing; micturition; postprandial; deglutition); **F)** Subclavian steal syndrome

**DDX OF CARDIOGENIC SYNCOPE:** Bradyarrhythmia / Block (AV block; SSS; pause following conversion of supraventricular tachyarrhythmia); Tachyarrhythmia (supraventricular; AF; WPW syndrome; VT; channelopathy; arrhythmogenic drugs; idiopathic VF); Obstructive valvular heart disease; Aortic dissection; Myxoma; Tamponade; HCM; Infarction / Ischemia; Congenital coronary artery anomalies; Massive pulmonary embolism; PHT; Pacemaker dysfunction

## ASSESSMENT

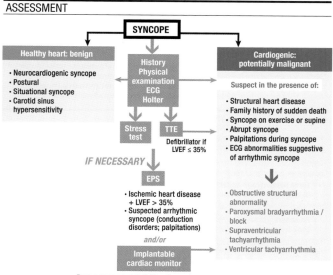

Rare syncope and definitive diagnosis necessary

**ASSESSMENT:** History of the present illness; Physical examination; BP supine - standing; carotid sinus massage; ECG; Holter (weekly syncope) or Loop recorder (monthly syncope); TTE

**ECG ABNORMALITIES SUGGESTIVE OF ARRHYTHMIC SYNCOPE:** diurnal sinus bradycardia < 40 bpm or diurnal sinus pauses ≥ 3 s; bifascicular block; QRS > 120 ms; Mobitz II or 3rd degree AV block; pre-excitation; NSVT; long QT; short QT; Brugada pattern; epsilon wave / T wave inversion in V1-V2-V3; early repolarization; LVH (dilated cardiomyopathy or HCM); Q waves

ELECTROPHYSIOLOGICAL STUDY: placement of intracardiac catheters to evaluate: **A)** sinoatrial node function (rule out SSS); **B)** AV node and His-Purkinje system function (rule out AV block); **C)** susceptibility to supraventricular and ventricular tachyarrhythmias

> **Indications (syncope): A)** Ischemic heart disease not meeting the criteria for ICD; **B)** Conduction disorder with suspected arrhythmic syncope (not meeting the criteria for permanent pacemaker); **C)** Abrupt syncope or preceded by palpitations with suspicion of an arrhythmic cause

> **Look for: A)** CSNRT > 525 ms; **B)** HV interval > 100 ms; **C)** Infra-His block during RA stimulation; **D)** Induced supraventricular tachycardia with hypotension; **E)** Monomorphic VT induced during programmed ventricular stimulation in the presence of ischemic heart disease

> **Programmed ventricular stimulation**: runs of 8 successive impulses (CL between 600 and 400 ms) then 1 or 2 or 3 premature complexes (minimal coupling interval of 200 ms)

## ORTHOSTATIC HYPOTENSION (OH)

DEFINITION: **reduction of SBP > 20 mmHg or DBP >10 mmHg on standing up (< 3 min)**    +

ETIOLOGIES: Drugs; Dehydration / Hemorrhage; Postprandial; Dysautonomia

> **Primary dysautonomia: A)** Pure dysautonomia (Bradbury-Eggleston syndrome); **B)** Multi-system atrophy (Shy-Drager syndrome); **C)** Parkinson's disease

> **Secondary dysautonomia**: DM; amyloidosis; alcohol; CRF; age; Guillain-Barré; mixed connective tissue disease; RA; Eaton-Lambert syndrome; SLE; carcinomatous autonomic neuropathy; multiple sclerosis; Wernicke's encephalopathy; hypothalamic or mesencephalic neoplastic or vascular disease; hereditary neuropathy; HIV; Chagas; Syphilis; botulism; Fabry; Tangier; vitamin B12 deficiency; porphyria; spinal cord lesion

MANAGEMENT: education; stand up slowly; lie down in the case of symptoms; sodium supplement (NaCl 1-2 g tid) and adequate hydration (2-3 L per day); avoid hypotensive drugs / alcohol; elastic compression stockings; Midodrine (alpha-agonist; 2.5-10 mg tid); Fludrocortisone (mineralocorticoid; 0.1-0.3 mg qd); raise the head of the bed by 10° to decrease nocturnal diuresis

## NEUROCARDIOGENIC SYNCOPE (VASOVAGAL)

PRESENTATION: Trigger factor (prolonged standing or emotional stress) → prodromal symptoms preceding syncope (nausea; diaphoresis; blurred vision; palpitations; faintness) → brief syncope

MECHANISM: vigorous ventricular contraction in the presence of low preload (secondary to venous pooling) → activation of cardiac mechanoreceptors → vagal hypertonia

> **Three responses to vagal hypertonia: A)** Cardioinhibitory (sinus pause and/or AV block); **B)** Vasodepressor; **C)** Mixed

TILT TABLE TEST: indication → to confirm the diagnosis of neurocardiogenic syncope when in doubt

> **Procedure**: 20 min in horizontal supine position → 30 to 45 min at 70° (± Isoproterenol or TNT)

> **Look for**: syncope + type of response following vagal hypertonia

MANAGEMENT: education; avoid trigger factors; sodium supplement (1-2 g NaCl tid) and adequate hydration; elastic compression stockings (30 mmHg); avoid hypotensive drugs / alcohol; isometric counterpressure maneuvers (handgrip for 2 min; leg crossing) or supine position in the case of prodromal symptoms; orthostatic training; raise the head of the bed by 10°; Midodrine / BB / Fludrocortisone / SSRI (Fluoxetine; Paroxetine; Venlafaxine); consider DDD pacemaker in the case of refractory syncope with dominant cardioinhibitory response (no benefit in ★ VPS-II; positive results in ★ ISSUE-3)

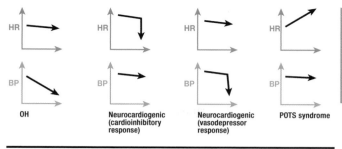

| OH | Neurocardiogenic (cardioinhibitory response) | Neurocardiogenic (vasodepressor response) | POTS syndrome |

## CAROTID SINUS HYPERSENSITIVITY

**CAROTID SINUS MASSAGE**: Apply pressure with 2 fingers (circular movements) for 10 s over the carotid pulse (at the level of the cricoid cartilage) with cardiac monitor

> **Contraindications**: carotid murmur; history of TIA - stroke
> **Cardioinhibitory response**: ventricular asystole > 3 s during massage → indication for DDD or VVI pacemaker in a patient with syncope

# 6.8/ ANTIARRHYTHMIC DRUGS (AAD)

| VAUGHAN WILLIAMS CLASSIFICATION | | |
|---|---|---|
| **CLASS IA – SODIUM CHANNEL BLOCKING AGENTS** | | |
| | • Slow phase 0 (↘ conduction velocity)<br>• Prolong the duration of the action potential (↗ QT)<br>• Intermediate kinetics<br>• Act on atria / ventricles / accessory pathway | |
| **Quinidine** | • **Indications**: Atrial and ventricular arrhythmias; Brugada; short QT syndrome; Idiopathic VF<br>• **Dose**: 6 to 10 mg/kg IV (0.3-0.5 mg/kg/min); 300 to 600 mg PO qid | • ↗ QRS (avoid ↗ > 25 %)<br>• ↗ QT (TdP)<br>• Hypotension; Nausea; Vomiting; Diarrhea; Thrombocytopenia; Lupus; Fever; Arrhythmogenic |
| **Procainamide** | • **Indications**: Atrial and ventricular arrhythmias; CCV AF (combined with AV node blocking agent); Pre-excited AF<br>• **Dose**: 15-20 mg/kg IV x 60 min (max 1 g) then 2 to 6 mg/min IV; stop if hypotension / ↗ QRS > 50 % / arrhythmia controlled | • **Metabolite**: N-acetylprocainamide (class III effect; renal elimination)<br>• **Adverse effects**: ANA+; drug Lupus; Arrhythmogenic; Infra-His block; ↗ QT (torsade de pointes); Negative inotropic agent with high-dose; Hypotension |
| **Disopyramide** | • **Indications**: Atrial and ventricular arrhythmias; HCM<br>• **Dose**: 100-300 mg PO tid to qid | • Negative inotropic agent<br>• Vagolytic effect (↗ heart rate)<br>• Urinary retention; constipation; ↗ QT (TdP) |

## CLASS IB – SODIUM CHANNEL BLOCKING AGENTS

- Decrease the duration of the action potential
- Rapid kinetics
- Main effect: ventricular

| Lidocaine | • **Indications**: Ventricular arrhythmias; (enhanced effect in ischemic tissues) <br> • **Dose**: 1 to 3 mg/kg IV (20-50 mg/min) then 1-4 mg/min (dilution: 2 g / 500 mL D5%) | • CNS toxicity (faintness; paresthesia; confusion) |
|---|---|---|
| Mexiletine | • **Indications**: Ventricular arrhythmias; long QT syndrome 3 <br> • **Dose**: 150 to 300 mg PO bid to tid | • Sinus bradycardia; hypotension <br> • CNS toxicity (dysarthria; faintness; paresthesia; confusion) |

## CLASS IC – SODIUM CHANNEL BLOCKING AGENTS

- Slow phase 0 (↘ conduction velocity)
- Slow kinetics
- **Use-dependent effect**: maximum antiarrhythmic effect at high HR (receptor open or inactivated)
- ↗ **QRS duration** (avoid ↗ > 25 %) especially at high HR

| Flecainide | • **Indications**: AF; Flutter; PSVT; catecholaminergic polymorphic VT <br> • **Dose**: 50 to 200 mg bid (combine with AV node blocking agent) | • Avoid in patients with CAD (★ CAST) / LV dysfunction <br> • Risk of organization of AF into flutter with 1:1 AV conduction <br> • Negative inotropic agent <br> • ↗ pacemaker stimulation threshold |
|---|---|---|
| Propafenone | • **Indications**: AF; Flutter; PSVT <br> • **Dose**: 150 to 300 mg PO bid to tid (in combination with AV node blocking agent) | • Avoid in CAD / LV dysfunction <br> • Hepatic metabolism (7% of patients are slow metabolizers) <br> • Negative inotropic agent <br> • ↗ pacemaker stimulation threshold |

## CLASS II – BETA–BLOCKERS

| Beta-blockers | • Block beta-adrenergic receptors <br> • **Indications**: supraventricular and ventricular arrhythmias <br> • **Metoprolol**: 2.5 to 5 mg IV every 5 min x 3 <br> • **Esmolol**: 0.5 kg /mg IV bolus then 50-200 µg/kg/min (dilution: 2500 mg/250 mL) | • **Adverse effects**: Negative inotropic agent; bronchospasm; hypotension; bradycardia; block; rebound effect on discontinuation; depression; exacerbation of severe PAD; masking of hypoglycemia symptoms; nightmares; erectile dysfunction |
|---|---|---|

## CLASS III – POTASSIUM CHANNEL BLOCKING AGENTS

- Increase the duration of the action potential; minimal effect on phase 0
- ↗ QT interval (risk of TdP)

| | | |
|---|---|---|
| **Amiodarone** | • **Indications**: AF; Flutter; VT; VF; PSVT<br>• **Dose**: 150 mg IV x 10 min then 1 mg/min IV x 6 h then 0.5-1 mg/min thereafter (dilution: 450 mg/250 mL D5%)<br>• **PO**: 800 to 1600 mg PO daily x 7-14 days (10 g) then 100 to 600 mg daily<br>• **Adverse effects**: ▶▶❘ Amiodarone | |
| **Sotalol** | • **Indications**: AF; PSVT; ventricular arrhythmias<br>• **Dose**: 80 to 160 mg bid | • ↗ QT (TdP)<br>• **Inverse use-dependent**: maximum antiarrhythmic effect at lower HR (resting receptors); ↗ QT at low HR<br>• ★ **SWORD**: ↗ mortality post-myocardial infarction with LVEF ≤ 40% with d-Sotalol (without BB effect)<br>• Renal excretion |
| **Dronedarone** | • **Indications**: Paroxysmal AF (★ ATHENA)<br>• **Dose**: 400 mg bid | • **Contraindication**: NYHA III-IV heart failure (★ ANDROMEDA); permanent AF (★ PALLAS); liver disease |
| **Dofetilide** | • **Indications**: AF and Flutter<br>• **Dose**: 0.125 to 0.5 mg PO bid | • ↗ QT (initiate in hospital; avoid if baseline QTc ≥ 440 ms)<br>• Renal excretion<br>• Safe in CAD or LV dysfunction (★ DIAMOND) |
| **Ibutilide** | • **Indications**: CCV of AF and Flutter (success: 70%)<br>• **Dose**: 1 mg x 10 min (with MgSO₄; repeat x 1 PRN) | • ↗ QT - TdP; Monitoring x 8 h post-dose<br>• Contraindicated if QTc > 440 ms or hypokalemia |

## CLASS IV – CALCIUM CHANNEL BLOCKING AGENTS

- Decrease conduction velocity (phase 0) of SA and AV nodes

| | | |
|---|---|---|
| **Verapamil and Diltiazem** | • **Indications**: PSVT; AF Flutter (rate control); fascicular VT<br>• **Diltiazem**: 0.25 mg/kg IV x 2 min (2ⁿᵈ bolus after 15 min); 120-360 mg PO daily | • Negative inotropic agent (avoid in the presence of LV dysfunction)<br>• Hypotension; Bradycardia; Leg edema; Drug interactions |

| OTHER AAD | | |
|---|---|---|
| **Digoxin** | • ↗ Vagal tone<br>• **Indications**: Rate control of HR in AF (at rest)<br>• **Dose**: loading dose of 0.5 to 1 mg x 24 h (PO or IV) then 0.0625 to 0.25 mg PO daily | • **Toxicity**: calcium overload → delayed afterdepolarization / ↗ automaticity<br>• ▶▶❙ Chapter 9 - Digoxin poisoning<br>• Renal excretion |
| **Adenosine** | • Brief inhibition of AV conduction<br>• **Indications**: PSVT; VT RVOT<br>• **Dose**: Adenosine: 6 to 12 mg rapid IV | • **Adverse effects**: precipitates AF (1-15%); flushing; dyspnea; retrosternal chest pain<br>• **Contraindications**: asthma; theophylline<br>• **Transplant recipient or Dipyridamole**: use a dose of 3 mg |
| **Atropine** | • Vagolytic<br>• **Indications**: symptomatic bradycardia<br>• **Dose**: 0.5 to 1 mg IV (up to 2 mg) | |

# 6.9/ AMIODARONE

## ADVERSE EFFECTS

| **Pulmonary toxicity (2%)** | **Toxicity correlated with cumulative dose**<br>• Interstitial lung disease; Organizing pneumonia / BOOP; ARDS<br>• Cough; Dyspnea; Fever<br>• **PFT**: ↘ DLCO / restrictive pattern<br>• **HDCT**: Interstitial / alveolar opacities; Ground glass; Fibrosis<br>• **Diagnosis of exclusion** (rule out infection and heart failure) | • Permanently discontinue Amiodarone<br>• Corticosteroids if severe<br>• Slow improvement (long half-life of amiodarone) |
|---|---|---|
| **GI toxicity (30%)** | • Nausea; Anorexia; Constipation<br>• ↗ AST ALT 2 x ULN<br>• Symptomatic hepatitis (3%) - Cirrhosis | • Rule out DDx<br>• Consider discontinuation |
| **Hypothyroidism (20%)** | • ↗ TSH and ↘ Free T4<br>• **Risk factors**: Female; underlying autoimmune thyroid disease (positive antibody); failure to escape from the Wolff-Chaikoff effect | • L-Thyroxine<br>• Continue Amiodarone |
| **Hyperthyroidism (10 %)** | • ↘ TSH and ↗ Free T4<br>• ↗ INR if treated with warfarin<br>• Thyroid scintigraphy falsified by the iodine load of Amiodarone<br>**Etiologies**<br>a) ↗ **T4 synthesis**: Underlying thyroid disease (Graves; multinodular goiter) exacerbated by iodine load<br>b) ↗ **T4 release**: Destructive thyroiditis (fever; painful gland); hypothyroid phase several weeks or months later<br>c) **Mixed** (majority) | **According to etiology**<br>**a)** PTU or Methimazole; Discontinue Amiodarone once hyperthyroid symptoms have been controlled (as Amiodarone blocks conversion of T4→T3)<br>**b)** Prednisone; ± Discontinue Amiodarone<br>**c)** Corticosteroids + antithyroid drugs (then stop antithyroid drugs if good response to corticosteroids in ≤ 1 week of treatment) |

| | | |
|---|---|---|
| **Skin** | • Photosensitivity (up to 75%)<br>• Blue discolouration (< 10%) | • Avoid exposure to sunlight |
| **CNS** | Ataxia; Paresthesia; Polyneuritis; Tremor | Dose-dependent effect |
| **Ophtalmic** | Halo; Optic neuropathy; Photophobia;<br>Blurred vision; Corneal microdeposits | Discontinue Amiodarone in the<br>presence of optic neuropathy |
| **Cardiac** | Bradycardia; Block; Arrhythmogenic (< 1%); ↗ **defibrillation threshold**;<br>↘ tachycardia CL | |

**MAJOR DRUG INTERACTIONS**: Digoxin; Procainamide; Disopyramide; Diltiazem; Flecainide;
Phenytoin; Cyclosporine; Simvastatin; Atorvastatin

> **Warfarin**: it is recommended to decrease the dose of warfarin by 30-50% on
> initiation of Amiodarone                                                          +

**WORK-UP BEFORE STARTING AMIODARONE**: TSH - Free T4 - T3; LFTs; CXR; Ophthalmological
examination if underlying abnormalities; renal function; ECG

**FOLLOW-UP ANALYSES**: TSH - Free T4 every 6 months; AST / ALT every 6 months; annual CXR

# 6.10/ PERMANENT PACEMAKER (PPM)

## INDICATIONS

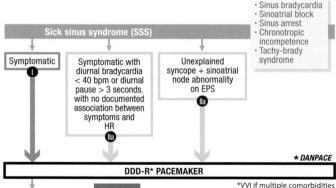

- Sinus bradycardia
- Sinoatrial block
- Sinus arrest
- Chronotropic incompetence
- Tachy-brady syndrome

Sick sinus syndrome (SSS)

| Symptomatic | Symptomatic with diurnal bradycardia < 40 bpm or diurnal pause > 3 seconds, with no documented association between symptoms and HR | Unexplained syncope + sinoatrial node abnormality on EPS |
|---|---|---|
| **I** | **IIa** | **IIa** |

★ *DANPACE*

**DDD-R\* PACEMAKER**

\*VVI if multiple comorbidities

Minimal RV pacing    ↗ **AV delay Algorithms**

↘ Atrial fibrillation
↘ Heart failure

★ *MOST;* ★ *CTOPP;* ★ *Danish;* ★ *DAVID*

## AV node disease - AV block

| 2nd or 3rd degree with bradycardia + symptoms **I** | Mobitz II with wide QRS **I** | AF and AV block with pause > 5 s **I** | High-grade 2nd degree or 3rd degree + (asystole > 3 s or escape < 40 bpm or infranodal escape) **I** | High-grade 2nd degree or 3rd degree with neuromuscular disease **I** | 2nd or 3rd degree on exercise **I** |

### DDD* PACEMAKER

*VVI if permanent AF

* VVI as alternative if multiple comorbidities

* CRT if LVEF < 35% and %V-Pace > 40%

* Consider VDD if normal sinoatrial node

| Mobitz II with narrow QRS **IIa** | 3rd degree with escape > 40 bpm **IIa** | 2nd degree intra-His or infra-His on EPS **IIa** |

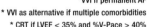

· RBBB + LAHB
· RBBB + LPHB
· LBBB

## AV node disease - Bifascicular block

| Mobitz II or high grade 2nd degree or 3rd degree **I** | Alternating RBBB and LBBB **I** | Unexplained syncope **IIa** | HV > 100 ms on EPS **IIa** | Infra-His block during RA stimulation on EPS **IIa** |

### DDD* PACEMAKER

* VVI if permanent AF

* VVI as alternative if multiple comorbidities

* CRT if LVEF < 35% and %V-Pace > 40%

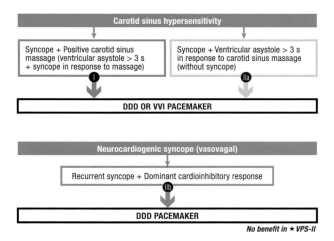

## TYPES OF PERMANENT PACEMAKERS

| NBG CODE | | | | |
|---|---|---|---|---|
| -1-<br>**Chamber paced** | -2-<br>**Chamber sensed** | -3-<br>**Response to sensing** | -4-<br>**Rate modulation** | -5-<br>**Multisite pacing** |
| • O = None<br>• A = Atrium<br>• V = Ventricle<br>• D = Dual (A + V) | • O = None<br>• A = Atrium<br>• V = Ventricle<br>• D = Dual (A + V) | • O = None<br>• T = Triggered<br>• I = Inhibited<br>• D = Dual (T + I) | • O = None<br>• R = Rate modulation | • A = Atrium<br>• V = Ventricle<br>• D = Dual (A + V) |

**AAI:** atrial pacing at the lower rate limit in the absence of sensing of an atrial event; indicated in sick sinus syndrome with preserved AV conduction

**VVI:** ventricular pacing at the lower rate limit in the absence of sensing of a ventricular event; absence of atrioventricular synchrony; indicated in AV block with permanent AF

**DDD:** atrial and ventricular pacing; atrial and ventricular sensing; indicated in AV block

> **4 possibilities**: **A)** A-Sense / V-Sense; **B)** A-Sense / V-Pace (at the end of the AV interval in the absence of sensing of a ventricular event); **C)** A-Pace / V-sense (A-Pace at the end of the atrial escape interval in the absence of sensing of an atrial event); **D)** A-Pace / V-Pace
> **AV delay**: set a long AV delay (not exceeding 250-300 ms) to promote intrinsic AV conduction and minimize ventricular pacing
> • **A-Pace / V-Pace delay > A-Sense / V-Pace delay** (A-Sense: part of the atrium is already + depolarized)

**VOO:** asynchronous ventricular pacing; mode used in pacemaker-dependent patients submitted to a source of electromagnetic interference (e.g.: electrocautery)

**VDD**: ventricular pacing with preserved atrioventricular synchrony on sensing of intrinsic P waves; requires a single lead (proximal atrial sensing by a ring; bipolar distal ventricular lead); consider in AV block in the absence of sick sinus syndrome

**DDI**: absence of "tracking" of sensed atrial events; V-Pace when the "lower rate interval" is reached (and A-Pace when the atrial escape interval is reached in the absence of a sensed event); indicated for atrial tachyarrhythmia with ineffective "mode-switch"

## DDD PACEMAKER INTERVALS

**PVAB**: Post-ventricular atrial blanking
**PVARP**: Post-ventricular atrial refractory period
**TARP**: Total atrial refractory period

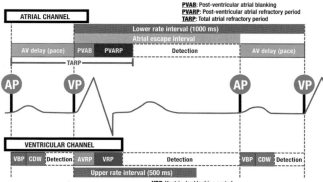

**VBP**: Ventricular blanking period
**CDW**: Crosstalk detection window (ventricular safety pacing)
**AVRP**: Absolute ventricular refractory period
**VRP**: Ventricular refractory period

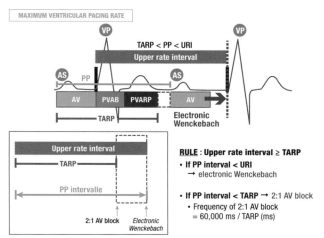

**RULE**: Upper rate interval ≥ TARP

- If PP interval < URI
  → electronic Wenckebach

- If PP interval < TARP → 2:1 AV block
  - Frequency of 2:1 AV block
    = 60,000 ms / TARP (ms)

## SPECIAL FUNCTIONS / ALGORITHMS

**RATE ADAPTIVE:** DDD-R or AAI-R or VVI-R; increased pacing rate when the patient is active (via activity sensor); activate in the case of symptomatic chronotropic incompetence / sick sinus syndrome

**HYSTERESIS:** **lower rate interval following V-Sense longer than lower rate interval following V-Pace (e.g.: 50 bpm vs 70 bpm);** promotes intrinsic rhythm

**AAI ⟷ DDD MODE (MVP MODE):** AAI mode switches to DDD mode when ≥ 2 of the previous 4 A-A intervals do not contain V-Sense

**DYNAMIC AV DELAY:** AV delay decreases at higher HR **(= ↘ TARP);** useful in patients with AV block and risk of 2:1 block on exercise

**MODE SWITCH:** DDD mode switches to DDI mode following atrial tachyarrhythmia to prevent tracking of this tachyarrhythmia

**VENTRICULAR SAFETY PACING: following A-Pace →** early ventricular pacing (AV delay: 100 ms) in the presence of a ventricular event detected inside the cross-talk detection window (preventing asystole in the presence of cross-talk or preventing R on T in the presence of a PVC)

**POST-PVC EXTENSION OF PVARP:** extension to 400 ms; prevents detection of a post-PVC retrograde P wave and therefore **the development of PMT**

**RATE SMOOTHING:** prevents an abrupt change of HR (during paroxysmal sinus arrest or following a mode switch)

**RATE DROP RESPONSE:** pacing at a higher rate (100-120 bpm) following an abrupt drop in HR (due to neurocardiogenic syncope)

**NOISE RESPONSE:** VOO or DOO mode activated following noise (nonphysiological signals)

## PACEMAKER MONITORING

| | |
|---|---|
| **Battery** | • ↘ Voltage and ↗ Impedance with time<br>• **ERI**: Elective replacement indicator (< 3 months) |
| **Lead** | • **Impedance**: significant change > 200 ohms<br>• **Low impedance (< 250 Ohms)**: insulation defect<br>• **Increased impedance (> 1000 Ohms)**: short circuit (lead fracture; loose set screw)<br>• Chest x-ray PRN |
| **Events** | • % A-Pace; % V-Pace; Frequency histogram<br>• Saved episodes; AT/AF; Mode switch; Ventricular high rate; PMT |
| **Sensitivity** | • **Atrial**: from 0.3 to 0.6 mV<br>• **Ventricular**: from 2 to 3.5 mV |
| **Pacing** | • **Safety margin**: programmed amplitude → twice the pacing threshold (or automatic capture)<br>• **Pulse width**: 0.4 to 0.5 ms |

| MINIMUM FOLLOW–UP FREQUENCY FOR PPM, CRT, OR ICD | |
|---|---|
| Post-implantation follow-up | • < 72 h post-implant (in person)<br>• 2 to 12 weeks post-implant (in person) |
| PPM or CRT follow-up | • 3 to 12 months (in person or by remote monitoring)<br>• At least once a year in person |
| ICD follow-up | • 3 to 6 months (in person or by remote monitoring)<br>• At least once a year in person |
| Signs of battery depletion | • Every 1 to 3 months (in person or by remote monitoring) |

## PACEMAKER DYSFUNCTION

| | |
|---|---|
| Capture failure | • **Early post-implant:** lead migration; myocardial perforation; maturation (inflammatory reaction)<br>• **Late lead maturation:** exit block<br>• **Modified threshold:** myocardial infarction; cardiomyopathy; acidosis; electrolyte disorders; drugs (class IC AAD; Sotalol)<br>• **Ineffective autocapture algorithm**<br>• **Inadequate programming:** insufficient pacing amplitude safety margin<br>• **Lead:** insulation defect; lead fracture; loose set screw<br>• **Battery depletion**<br>• **Failure to capture:** pacing during the refractory period; ± associated undersensing |
| Output failure | • **Oversensing** (inhibition)<br>• **Lead:** insulation defect; short circuit (lead fracture; loose set screw)<br>• **Hysteresis**<br>• **Battery depletion**<br>• **Post-PVC extension of PVARP**<br>• **Generator dysfunction** (rare) |
| Undersensing | • **Inadequate intrinsic signal:** PVC or APC<br>• **Signal modification:** myocardial infarction; cardiomyopathy; conduction disorder; metabolic disorder<br>• **Programming:** high sensitivity<br>• **Lead:** migration; maturation; insulation defect; lead fracture; loose set screw<br>• **Magnet**<br>• **Noise response**<br>• **Safety pacing function**<br>• **Battery depletion**<br>• **Pseudofusion**<br>• **Functional undersensing** (refractory period) |
| Oversensing | • **Cross-talk:** pacing of one chamber induces sensing of an event in the other chamber; minimized by blanking<br>• **Far-field:** QRS detected as atrial event<br>• **Oversensing of T wave**<br>• **Electromagnetic interference:** electrocautery; MRI<br>• **Myopotentials (unipolar electrode)**<br>• **Lead:** insulation defect (internal contact of the two conductors); short circuit (lead fracture; loose set screw) |

| Pacing at a rate different from programmed rate | **High heart rate**<br>• **Rate-adaptive:** R<br>• **Undersensing**<br>• **Tracking** of intrinsic atrial rhythm (or atrial oversensing)<br>• **Rate smoothing**<br>• **Rate drop**<br>• **Pacemaker-mediated tachycardia**<br>• **Runaway pacemaker** (battery depletion) | **Low heart rate**<br>• **Oversensing**<br>• **Hysteresis**<br>• **AAI ⟷ DDD**<br>• **Sleep mode**<br>• **Battery depletion** |
|---|---|---|

### PACEMAKER-MEDIATED TACHYCARDIA (PMT)

> **Risk factors**: A) PVC with retrograde conduction; B) Atrial capture failure; C) Very long programmed AV delay; D) Atrial oversensing or undersensing

> **Mechanism**: Retrograde V-A conduction (often post-PVC) → A-Sense (outside of the PVARP) → V-Pace → retrograde V-A conduction → A-Sense (and so on)

> **Diagnosis**: A) A-Sense / V-Pace at the maximum pacing rate; B) A-Sense following V-Pace with V-A interval < 400 ms; C) Discordance between pacing rate and activity sensor; D) Modulation of P-V period

> **Prevention / Termination**: A) PVARP > retrograde V-A conduction time (while avoiding excessively prolonged TARP, which would lead to low frequency 2:1 block); B) Extension of post-PVC PVARP; C) 1 cycle without V-Pace following A-Sense during PMT

PACEMAKER SYNDROME: **secondary to loss of AV synchrony** (± atrial contraction on closed AV valve) with VVI pacemaker; tiredness / retrosternal chest pain / dyspnea / cough / confusion / faintness / syncope

DIAPHRAGMATIC STIMULATION: lead close to phrenic nerve; incorrectly positioned lead (cardiac vein; myocardium perforation; migration); high stimulation amplitude

## 6.11/ CARDIAC RESYNCHRONIZATION THERAPY (CRT)

HEART FAILURE: altered electromechanical coupling → inter- and intraventricular delays → ventricular asynchrony → ↗ systolic dysfunction → altered myocardial metabolism / functional MR / ventricular remodeling / LV dilatation

| SCIENTIFIC EVIDENCE | |
|---|---|
| • ★ **COMPANION**: LVEF ≤ 35% + NYHA III or IV (ambulant) + SR + QRS ≥ 120 ms + Hospitalization for heart failure during the previous year<br>• ★ **CARE-HF**: LVEF ≤ 35% + NYHA III or IV (ambulant) + SR + QRS ≥ 150 ms (120-149 ms with TTE criteria of asynchrony) | • ★ **MADIT-CRT**: LVEF ≤ 30% + NYHA I (15%) or NYHA II (85%) + SR + QRS ≥ 130 ms<br>• ★ **RAFT**: LVEF ≤ 30% + NYHA II (80%) or NYHA III (20%) + QRS ≥ 130 ms |
| • ↘ All-cause mortality<br>• ↘ Hospitalization<br>• Improvement of quality of life<br>• Reverse remodeling | • ↘ All-cause mortality (★ RAFT)<br>• ↘ Hospitalization<br>• Improvement of quality of life<br>• Reverse remodeling |
| **MAINLY BENEFICIAL IN LBBB WITH QRS ≥ 150 MSEC** | |

## INDICATIONS

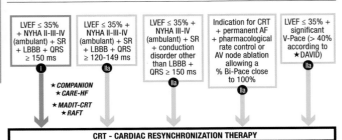

| | | | | |
|---|---|---|---|---|
| LVEF ≤ 35% + NYHA II-III-IV (ambulant) + SR + LBBB + QRS ≥ 150 ms | LVEF ≤ 35% + NYHA II-III-IV (ambulant) + SR + LBBB + QRS ≥ 120-149 ms | LVEF ≤ 35% + NYHA III-IV (ambulant) + SR + conduction disorder other than LBBB + QRS ≥ 150 ms | Indication for CRT + permanent AF + pharmacological rate control or AV node ablation allowing a % Bi-Pace close to 100% | LVEF ≤ 35% + significant V-Pace (> 40% according to ★DAVID) |

★ **COMPANION**
★ **CARE-HF**

★ **MADIT-CRT**
★ **RAFT**

**CRT - CARDIAC RESYNCHRONIZATION THERAPY**

\* Life expectancy with satisfactory functional capacity > 1 year

## PROGRAMMING

| | |
|---|---|
| **RA pacing** | • **Minimal** to avoid interatrial asynchrony<br>• Minimum rate: 50 bpm<br>• Do not activate "R" |
| **AV delay** | • **100-120 ms (minimize intrinsic AV conduction; ensure adequate duration of atrial kick)**<br>• Consider echocardiography-guided optimization in the presence of a pseudonormal (grade II) or restrictive (grade III) mitral diastolic pattern |
| **LV lead position** | • **Basal posterolateral wall** (site of maximum electromechanical delay)<br>• Avoid scars whenever possible (LGE on MRI); target adequate threshold; avoid phrenic nerve stimulation (electronic reprogramming of vectorial stimulation configuration PRN) |
| **V-V delay** | • **Simultaneous or pre-excitation of LV stimulation (30 ms)**<br>• Echocardiographic optimization PRN in non-responders (using aortic VTI and/or deformation imaging and/or RV - LV pre-ejection intervals) |
| **Maximize Bi-Pace** | • **Target Bi-Pace > 98%**<br>• AF → AV node blocking agent or RF ablation of AV node<br>• Frequent PVCs → AAD or RF ablation |
| **ECG** | • **V1: dominant R wave**<br>• **I: negative**<br>• V4-V5: positive in the case of basal LV stimulation (negative if apical)<br>• Frontal axis: -90° to 180° |

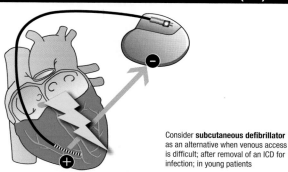

| V1 | I | FRONTAL AXIS |
|---|---|---|
| **RV apical stimulation** | | |
| | | 0 to -90° |
| **Resynchronization therapy** | | |
| | | -90 to 180° |

# 6.12/ IMPLANTABLE CARDIOVERTER-DEFIBRILLATOR (ICD)

Consider **subcutaneous defibrillator** as an alternative when venous access is difficult; after removal of an ICD for infection; in young patients

## SCIENTIFIC EVIDENCE

**SECONDARY PREVENTION**: ★ AVID; ★ CIDS; ★ CASH

> Reduction of the absolute mortality (vs Amiodarone): 10.5% at 36 months **(NNT 10 patients)** +

**PRIMARY PREVENTION**: reduction of absolute mortality of 5-8% at 36 months **(NNT 14-18** +
**patients)**

> ★ **MADIT-I**: Ischemic heart disease; LVEF ≤ 35%; NYHA I-II-III, NSVT; inducible VT
  → ↘ all-cause mortality
> ★ **MUSTT**: Ischemic heart disease; LVEF ≤ 40%; NYHA I-II-III, NSVT; inducible VT
  → ↘ all-cause mortality
> ★ **MADIT-II**: Ischemic heart disease; LVEF ≤ 30%; NYHA I-II-III → ↘ all-cause mortality
> ★ **DEFINITE**: Nonischemic heart disease; LVEF ≤ 35%; NYHA I-II-III, NSVT (or ≥ 10 PVCs / h)
  → trend to ↘ all-cause mortality
> ★ **SCD-HeFT**: LVEF ≤ 35%; (ischemic or nonischemic heart disease); NYHA II-III
  → ↘ all-cause mortality
> ★ **DINAMIT**: LVEF ≤ 35%; **< 40 days post-MI**; decreased HR variability or high resting HR
  → no benefit
> ★ **IRIS**: LVEF < 40%; **< 30 days post-MI**; HR > 90 bpm or NSVT > 150 bpm → no benefit

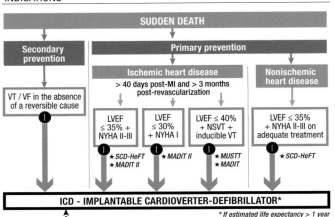

**SUDDEN DEATH**

| Secondary prevention | Primary prevention | | |
|---|---|---|---|

**Secondary prevention**

VT / VF in the absence of a reversible cause
**I**

**Primary prevention**

**Ischemic heart disease**
> 40 days post-MI and > 3 months post-revascularization

**Nonischemic heart disease**

LVEF ≤ 35% + NYHA II-III
**I**
★ SCD-HeFT
★ MADIT II

LVEF ≤ 30% + NYHA I
**I**
★ MADIT II

LVEF ≤ 40% + NSVT + inducible VT
**I**
★ MUSTT
★ MADIT

LVEF ≤ 35% + NYHA II-III on adequate treatment
**I**
★ SCD-HeFT

**ICD - IMPLANTABLE CARDIOVERTER-DEFIBRILLATOR***

CONSIDER

*\* If estimated life expectancy > 1 year*

**OTHER CONDITIONS** HCM + risk factors · ARVD + risk factors · Long QT syndrome with syncope or VT on beta-blockers · Brugada with syncope or VT · Catecholaminergic polymorphic VT with syncope or VT on beta-blockers · Sarcoidosis or giant cell myocarditis or Chagas · LV noncompaction · Congenital heart disease

## PROGRAMMING – PRIMARY PREVENTION

| ZONE #1: SLOW VT | ZONE #2: FAST VT | ZONE #3: VF |
|---|---|---|
| 150 to 188-200 bpm (400 to 320-300 ms) | 188-200 to 250 bpm (320-300 to 240 ms) | > 250 bpm (< 240 ms) |
| · Monitor (at user discretion) | a) ≥ 1 ATP (**burst**) attempt (8 impulses at 84-88% of tachycardia CL) <br> b) Maximum energy shock | · Maximum energy shock (> 30 J) x 6 (ATP during charge) |

- **Detection duration**: ≥ 30 intervals (≥ 6-12 sec)
- **VT/VF discriminators vs supraventricular arrhythmia (up to 230 bpm)**: A) V > A / A-V dissociation; B) EGM morphology (vs baseline template); C) Abrupt onset; D) Stable R-R interval

**ANTI-TACHYCARDIA PACING (ATP)**: interrupt the reentry circuit of monomorphic VT; effective in 70-80% of patients with fast VT (★ PainFREE Rx II)

> **Burst**: 8 impulses with constant inter-stimulus interval (at 88% of tachycardia CL)
> **Ramp**: 8 impulses with decreasing inter-stimulus interval

★ **MADIT-RIT**: primary prevention; administration of therapy only during fast VT (≥ 200 bpm) or following a period of prolonged detection (> 60 s for 170-199 bpm or > 12 s for 200-249 bpm or > 2.5 s for 250 bpm) associated with ↘ **all-cause mortality / ↘ inappropriate ICD +  therapies**

06

Arrhythmias

# PROGRAMMING – SECONDARY PREVENTION

DETECTION DURATION: ≥ 30 intervals (≥ 6-12 sec)

SLOWEST ZONE: at least 10 bpm below the documented tachycardia rate (but not faster than 200 bpm except for some young patients) → ATP (≥ 1 burst attempt - 8 impulses at 88% of VT CL; 10 ms scan decrement) → Shock

VF: > 250 bpm → ATP while charging → Shock (full output)

# MANAGEMENT FOLLOWING AN ICD SHOCK

MEDICAL ASSESSMENT: < 24 h (urgent if multiple shocks or symptoms)

APPROPRIATE SHOCK: VF; monomorphic VT; polymorphic VT

INAPPROPRIATE SHOCK: apply a magnet over the device; reprogram treatment / parameters

> **Supraventricular tachycardia** → modify therapy zones; optimize discriminator programming; AV node blocking agent / AAD; RF ablation
> **T wave oversensing (and small R wave)** → decrease ventricular sensitivity (however, must be sufficient to detect VF; defibrillator test PRN); prolong the ventricular refractory period; modify sensing decay; lead repositioning
> **Atrial far-field** (distal coil of an integrated bipolar electrode close to the tricuspid valve)
> **R-wave double counting** → modify sensing decay; prolong the refractory period; decrease ventricular sensitivity (however, must be sufficient to detect VF; defibrillator test PRN)
> **Electromagnetic interference**
> **Myopotentials**
> **Lead** (insulation defect; lead fracture; loose set screw)

ELECTRICAL STORM: ▶▶| Ventricular fibrillation

PREVENTION OF NEW SHOCKS: BB; Amiodarone; Sotalol; therapy reprogramming; RF ablation

SHOCK APPROPRIATE BUT INEFFECTIVE

> **Increased defibrillation threshold**: ischemia; progressive heart failure; AAD (sodium channel blocking agents; Amiodarone); electrolyte / metabolic disorders; pleural / pericardial effusion
> **Secondary to defibrillator**: insufficient programmed shock amplitude; battery depletion; lead (insulation defect; lead fracture; loose set screw; migration)

- Bonow RO, Mann DL, Zipes DP, Libby P. *Braunwald's Heart Disease. A textbook of cardiovascular medicine.* Elsevier. 2012. 1961 p.
- Ellenbogen KA. Kay GN. Lau CP. Wilkoff BL. *Clinical cardiac pacing, defibrillation, and resynchronization therapy.* Fourth Edition. Elsevier. 2011. 1085 p.
- 2015 ACC/AHA/HRS Guideline for the Management of Adult Patients With Supraventricular Tachycardia. *JACC* 2016; In press.
- ACC/AHA/ESC Guidelines for the Management of Patients With Supraventricular Arrhythmias. *JACC* 2003; *42;* 1493-1431
- Link MS. Evaluation and Initial Treatment of Supraventricular Tachycardia. *NEJM* 2012; *367;* 1438-48.
- Delacrétaz E. Supraventricular Tachycardia. *NEJM* 2006; *354;* 1039-1051.
- 2014 AHA/ACC/HRS Guideline for the Management of Patients With Atrial Fibrillation. *JACC* 2014; *64;* e1-e76.
- 2014 Focused Update of the Canadian Cardiovascular Society Guidelines for the Management of Atrial Fibrillation. *CJC* 2014; 30; 1114-1130.
- Focused 2012 Update of the Canadian Cardiovascular Society Atrial Fibrillation Guidelines: Recommendations for Stroke Prevention and Rate/Rhythm Control. *CJC* 2012; *28;* 125-136.
- 2012 focused update of the ESC Guidelines for the management of atrial fibrillation. *EHJ* 2012; *33;* 2719-2747.
- Canadian Cardiovascular Society Atrial Fibrillation Guidelines 2010: Etiology and Initial Investigations. *CJC* 2011; *27;* 31-37.
- Canadian Cardiovascular Society Atrial Fibrillation Guidelines 2010: Management of Recent-Onset Atrial Fibrillation and Flutter in the Emergency Department. *CJC* 2011; *27;* 38-46.
- Canadian Cardiovascular Society Atrial Fibrillation Guidelines 2010: Rate and Rhythm Management. *CJC* 2011; *27;* 47-59.
- Canadian Cardiovascular Society Atrial Fibrillation Guidelines 2010: Catheter Ablation for Atrial Fibrillation/Atrial Flutter. *CJC* 2011; *27;* 60-66.
- Canadian Cardiovascular Society Atrial Fibrillation Guidelines 2010: Surgical Therapy. *CJC* 2011; *27;* 67-73.
- Canadian Cardiovascular Society Atrial Fibrillation Guidelines 2010: Prevention of Stroke and Systemic Thromboembolism in Atrial Fibrillation and Flutter. *CJC* 2011; *27;* 74-90.
- Canadian Cardiovascular Society Atrial Fibrillation Guidelines 2010: Prevention and Treatment of Atrial Fibrillation Following Cardiac Surgery. *CJC* 2011; *27;* 91-97.
- Antithrombotic Therapy for Atrial Fibrillation. Antithrombotic Therapy and Prevention of Thrombosis, 9th ed: American College of Chest Physicians Evidence-Based Clinical Practice Guidelines. *CHEST* 2012; *141;* e531S-e575S.
- Bassand J-P. Review of atrial fibrillation outcome trials of oral anticoagulant and antiplatelet agents. *Europace* 2012; *14;* 312–324.
- Updated EHRA Practical Guide on the use of non-vitamin K antagonist anticoagulant in patients with non-valvular atrial fibrillation. *Europace* 2015; *17;* 1467-1507.
- Management of antithrombotic therapy in atrial fibrillation patients presenting with acute coronary syndrome and/or undergoing percutaneous coronary or valve interventions: a joint consensus document of the European Society of Cardiology Working Group on Thrombosis, EHRA, EAPCI and ACCA endorsed by the Heart Rhythm Society (HRS) and Asia-Pacific Heart Rhythm Society (APHRS). *EHJ* 2014; *35;* 3155-3179.
- Wazni O. Wilkoff B. Saliba W. Catheter Ablation for Atrial Fibrillation. *NEJM* 2011; *365;* 2296-2304.
- Michaud GF, John R. Percutaneous Pulmonary Vein Isolation for Atrial Fibrillation Ablation. *Circulation* 2011; *123;* e596-e601.
- Lamas G. How Much Atrial Fibrillation Is Too Much Atrial Fibrillation? *NEJM* 2012; *366;* 178-180.

- ACC/AHA/ESC 2006 Guidelines for Management of Patients With Ventricular Arrhythmias and the Prevention of Sudden Cardiac Death. *JACC* 2006; *48;* e248-e346.
- Prystowsky E, Padanilam BJ, Joshi S et al. Ventricular Arrhythmias in the Absence of Structural Heart Disease. *JACC* 2012; *59;* 1733-1744.
- Alzand B, Crijns H. Diagnostic criteria of broad QRS complex tachycardia: decades of evolution. *Europace* 2011; *13;* 465–472
- Pellegrini CN. Scheinman MM. Clinical Management of Ventricular Tachycardia. *Curr Probl Cardiol* 2010; *35:* 453-504.
- EHRA/HRS/APHRS expert consensus on ventricular arrhythmias. *Europace* 2014; *16;* 1257-1283.
- HRS/EHRA/APHRS expert consensus statement on the diagnosis and management of patients with inherited primary arrhythmia syndromes. *Europace* 2013; *15;* 1389-1406
- Webster G, Berul CI. An Update on Channelopathies: From Mechanisms to Management. *Circulation* 2013; *127:* 126-140.
- Roden DM. Long-QT Syndrome. *NEJM* 2008; *358;* 169-176.
- Schwartz PJ, Moss AM, Vincent GM, et al. Diagnostic criteria for the long QT syndrome. *Circulation* 1993; *88:* 782-784.
- Gollob MH, Redpath CJ, Roberts JD et al. The short QT syndrome. Proposed diagnostic criteria. *JACC* 2011; *57:* 802-812
- Brugada Syndrome: Report of the Second Consensus Conference. *Circulation.* 2005; *111:* 659-670.
- Van der Werf C, Zwinderman AH, Wilde A. Therapeutic approach for patients with catecholaminergic polymorphic ventricular tachycardia: state of the art and future developments. *Europace* 2012; *14;* 175–183
- Recommendations for the Use of Genetic Testing in the Clinical Evaluation of Inherited Cardiac Arrhythmias Associated with Sudden Cardiac Death: Canadian Cardiovascular Society/Canadian Heart Rhythm Society Joint Position Paper. *CJC* 2011; *27;* 232-245.
- Guidelines for the diagnosis and management of syncope (version 2009). *EHJ* 2009; *30;* 2631-2671.
- Standardized Approaches to the Investigation of Syncope: Canadian Cardiovascular Society Position Paper. *CJC* 2011; *27;* 246-253.
- AHA/ACCF Scientific Statement on the Evaluation of Syncope. *JACC* 2006; *47;* 473-484.
- Grubb BP. Neurocardiogenic Syncope. *NEJM* 2005; *352;* 1004-1010.
- Benditt DG. Nguyen JT. Syncope: Therapeutic Approaches. *JACC* 2009; *53;* 1741-1751.
- Goldschlager N. Epstein AE. Naccarelli GV. A Practical Guide for Clinicians Who Treat Patients with Amiodarone: 2007. *Heart Rhythm* 2007; *4;* 1250-1259.
- ACC/AHA/HRS 2008 Guidelines for Device-Based Therapy of Cardiac Rhythm Abnormalities. *JACC* 2008; *51;* e1-e62.
- 2012 ACCF/AHA/HRS Focused Update of the 2008 Guidelines for Device-Based Therapy of Cardiac Rhythm Abnormalities. *JACC* 2012; *60;* 1297-1313.
- HRS/ACCF Expert Consensus Statement on Pacemaker Device and Mode Selection. *JACC* 2012; *60;* 682-703.
- Canadian Cardiovascular Society Guidelines on the Use of Cardiac Resynchronization Therapy: Evidence and Patient Selection. *CJC* 2013; *29;* 182-195.
- 2012 EHRA/HRS expert consensus statement on cardiac resynchronization therapy in heart failure: implant and follow-up recommendations and management. *Europace* 2012; *14;* 1236-1286.
- Moss AJ., Schuger C., Beck CA. et al. Reduction in Inappropriate Therapy and Mortality through ICD Programming. *NEJM* 2012; *367;* 2275-2283
- 2015 HRS/EHRA/APHRS/SOLAECE Expert Consensus Statement on Optimal Implantable Cardioverter-Defibrillator Programming and Testing. *H Rhythm* 2016; In press.
- Management of patients receiving implantable cardiac defibrillator shocks. *Europace* 2010; *12;* 1673-1690.
- UpToDate 2015

| 7.1/ | Segmental assessment & Fetal circulation | 248 |
|------|------------------------------------------|-----|
| 7.2/ | Atrial septal defect (ASD) | 248 |
| 7.3/ | Patent foramen ovale (PFO) | 250 |
| 7.4/ | Ventricular septal defect (VSD) | 250 |
| 7.5/ | Atrioventricular canal defect | 251 |
| 7.6/ | Patent ductus arteriosus | 252 |
| 7.7/ | Left ventricular outflow tract obstruction | 253 |
| 7.8/ | Coarctation of the aorta (CoA) | 254 |
| 7.9/ | Right ventricular outflow tract obstruction | 256 |
| 7.10/ | Tetralogy of Fallot (TOF) | 257 |
| 7.11/ | Transposition of the great arteries (D-TGV) | 259 |
| 7.12/ | Congenitally corrected transposition of the great arteries (L-TGV) | 261 |
| 7.13/ | Ebstein's anomaly | 262 |
| 7.14/ | Marfan syndrome | 263 |
| 7.15/ | Fontan procedure | 265 |
| 7.16/ | Eisenmenger syndrome | 266 |
| 7.17/ | Cyanotic heart disease | 267 |
| 7.18/ | Anomalous pulmonary venous connection | 268 |
| 7.19/ | Congenital coronary artery anomalies | 268 |
| 7.20/ | Vascular annulus | 269 |
| 7.21/ | Cor triatriatum | 270 |
| 7.22/ | Heart disease in pregnant women | 270 |

# 7.1/ SEGMENTAL ASSESSMENT & FETAL CIRCULATION

## SEGMENTAL ASSESSMENT

**POSITION OF THE APEX: A)** Levocardia (apex points to the left); **B)** Dextrocardia (apex points to the right); **C)** Mesocardia (apex in the middle)

**ATRIAL SITUS (solitus; inversus; ambiguus)**: according to the position of the atrial appendages, IVC (which drains into the RA) and visceral situs

> **Right atrial appendage morphology:** large base, triangular shape, contains numerous pectinate muscles
> **Left atrial appendage morphology:** narrow base, finger-shaped

**AV CONNECTION: A)** Concordance: morphological LA connected to morphological LV (and RA connected to RV); **B)** Discordance

> **Right ventricle morphology:** moderator band, extensive trabeculations, infundibulum, tricuspid valve
> • **Tricuspid valve:** 3 leaflets - septal attachments - closer to apex than M valve - absence of distinct papillary muscles
> **Left ventricle morphology:** fine trabeculations; mitral valve
> • **Mitral valve:** 2 leaflets - mitro-aortic continuity - 2 papillary muscles - less apical than the T valve

**VENTRICULO-ARTERIAL CONNECTION: A)** Concordance: Morphological LV connected to the aorta; morphological RV connected to the PA; **B)** Discordance; **C)** Double-outlet (> 50 % of the aorta and PA arise from the same ventricle)

> **Aorta:** "Candy cane"; 3 vessels (innominate artery, left carotid artery, left subclavian artery); always associated with its aortic valve
> **Pulmonary trunk:** rapidly divides into RPA and LPA; always associated with its pulmonary valve

## FETAL CIRCULATION

1. **DUCTUS VENOSUS:** allows oxygenated umbilical blood to short-circuit the liver and reach the IVC

2. **FORAMEN OVALE:** allows blood derived from the IVC (part of which is derived from the placenta and is oxygenated) to go directly to the left heart (preferentially perfusing the coronary arteries and CNS)

3. **PATENT DUCTUS ARTERIOSUS:** allows blood (predominantly derived from the SVC) to go from the right heart to the descending aorta (to the placenta)

# 7.2/ ATRIAL SEPTAL DEFECT (ASD)

## 4 TYPES

1. **SECUNDUM ASD (80 %):** in the fossa ovale

2. **PRIMUM ASD (15 %):** close to AV valves; associated with AV canal defect

3. **SINUS VENOSUS ASD (5 %):** close to the origin of the SVC (exceptionally IVC); associated with anomalous pulmonary venous connection (R > L)

4. **CORONARY SINUS ASD (1 %):** communication between the coronary sinus and the LA; associated with persistent left SVC

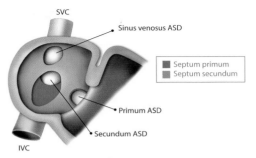

SVC

Sinus venosus ASD

■ Septum primum
■ Septum secundum

Primum ASD

Secundum ASD

IVC

**SIGNIFICANT ASD**: generally **> 10 mm with Qp/Qs > 1.5 : 1**

**ACCENTUATION OF L → R SHUNT**: in the presence of ↘ LV compliance or ↗ LA pressure (age; LVH; HTN; cardiomyopathy; myocardial infarction; MR...)

**LUTEMBACHER SYNDROME**: ASD + rheumatic MS

**HOLT-ORAM SYNDROME**: autosomal dominant; TBX5 mutation; abnormalities of hands; secundum ASD

**FEATURES**: left parasternal heave; palpable dilated PA (2ⁿᵈ left intercostal space); **fixed split S2**; pulmonary ejection murmur (↗ flow); tricuspid diastolic rumble in the presence of significant shunt; TR murmur in the presence of right heart failure

**ECG**

> **Secundum ASD: Incomplete RBBB; right axis deviation; RAH; Notch on R wave in inferior leads**                                                          +

> **Primum ASD: RBBB; left axis deviation; RAH**

> **Sinus venosus ASD: non-sinus rhythm (negative P wave in inferior leads)**

**CXR**: RA-RV dilatation; ↗ vascularization; prominent central PA

**TEE**: evaluate pulmonary venous return; ASD dimensions; possibility of percutaneous closure; agitated-saline PRN (R→L shunt = contrast in left chambers; L→R shunt = negative contrast in right chambers)

---

**COMPLICATIONS**

**a) Right heart failure (± TR) (volume overload)**

b) Atrial arrhythmias: typical flutter; IART; AF; SSS after repair

c) Paradoxical embolism

d) PHT (5-9%) (rarely severe)

**INDICATIONS FOR ASD CLOSURE**

**a) Dilatation of right chambers** (I;B)

**b) Paradoxical embolism** (IIa;C)

**c) Platypnea-orthodeoxia** (IIa;C)

d) PHT with marked L→R shunt > 1.5 : 1 or with significant reactivity to vasodilator (IIb;C)

e) Do not close if **irreversible PHT** with sPAP > 2/3 SBP or PVR > 2/3 SVR (III;C)

---

**PERCUTANEOUS CLOSURE:** possible if **secundum ASD < 38 mm with adequate margins** +
**(distance > 5 mm** from AV valves, coronary sinus, origin of SVC / IVC and right pulmonary veins)
**and with normal pulmonary venous return**

> ASA for 6 months after ASD closure; **complications** (1 %) → prosthesis embolization; erosion
(atrial wall or Ao); thromboembolism; arrhythmia - AF; endocarditis; tamponade

**PACEMAKER LEADS:** risk of paradoxical embolism if ASD not repaired

**PREGNANCY:** generally well tolerated; risk of paradoxical embolism

# 7.3/ PATENT FORAMEN OVALE (PFO)

**Absence of fusion of septum secundum and septum primum at birth**

25% of adults

**ASSOCIATION WITH CRYPTOGENIC STROKE:** possibility of paradoxical embolism

> **Risk factors:** PFO > 5 mm or spontaneous R→L shunt or atrial septal aneurysm or prominent
Eustachian valve

**DIAGNOSIS:** TEE with bubbles: **bubbles in ≤ 3 beats in left chambers;** facilitated by Valsalva +
maneuver

**TREATMENT OF CRYPTOGENIC STROKE:** highly controversial

1) First-line ASA; Warfarin if documented DVT (± closure of PFO)

2) If recurrence: anticoagulation vs percutaneous closure
   - No convincing evidence for the superiority of percutaneous closure versus medical
     treatment (equivocal results in ★ CLOSURE-I, ★ RESPECT and ★ PC)

**ANEURYSM OF INTERATRIAL SEPTUM: redundant and mobile portion of the atrial** +
**septum with excursion ≥ 15 mm** from the midline

# 7.4/ VENTRICULAR SEPTAL DEFECT (VSD)

## 4 TYPES

1) **SUBARTERIAL** (5%): below the Ao and P valves; associated with AR (due to leaflet prolapse);
   numerous synonyms (outlet; conal; subpulmonary; subaortic; infundibular; supracristal)

2) **MEMBRANOUS** (80%): membranous septum; adjacent to Ao and T valves

3) **AV CANAL (INLET):** below the AV valve (see AV canal defect)

4) **MUSCULAR** (15-20%): completely surrounded by muscle

| SUBARTERIAL VSD | MEMBRANOUS VSD | INLET VSD | MUSCULAR VSD |
|---|---|---|---|

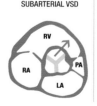

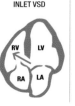

CLINICAL FEATURES AND SEVERITY: **Restrictive VSD** (RV pressure << LV pressure) or **nonrestrictive VSD** (RV pressure similar to LV pressure)

> **Small VSD**: normal LV dimensions; absence of PHT; **holosystolic murmur in left parasternal region (3rd-4th left intercostal spaces) with spoke-wheel radiation ± palpable thrill**; spontaneous closure is possible

> **Moderate VSD**: LA and LV dilatation (volume overload); PHT (reversible); ± mitral diastolic rumble; S3; lateralized apex

> **Large VSD**: Progressive PHT then Eisenmenger; **absence of VSD murmur; signs of PHT (left parasternal heave; ↗ and palpable P2; right S4; ejection click; Graham-Steel murmur and TR)**

---

### COMPLICATIONS

**a) Left heart failure (volume overload)**

b) PHT (± right heart failure due to pressure overload)

c) Progressive AR due to leaflet prolapse (subarterial VSD or membranous VSD)

d) Double chamber RV (muscle band develops as a result of the VSD jet, inducing subpulmonary stenosis)

e) Progressive subaortic stenosis

f) Arrhythmia: AF; PVCs; NSVT; postoperative AV block

g) Endocarditis

### INDICATIONS FOR VSD CLOSURE

**a) Significant VSD**: symptoms or progressive left ventricular dysfunction (volume overload) or right ventricular dysfunction (pressure overload) or Qp:Qs > 2:1 or sPAP > 50 mmHg (I;B)

b) Subarterial or membranous VSD with **AR ≥ moderate** (I;B)

c) In the presence of **severe PHT** (sPAP > 2/3 SBP or PVR > 2/3 SVR), closure should only be considered in the case of L→R shunt > 1.5:1 or significant reactivity to vasodilators (I;B)

d) **Double chamber RV**: significant obstruction (mean gradient > 40 mmHg or > 30 mmHg with symptoms)

e) Endocarditis (IIa;B)

---

**PERCUTANEOUS CLOSURE IS POSSIBLE: A)** Trabecular muscle VSD situated away from T or Ao valves; **B)** Membranous VSD situated away from the Ao valve

**PREGNANCY**: a small VSD is well tolerated in the absence of associated PHT or LV dysfunction

## 7.5/ ATRIOVENTRICULAR CANAL DEFECT

Developmental anomaly of endocardial cushions

a) **Partial atrioventricular canal defect:** intact interventricular septum; primum ASD; mitral cleft; AV valves inserted at same level (common annulus)

b) **Complete atrioventricular canal defect:** defect of the septum on either side of the cardiac crux: non-restrictive VSD (inlet VSD) and primum ASD; common atrioventricular orifice (one common AV valve with 5 leaflets)

> **Associated Down syndrome** (Trisomy 21): small stature, typical facies, mental retardation, brachydactyly, atlanto-axial instability, hypothyroidism, propensity to PHT, OSAHS

**ECG**: Complete or incomplete RBBB; **left axis deviation; spontaneous or postoperative AV block;** atrial arrhythmia

**VENTRICULOGRAPHY**: Elongated LVOT (goose neck deformity)

### COMPLICATIONS

   a) **Left and right AV valve regurgitation**
   b) **Left heart failure** (secondary to VSD and left AV valve regurgitation)
   c) **Right heart failure** (secondary to ASD and right AV valve regurgitation)
   d) PHT; Eisenmenger if not operated
   e) **Arrhythmias: AF; flutter; AV block**
   f) Progressive subaortic stenosis
   g) Paradoxical embolism
   h) Postoperative residual shunt
   i) Postoperative mitral stenosis

### INDICATIONS FOR SURGERY

#### Patient already operated

   a) **Hemodynamically significant** persistent or *de novo* defect (I;B)
   b) **Deterioration of LV function** (I;B)
   c) **Symptomatic left AV valve regurgitation** (I;B)
   d) **Symptomatic left AV valve stenosis** (post-repair) (I;B)
   e) **Subaortic obstruction** with mean gradient > 50 mmHg (I;B)
   f) Do not operate if **severe, irreversible PHT** (sPAP > 2/3 SBP or PVR > 2/3 SVR) (III;C)

# 7.6/ PATENT DUCTUS ARTERIOSUS

Connection between proximal pulmonary artery and descending aorta (distal to the left subclavian artery)

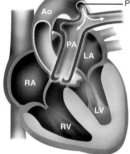

Patent ductus arteriosus

A) **SILENT DUCTUS ARTERIOSUS:** incidental finding on TTE

B) **SMALL PATENT DUCTUS ARTERIOSUS:** continuous murmur; minimal hemodynamic impact; Qp/Qs < 1.5:1

C) **MODERATE PATENT DUCTUS ARTERIOSUS: continuous machinery murmur in 2nd left intercostal space ± thrill; increased pulse pressure**; bounding pulse; LV dilatation (lateralized, hyperdynamic apex); S3; reversible PHT (induces ↘ duration of the murmur)

D) **LARGE PATENT DUCTUS ARTERIOSUS:** Severe PHT; Eisenmenger physiology; absence of continuous murmur; **differential hypoxemia and cyanosis (lower limbs cyanosed; clubbing of the toes)**       +

TTE: flow from aorta to PA visible on PLAX (RVOT/PA view); **diastolic flow reversal** in descending aorta

---

COMPLICATIONS

   a) **Left heart failure (volume overload)**

   b) Progressive PHT

   c) Arrhythmias (AF)

   d) Endarteritis / Ductus aneurysm

INDICATIONS FOR SURGERY

   a) **All cases of patent ductus arteriosus** except when silent or large with irreversible PHT (IIa;B)

   b) **Endarteritis** (IIa;B)

   c) In the presence of **severe PHT** (sPAP > 2/3 SBP or PVR > 2/3 SVR), closure should only be considered in the case of L→R shunt > 1.5:1 or significant reactivity to vasodilators (IIa;B)

---

PERCUTANEOUS CLOSURE: preferable in the case of ductus arteriosus < 8 mm (without aneurysm) or in the presence of calcification

PREGNANCY: similar considerations to those of VSD

# 7.7/ LEFT VENTRICULAR OUTFLOW TRACT OBSTRUCTION

## SUPRAVALVULAR AORTIC STENOSIS

**Fixed obstruction above the sinus of Valsalva**

CORONARY ARTERIES submitted to high pressures; risk of dilatation / ostial stenosis / early CAD; requires regular screening for CAD

WILLIAMS SYNDROME: autosomal dominant; 7q11.23 deletion; supravalvular aortic stenosis, peripheral pulmonary artery stenosis, renal artery stenosis, HTN, hypercalcemia, cognitive deficits, "cocktail" personality, elf-like facies

CLINICAL FEATURES: **BP right arm >> BP left arm (Coanda effect with preferential jet to innominate artery)**; crescendo-decrescendo systolic murmur; suprasternal thrill; **increased A2**; absence of ejection click; S4; peripheral PA stenosis can cause end-systolic or continuous posterior murmur

VENTRICULOGRAPHY: **"ballerina foot" pattern of LV**

---

INDICATIONS FOR SURGERY (patch aortoplasty or ascending aorta replacement or resection with end-to-end anastomosis)

   a) **Symptoms and/or mean gradient > 50 mmHg** (I;C)

   b) **Doppler instantaneous maximum gradient > 70 mmHg** if mild obstruction (I;C)

---

## VALVULAR AORTIC STENOSIS

BICUSPID AORTIC VALVE (▶▶| Chapter 4 - Valvular heart disease)

ASSOCIATED WITH: CoA; patent ductus arteriosus; ascending aortopathy

**ROSS PROCEDURE:** replace the aortic valve by the patient's pulmonary valve and replace the pulmonary valve by a cadaveric homologous graft; reimplantation of coronary arteries

> **Complications:** structural deterioration of the homologous P graft; aortopathy (specific to bicuspid aortic valve); AR; coronary stenosis

## SUBVALVULAR AORTIC STENOSIS

Discrete membrane or tunnel-shaped LVOT stenosis

**ASSOCIATED WITH:** AR (valvular damage caused by the high velocity jet); VSD; AV canal defect; Shone complex

> **Shone complex:** multiple stenoses at different levels: **A)** Supravalvular mitral annulus or parachute mitral valve; **B)** Subvalvular aortic stenosis; **C)** Bicuspid aortic valve; **D)** CoA

**DDX:** HCM (absence of SAM in subaortic stenosis)

**CLINICAL FEATURES:** crescendo-decrescendo systolic murmur ± thrill; **no radiation to the** +
**carotids; absence of ejection click; AR diastolic murmur**

---

INDICATIONS FOR SURGERY

  a) **Symptoms with Doppler instantaneous maximum gradient > 50 mmHg** or mean gradient > 30 mmHg (I;C)

  b) **Associated progressive AR** (I;C)

---

**MEMBRANE:** resection of the membrane ± myomectomy ± AVR

**TUNNEL:** **Konno procedure** (aortoventriculoplasty ± AVR)

> Complications: recurrence; AV block; iatrogenic VSD

# 7.8/ COARCTATION OF THE AORTA (COA)

**Stenosis in the region of the ligamentum arteriosum** (distal to the left subclavian artery)

**ASSOCIATED ABNORMALITIES:** Bicuspid aortic valve (80% of cases); aneurysm of the circle of Willis; collateral circulation (intercostal and mammary arteries); aortopathy; anomalous brachiocephalic circulation; aortic arch hypoplasia; VSD; Shone complex

> **Turner Syndrome** (45, X): CoA (35%); bicuspid aortic valve; ASD; VSD

**SIGNIFICANT COA (IN THE ABSENCE OF COLLATERAL):** **HTN in arms with trans-CoA** +
**gradient on catheterization > 20 mmHg or with SBP in arms ≥ 20 mmHg higher than SBP**
**in legs**

CLINICAL FEATURES

> **In the absence of collaterals:** HTN in arms; SBP in arms higher than in legs; radiofemoral delay on palpation of pulse; interscapular ejection murmur (rarely continuous); S4; ↗ A2; systolic click / systolic murmur in the presence of bicuspid aortic valve

> **In the presence of collaterals:** continuous crescendo-decrescendo murmur in left parasternal region or left scapula

**CXR: A) "3" sign:** indentation of the aorta at the site of CoA with distal and proximal dilatation; +
**B) Erosion of the ribs:** intercostal collaterals

**TTE:** turbulence and ↗ velocity in descending Ao (suprasternal view) with diastolic extension of anterograde flow

> **Abdominal aorta:** ↘ velocity of systolic flow and diastolic extension of anterograde flow

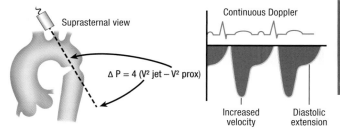

Suprasternal view

$$\Delta P = 4 (V^2 \text{ jet} - V^2 \text{ prox})$$

Continuous Doppler

Increased velocity

Diastolic extension

**MANAGEMENT**

a) Congenital cardiology follow-up for life

b) Control of BP (at rest and on exercise) and cardiovascular risk factors

c) BB if aortopathy

d) Imaging of the entire aorta (MRI) with regular follow-up (by TTE for ascending Ao / Ao valve and MRI for entire Ao)

e) Brain MRI (rule out aneurysm of the circle of Willis)

f) Avoid contact sports / isometric exercises if residual CoA or associated aortopathy

**COMPLICATIONS**

a) **Left heart failure (pressure overload)**

b) Persistent HTN

c) Aortopathy / Aortic dissection

d) Aortic valve disease

e) Early CAD and PAD

f) Intracranial aneurysms / Hemorrhage

g) Endarteritis

**INDICATIONS FOR SURGERY**

> **In the presence of significant CoA: peak-to-peak gradient ≥ 20 mmHg** on catheterization or less in the presence of collaterals (I;C)

**PERCUTANEOUS APPROACH** (dilatation + stenting): preferable in the majority of cases (except in the case of a long or tortuous lesion) and preferred technique in the presence of re-coarctation

> **Complications:** aortic dissection / rupture; stroke; aneurysm or pseudoaneurysm; aortobronchial fistula; re-CoA; persistent HTN

**SURGICAL OPTIONS:** resection with end-to-end anastomosis or graft placement; patch aorto-plasty; subclavian flap aortoplasty; bypass graft

> **Complications:** paraplegia; recurrent laryngeal nerve or phrenic nerve paralysis; dissection; aneurysm (post-patch aortoplasty); pseudoaneurysm; claudication of arms (subclavian flap aortoplasty); re-CoA; persistent HTN; endarteritis

**POST-REPAIR FOLLOW-UP:** Regular MRI and regular TTE

> Consider screening for intracranial aneurysms in the circle of Willis

**PREGNANCY:** pregnancy contraindicated if CoA not repaired (risk of IUGR - fetal loss - HTN); imaging of the entire Ao is necessary

# 7.9/ RIGHT VENTRICULAR OUTFLOW TRACT OBSTRUCTION

## SEVERITY

|  | MILD | MODERATE | SEVERE |
|---|---|---|---|
| Doppler instantaneous maximum gradient (mmHg) | < 36 | 36 - 64 | > 64 |
| Peak velocity (m/s) | < 3 | 3 - 4 | > 4 |

\* Doppler measurements not valid in the presence of long stenosis / tunnel stenosis

## SUPRAVALVULAR PULMONARY STENOSIS / PERIPHERAL PULMONARY ARTERY STENOSIS

**ASSOCIATED WITH**: TOF; Williams syndrome; Noonan syndrome; Alagille syndrome; VSD; Congenital rubella

**CLINICAL FEATURES: systolic ejection murmur (left parasternal region and posterior; increased by inspiration; sometimes continuous in peripheral pulmonary artery stenosis); absence of ejection click; increased or preserved P2; left parasternal heave**

## SUBVALVULAR PULMONARY STENOSIS

**Associated with VSD or TOF**

**DOUBLE CHAMBER RV:** mid-chamber obstruction secondary to a prominent muscle band; associated with VSD

## VALVULAR PULMONARY STENOSIS

**2 TYPES**

1) **Dome-shaped**: thin, pliable, mobile valve; fusion of commissures; post-stenotic dilatation of the PA
2) **Dysplastic (10-15%)**: thickened, immobile leaflets; associated with Noonan syndrome; absence of post-stenotic dilatation

**CLINICAL FEATURES:** Prominent a wave in jugular vein; left parasternal heave; crescendo-decrescendo systolic murmur ± thrill; **ejection click if the valve is pliable** (early if severe PS; absent in the presence of a dysplastic valve; ↘ **during inspiration** due to premature valve opening); delayed and decreased P2 (absent if severe PS); right S4; ± cyanosis (if ASD or PFO)

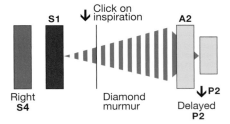

**Noonan syndrome**: autosomal dominant; dysplastic pulmonary valve, pulmonary artery stenosis, ASD, HCM, developmental delay, facial dysmorphism, small stature, congenital lymphedema

**LEOPARD syndrome**: autosomal dominant; lentigines, ECG abnormalities, ocular hypertelorism, pulmonary stenosis, abnormal genital organs, growth retardation, deafness, LVH

---

**POSSIBLE COMPLICATIONS**

> **RVH**
> Right heart failure ± TR
> Pulmonary regurgitation (postoperative)
> Pulmonary artery dilatation (post-stenotic)
> Cyanosis in the presence of associated ASD or VSD
> Atrial arrhythmia (AF / flutter) or ventricular arrhythmia

**INDICATIONS FOR SURGERY**

a) Balloon valvuloplasty for **dome-shaped valvular stenosis with symptoms and maximum Doppler gradient > 50 mmHg** or mean gradient > 30 mmHg (I;C)

b) Balloon valvuloplasty for **asymptomatic dome-shaped valvular stenosis and maximum Doppler gradient > 60 mmHg** or mean gradient > 40 mmHg (I;C)

c) **Surgery if significant RVOT obstruction with:** dysplastic valve or supravalvular stenosis or subvalvular stenosis or associated pulmonary hypoplasia or severe associated PR (I;C)

d) **Severe postoperative PR:** deterioration of functional class or deterioration of RV function or significant TR or flutter / AF or sustained ventricular arrhythmia (I;C)

e) **Valvular stenosis with**: significant arrhythmia or ASD / VSD (with R→L shunt) or recurrent endocarditis (IIa;C)

f) **Double chamber RV** with significant mid-chamber obstruction (gradient > 50 mmHg on catheterization) (IIa;C)

---

**PREGNANCY**: well tolerated if RV pressure < 70% of LV pressure; valvuloplasty as required during pregnancy in the presence of severe refractory symptoms (ideally after first trimester)

# 7.10/ TETRALOGY OF FALLOT (TOF)

**COMBINATION OF: A) Non-restrictive** (subarterial) VSD; **B)** RVOT obstruction (infundibular, valvular or supravalvular); **C)** RVH; **D)** Aorta overriding the septum

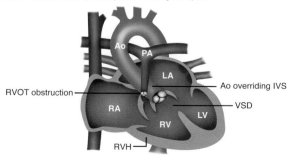

**CORRECTIVE SURGERY: A) Closure of the VSD; B) RVOT disobstruction; C)** ± infundibulectomy or subannular patch or transannular patch (induces significant PR) or RV - PA conduit (if congenital coronary artery anomalies crossing over the RVOT) or PVR or pulmonary valvotomy or pulmonary arterioplasty

**ASSOCIATED ABNORMALITIES:** right aortic arch; secundum ASD (pentalogy of Fallot); pulmonary trunk and peripheral pulmonary artery stenosis / hypoplasia; congenital coronary artery anomalies (LAD with ectopic origin crossing over the RVOT)

> **DiGeorge syndrome** (15% of TOF): 22q11 deletion; facial dysmorphism; hypocalcemia, thymus hypoplasia, immune deficit, psychiatric illness, truncus arteriosus, interrupted aortic arch, double outlet RV

**CLINICAL FEATURES (POST-CORRECTION):** left parasternal heave; soft ejection murmur (RVOT); subtle and soft diastolic pulmonary murmur (PR); ± absent P2; ± holosystolic murmur in the case of residual VSD; ± AR murmur

**ECG:** RBBB; wide QRS **(QRS > 180 ms is a risk factor for VT)**                  +

**INVESTIGATIONS: A)** TTE; **B)** MRI (RV and LV function and dimensions; PR; TR; RVOT; pulmonary arteries; shunt; Ao); **C)** Stress test (exercise capacity); **D)** Holter; **E)** Electrophysiological study PRN

**TTE:** Severe PR if **the continuous Doppler regurgitation envelope is dense and reaches**          +
**zero before the end of diastole** (equalization of pressures on either side of the valve) or if PHT
< 100 msec

---

**POST-CORRECTION COMPLICATIONS**

> **Pulmonary regurgitation**
> **RV dysfunction / RV dilatation (± TR)**
> Residual RVOT obstruction (subvalvular, valvular or supravalvular) / peripheral pulmonary artery stenosis (causing RV pressure overload)
> Residual VSD
> Infundibular aneurysm
> LV dysfunction
> Aortic root dilatation / Progressive AR
> Arrhythmia: atrial flutter; IART; AF; AV block
> VT (RVOT heavily scarred from surgical intervention); sudden death (0.2% year)
> Endocarditis

**INDICATIONS FOR POST-CORRECTION SURGERY (IIA;C)**

a) **Severe PR** with: symptoms or moderate-to-severe RV dilatation (**end-diastolic volume**        +
   **> 170 mL/m²; end-systolic volume > 85 mL/m²**) or moderate-to-severe RV dysfunction
   (**RVEF < 45 %**) or moderate-to-severe TR or atrial or ventricular arrhythmia

b) **Residual VSD** with shunt > 1.5:1

c) **Moderate to severe RVOT obstruction** (peak Doppler gradient > 50 mmHg)

d) **Severe AR** with symptoms or LV dysfunction

e) **Aortic root > 55 mm**

f) **RVOT aneurysm or false aneurysm**

g) **Combination** of residual VSD and/or residual PS and PR inducing RV dilatation / dysfunction
   or symptoms

---

**SURGICAL OPTIONS: A)** PVR (bioprosthesis or cadaver) ± tricuspid annuloplasty; **B)** Percutaneous pulmonary valve inserted into a pre-existing RV-PA conduit; **C)** Infundibular resection or RVOT patch or transannular patch or valved conduit if obstruction persists

**VENTRICULAR ARRHYTHMIA: Risk factors: A)** Inducible VT on EPS; **B)** QRS > 180 ms; **C)** History of palliative shunt; **D)** Significant PR or RVOT obstruction; **E)** Advanced age at the time of complete correction; **F)** NSVT on Holter; **G)** RV or LV dysfunction; **H)** Syncope; **I)** Severe RV dilatation (> 150-180 ml/m²)

> **Secondary prevention**: ICD indicated
> **Primary prevention**: indication for ICD determined on an individual basis according to the risk of sudden death (risk of frequent inappropriate shocks)

**PREGNANCY**: risk of right heart failure in the presence of RVOT obstruction and/or severe PR and/or RV dysfunction; screen for 22q11 deletion

# 7.11/ TRANSPOSITION OF THE GREAT ARTERIES (D-TGV)

Atrioventricular concordance and ventriculoarterial discordance (the RA is connected to the morphological RV which is connected to the Ao; the LA is connected to the morphological LV which is connected to the PA); incompatible with life in the absence of operation (2 parallel circuits)

**POSITION OF THE AORTA**: anterior and to the right of the PA (connected to the RV)

**ASSOCIATED ABNORMALITIES**: VSD; LVOT obstruction; ASD; CoA; congenital coronary artery anomalies

## ATRIAL SWITCH: MUSTARD (OR SENNING) PROCEDURE

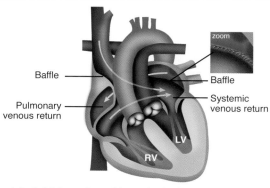

The majority of adults have undergone this procedure (but this operation was replaced by arterial switch in about 1990); the blood is redirected to the atria by means of a conduit (baffle) made from pericardium or Dacron allowing physiological correction (systemic venous blood is redirected towards the subpulmonary LV; pulmonary venous blood is redirected towards the subaortic RV)

**CLINICAL FEATURES:** Single S2 (loud A2; P2 is inaudible as the PA is posterior); left parasternal heave; holosystolic murmur of the systemic AV valve

**ECG**: RVH; block - bradycardia; atrial arrhythmia

**CXR**: Egg-shaped heart (narrow mediastinum due to parallel great vessels); retrosternal aorta (lateral view)

**TTE**: Ao and PA are parallel; phasic flow in the baffle with **peak velocity < 1 m/s**; agitated-saline to evaluate baffle leak or stenosis

## COMPLICATIONS

a) **Systemic RV failure (+ TR)**

b) Systemic RV ischemia (perfused only by the RCA)

c) Systemic AV valve regurgitation (abnormal septal geometry)

d) Obstruction of the baffle (SVC; IVC)

e) Baffle leak (paradoxical embolism; cyanosis)

f) Subpulmonary obstruction (abnormal LV geometry)

g) Arrhythmias: atrial flutter; IART; SSS; AV block

h) VT - Sudden death (risk factors: RV dysfunction; age; supraventricular arrhythmia; QRS > 140 ms)

### INDICATIONS FOR POST-MUSTARD SURGERY (IIA;C)

a) **Moderate-to-severe systemic AV valve regurgitation**

b) **SVC or IVC obstruction** (dilatation + stent in baffle)

c) **Pulmonary vein obstruction** (post-Senning procedure)

d) **Baffle leak with:** significant shunt (Qp:Qs > 1.5:1) or symptoms or PHT or progressive ventricular dilatation / dysfunction or need for pacemaker transvenous lead or R→L shunt with cyanosis (percutaneous closure of the leak)

e) **Symptomatic tachyarrhythmia:** ablation

f) **Bradyarrhythmia:** pacemaker with endovenous lead in the absence of baffle stenosis or baffle leak

g) **Consider transplant** if severe systemic RV dysfunction

**PREGNANCY:** avoid pregnancy in the presence of moderate-to-severe systemic RV dysfunction and/or severe systemic AV valve regurgitation

## ARTERIAL SWITCH: JATENE PROCEDURE

Switching of the Ao and PA; the PA is replaced anteriorly (Lecompte maneuver); the coronary arteries are reimplanted; the LV becomes subaortic

### COMPLICATIONS

a) Obstruction of the aorta and pulmonary artery at the sites of surgical anastomosis

b) Subpulmonary or PA or pulmonary arterial branch obstruction following Lecompte maneuver

c) Aortic root dilatation / AR

d) Stenosis of the coronary ostia (regular screening for CAD is indicated)

### INDICATIONS FOR POST-JATENE SURGERY (IIA;C)

a) **Significant PA obstruction (subvalvular, supravalvular or arterial branch)**

b) **Coronary artery obstruction**

c) **Severe AR**

d) **Severe Ao dilatation > 55 mm**

## RASTELLI PROCEDURE

For treatment of D-TGV with VSD and RVOT obstruction

**PROCEDURE: A)** LVOT tunneled to the Ao by an intracardiac patch through the VSD; **B)** RV - PA extracardiac valved conduit

**DOUBLE DISCORDANCE** (atrioventricular and ventriculoarterial): the circulation is corrected physiologically; the morphological RV is systemic (subaortic)

**POSITION OF THE AORTA:** anterior and to left of the PA

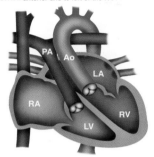

**ASSOCIATED ABNORMALITIES: abnormalities of the systemic T valve (Ebstein-like malformation);** VSD; PS; dextrocardia

**ECG:** AV block (fragile His bundle wich is displaced anteriorly and laterally); septal activation from R to L (septal Q waves absent on left precordial leads, but present on right precordial and inferior leads); accessory pathway

**CLINICAL FEATURES:** Palpable A2 (anterior Ao); inaudible P2 (posterior PA); holosystolic murmur due to systemic AV valve regurgitation

**COMPLICATIONS**

a) **Progressive systemic AV valve regurgitation (T valve)**

b) **Progressive systemic RV dysfunction**

c) Systemic RV ischemia (only perfused by the RCA)

d) **Complete AV block (2% / year)**

e) **Atrial arrhythmia:** AF; IART; accessory pathway

f) VT - sudden death

**INDICATIONS FOR SURGERY**

a) Moderate-to-severe systemic AV valve **regurgitation** (IIa;B)

b) **Deterioration of the systemic RV** (IIa;C): consider heart transplantation

**PREGNANCY:** avoid pregnancy if RVEF < 40% and/or moderate-to-severe TR

Apical displacement of the tricuspid valve **> 8 mm/m²** (septal and posterior leaflets) with     +
elongated / redundant anterior leaflet; atrialized RV (small volume functional RV)

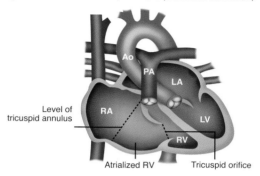

Level of
tricuspid annulus

Atrialized RV                    Tricuspid orifice

**ASSOCIATED ABNORMALITIES: A)** Accessory pathway(s) (25% of patients; 50% have multiple pathways); **B)** secundum ASD or PFO ± cyanosis (50% of patients); **C)** RVOT obstruction (by T valve); VSD; mitral valve disease

**CLINICAL FEATURES:** ± V wave in jugular veins (often absent due to severe RA dilatation); left parasternal heave; split S1 with ↗ T1; split S2 (RBBB); right S3; lower left parasternal holosystolic murmur (↗ on inspiration); systolic clicks; ± cyanosis; low output state; signs of right heart failure

**ECG: RA dilatation (Himalayan P waves)**; low voltage; ± pre-excitation; RBBB; Q waves in V1 (as far as V4) and inferior leads; AF - flutter

**CXR:** "water bottle heart": RA dilatation and left convexity (dilatation of the RV infundibulum); ↘ vascularization

---

**COMPLICATIONS**

a) **Severe TR**

b) **Right heart failure / Dilatation of right chambers**

c) Arrhythmias: flutter; AF; AT; accessory pathway(s)

d) Sudden death (pre-excited atrial arrhythmia or VT)

e) Cyanosis - paradoxical embolism in the presence of PFO or ASD

f) RVOT obstruction due to the abnormal tricuspid valve

g) Tricuspid stenosis or prosthetic valve dysfunction post-surgery

**INDICATIONS FOR SURGERY (I;B)**

a) **Severe TR** with NYHA III - IV or deterioration of functional class

b) **Progressive RV dysfunction or dilatation**

c) **Progressive cardiomegaly** on CXR (cardiothoracic ratio > 65%)

d) **Cyanosis** with resting SaO2 < 90% (closure of ASD)

e) **Paradoxical embolism** (closure of ASD)

f) **Arrhythmia / WPW**: ablation by catheter or surgical cryoablation

---

REPAIR: feasibility according to: **A) Length and mobility of the anterior leaflet (creation of a monoleaflet valve); B) Size of the residual RV > 1/3 of total RV**

OTHER SURGICAL OPTIONS
> **Conventional TVR**
> **Bidirectional cavopulmonary connection** (bidirectional Glenn): decreases preload and workload of the small RV
> **Fontan procedure in** the presence of a hypoplastic RV
> **Heart transplantation**

PREGNANCY: well tolerated in the absence of cyanosis / right heart failure / arrhythmia

# 7.14/ MARFAN SYNDROME

**Autosomal dominant; FBN1 gene mutation (> 1,000 mutations have been reported)**

COMPLICATIONS: Aortic root dilatation; aortic dissection; AR; MVP - MR; left heart failure; tricuspid valve prolapse - TR

MANAGEMENT

a) BB ($\searrow$ dP/dT) and ARB

b) Target SBP < 120 mmHg (BB; ARB)

c) Avoid isometric exercise - competitive / contact sports

d) MRI indicated to evaluate all of the aorta; regular follow-up is recommended

| TTE FOLLOW-UP | MRI OR CT ANGIOGRAPHY |
|---|---|
| Annually | Every 3 to 5 years (more frequent if dilatation / imminent indication for surgery / 1 year postop / recent dissection) |

INDICATIONS FOR SURGERY (I;B)

a) **Ascending aorta > 50 mm**

b) **Ao > 45 mm**: with: progression > 5 mm/year or progressive AR with probable valve preservation or family history of aortic dissection with Ao < 50 mm or severe MR requiring surgery

c) **Ao > 40 mm before pregnancy**

d) **Other regions of the Ao** between 50-60 mm or progressive dilatation

SURGICAL OPTIONS: **A) Bentall procedure**: replacement of ascending Ao with valved graft; **B) David procedure:** replacement of the ascending Ao with graft and resuspension of the native aortic valve (valve sparing)

PREGNANCY: risk of transmission (autosomal dominant); MRI imaging of the entire Ao; TTE every 4-8 weeks; BB; avoid $\nearrow$ dP/dT during delivery; cesarean section if unstable aorta (> 40-45 mm)
> **Pregnancy contraindicated if Ao > 45 mm** (risk of aortic dissection)                    +
> **If Ao ≥ 40 mm**: referral for sugery is recommended if contemplating pregnancy

| SYSTEM | MAJOR CLINICAL SIGNS | MINOR CLINICAL SIGNS | DEFINITION OF SYSTEM INVOLVEMENT |
|---|---|---|---|
| **Skeletal** | • *Pectus carinatum*<br>• Surgical *Pectus excavatum*<br>• Long limbs<br>  ➤ Arm span to height ratio > 1.05 or<br>  ➤ ↘ Upper segment to lower segment ratio<br>• Long fingers<br>  ➤ Wrist sign and thumb sign<br>• Scoliosis > 20° or spondylolisthesis<br>• Maximum elbow extension < 170°<br>• Flat foot<br>• Acetabular protrusion (hip x-ray) | • Moderate *Pectus excavatum*<br>• Joint hypermobility<br>• Arched palate with overlapping teeth<br>• Characteristic facies | **Major**<br>≥ 4 major signs<br><br>**Minor**<br>≥ 2 major signs<br>or<br>1 major and 2 minor signs |
| **Ocular** | • Lens dislocation | • Flat cornea<br>• Elongated eyeball<br>• Myopia | **Major**<br>1 major sign<br><br>**Minor**<br>≥ 2 minor signs |
| **Cardio-vascular** | • Aortic root dilatation<br>• Aortic dissection | • MVP<br>• Pulmonary trunk dilatation < 40 years<br>• MAC < 40 years<br>• Dilatation or dissection of the descending thoracic aorta or abdominal aorta < 50 years | **Major**<br>≥ 1 major sign<br><br>**Minor**<br>≥ 1 minor sign |
| **Pulmonary** | | • Spontaneous pneumothorax<br>• Apical bulla (CXR or CT) | **Minor**<br>≥ 1 minor sign |
| **Cutaneous** | | • *Striae atrophicae* (unexplained)<br>• Recurrent incisional herniae | **Minor**<br>≥ 1 minor sign |
| **Dura mater** | • Lumbosacral dural ectasia (CT or MRI) | | **Major**<br>1 major sign |
| **Genetic** | • 1 first-degree relative with diagnostic criteria<br>• FBN1 gene mutation causing Marfan | | |

**Diagnosis established:**
- 1 system with major involvement + 1 system with minor involvement + 1 genetic criterion
- 2 systems with major involvement + 1 system with minor involvement

*Lœys BL, Dietz HC, Braverman AC, et al. J Med Genet 2010; 47:476-485*

Palliative procedure in the presence of a single ventricle (anatomical or functional); systemic venous return redirected to PA, short-circuiting the subpulmonary ventricle

**PREREQUISITES:** **Mean PAP < 15 mmHg** with normal-sized PA, normal function of the single ventricle, absence of any significant AV valve regurgitation

**STEPS OF THE MODIFIED FONTAN PROCEDURE: 1) Bidirectional cavopulmonary connection (bidirectional Glenn):** connection between the SVC and R or L pulmonary arteries; **2) Connection of IVC to PA** (lateral conduit or extracardiac conduit or intracardiac conduit) with pulmonary trunk ligation

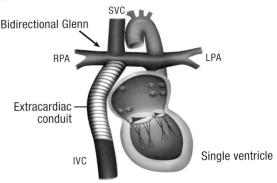

**FACTORS OF HEMODYNAMIC DETERIORATION**

a) Any ↗ filling pressure of the systemic ventricle
b) Obstruction to systemic venous return (thrombosis or obstruction of Fontan; ↗ PVR; pulmonary arteries stenosis; pulmonary vein compression)
c) Arrhythmia (risk of hemodynamic deterioration and thrombus)

**CLINICAL FEATURES:** JVD but nonpulsatile; single S1 and S2; absence of murmur (except in the case of AV valve regurgitation or subaortic obstruction); hepatomegaly / leg edema / ascites

---

**COMPLICATIONS**

a) **Intra-Fontan thrombus:** predisposed by stasis and atrial arrhythmia; leads to Fontan obstruction / pulmonary embolism / paradoxical embolism
b) **Fontan obstruction** (at anastomotic sites or by thrombus)
c) **Right pulmonary vein compression** by the interatrial septum or the dilated RA
d) **Arrhythmia:** IART; flutter; AF; SSS; AV block
e) **Cyanosis in the presence of a R→L shunt:** systemic venous collateral to pulmonary veins; pulmonary AVM; residual ASD; fenestrated Fontan; hepatopulmonary syndrome
f) **Ventricular dysfunction / systemic AV valve regurgitation**
g) **Protein-losing enteropathy:** anasarca; diarrhea; ↗ fecal alpha-1-antitrypsin and hypoalbuminemia
h) **Congestive hepatopathy** (or even cardiac cirrhosis)

---

## MANAGEMENT

a) **A/C** if thrombus or stasis or thromboembolism or ASD or fenestration or atrial arrhythmia

b) **Single-ventricle failure:** consider ACE inhibitors - BB; sildenafil; transplant; mechanical support

c) **Aggressive treatment of atrial arrhythmias:** look for a hemodynamic cause; TEE prior to ECV; AAD; A/C; catheter ablation; conversion to extracardiac Fontan with intraoperative Maze

d) **When a pacemaker is indicated:** epicardial ventricular lead

e) **Protein-losing enteropathy:** diuretics - aldactone; eliminate obstruction or arrhythmia; dietary support; IV albumin; corticosteroids; sildenafil; Fontan fenestration; transplant

## INDICATIONS FOR REOPERATION (I;C)

a) **Obstruction** to systemic venous return (revision of the Fontan or angioplasty / stenting or conversion of Fontan or thrombectomy)

b) **Obstruction** to pulmonary venous return (conversion to extracardiac Fontan)

c) Moderate-to-severe systemic AV valve **regurgitation**

d) **Symptomatic cyanosis** with venovenous collaterals or pulmonary AVM (catheter occlusion)

e) Residual ASD or fenestrated Fontan with significant R→L shunt (percutaneous closure)

f) **Subaortic stenosis** with peak-to-peak gradient > 30 mmHg

g) **Protein-losing enteropathy** with Fontan obstruction (revision of the Fontan or angioplasty / stenting) or with elevation of systemic venous pressures (consider fenestration)

h) **Symptomatic and refractory atrial arrhythmia** (conversion to extracardiac Fontan with intraoperative Maze)

**PREGNANCY:** increased risk of all Fontan-specific complications; risk of spontaneous abortion / IUGR / prematurity; follow-up by an experienced, multidisciplinary team

# 7.16/ EISENMENGER SYNDROME

Obstructive pulmonary vascular disease secondary to communication between pulmonary and systemic circulations (L→R shunt), leading in the long term to irreversible elevation of PAP and PVR (to systemic levels) and reversal of the shunt (R→L)

**CLINICAL FEATURES:** Central cyanosis (differential cyanosis in the presence of patent ductus arteriosus); clubbing; JVD (prominent A wave; prominent V wave in the presence of TR); signs of PHT

**ECG:** RAH; RVH; right axis deviation; atrial arrhythmia

**CXR:** dilatation of central pulmonary arteries ± calcification; dilatation of right chambers

## COMPLICATIONS

a) RV dysfunction

b) **Complications of cyanotic heart disease:** erythrocytosis; bleeding; CRF; hyperuricemia / gout; cholelithiasis

c) Intrapulmonary hemorrhage / hemoptysis

d) Pulmonary artery aneurysm

e) Pulmonary artery thrombosis / Pulmonary embolism

f) Stroke - TIA; paradoxical embolism

g) Brain abscess

h) Arrhythmias: AF; flutter; VT

i) Sudden death

j) Endocarditis

## MANAGEMENT

a) Correct iron deficiency, when present
b) Aggressive treatment of arrhythmia
c) Noncardiac surgery: multidisciplinary preoperative assessment in a tertiary institution
d) Pregnancy contraindicated
e) Avoid dehydration - hemorrhage - anemia
f) Avoid NSAID - vasoactive agents (which ↗ the shunt and cyanosis) - estrogens - nephrotoxins
g) Air filter on IV lines
h) Avoid vigorous physical exercise
i) Dental hygiene and prophylactic antibiotics
j) Investigate hemoptysis (CXR; CBC; CT scan; embolization PRN)
k) Influenza - pneumococcus vaccination

### TREATMENT OF PHT

a) First-line endothelin antagonists (Bosentan; Macitentan)
b) PDE-5 inhibitors or prostanoids

**LUNG ± HEART TRANSPLANT:** in the case of refractory symptoms with estimated 1-year survival < 50%; contraindicated in the presence of multiple pleuropulmonary collaterals

# 7.17/ CYANOTIC HEART DISEASE

R→L shunt (deoxygenated blood enters the systemic circulation); chronic hypoxemia

### SECONDARY ERYTHROCYTOSIS (↗ EPO)

> **Hyperviscosity (Hct > 65% and Hb > 20 g/dL):** headache; faintness; tiredness; disorders of concentration; visual disorders; paresthesia; tinnitus; myalgia; intraoperative bleeding
  • **Treatment:** phlebotomies (if patient is iron-repleted and well hydrated)
  • **Treat any iron deficiency** (as microcytosis can cause hyperviscosity and is a risk factor for stroke); beware of rebound effect
> **Bleeding / clotting abnormalities** (if severe bleeding: FFP; vitamin K; cryoprecipitates; DDAVP; platelets)

**OTHER COMPLICATIONS:** Stroke - TIA; cerebral hemorrhage; paradoxical embolism; brain abscess; CRF; proteinuria; hyperuricemia; gout; hypertrophic osteoarthropathy (arthralgia); scoliosis; cholelithiasis

> Beware of nephrotoxic agents, including contrast agents

**BASIC WORK-UP:** SaO₂; CBC; ferritin; transferrin; iron saturation; ± folate; ± vitamin B12; PT-PTT; renal function; uric acid

**PALLIATIVE SHUNTS** (systemic to pulmonary): objective: improve pulmonary blood flow and cyanosis

> **Blalock-Taussig:** subclavian artery to pulmonary artery (modern: graft connecting the two arteries, preserving perfusion of the upper limb)
> **Waterston:** Ascending Ao to right PA
> **Potts:** Descending Ao to left PA
> **Physical examination:** Continuous murmur (except in the presence of stenosis / occlusion / significant PHT)
> **Complications:** PHT; distortion of PAs; stenosis / aneurysm at the site of anastomosis; heart failure (volume overload); arrhythmias

## 7.18/ ANOMALOUS PULMONARY VENOUS RETURN

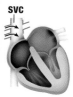

**SVC**

RPV TO SVC
(WITH SINUS
VENOSUS ASD)

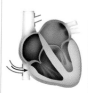

RPV TO IVC
(SCIMITAR)

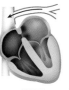

LPV TO
INNOMINATE VEIN

Coronary
sinus

LPV TO CORONARY
SINUS

**CONSEQUENCES AND CLINICAL FEATURES:** similar to ASD

**INDICATION FOR SURGERY:** dilatation of right chambers

**SCIMITAR SYNDROME: pulmonary veins (right lung) drain into the IVC; scimitar appearance on CXR;** ± hypoplasia of right lung

## 7.19/ CONGENITAL CORONARY ARTERY ANOMALIES

### ECTOPIC ORIGIN OF A CORONARY ARTERY

1 % of the population

**CLINICAL FEATURES:** sudden death; retrosternal chest pain; arrhythmia; LV dysfunction; syncope

**DETECTION:** coronary CT angiography (or cardiac MRI); cholelithiasis

> Look for ventricular arrhythmia during exercise testing

**INDICATIONS FOR SURGERY**
(reimplantation; marsupialization)

a) Coronary artery coursing between the great vessels with **documented ischemia** (I;B)
b) Ectopic origin of **LMCA** (opposite sinus) coursing between the Ao and the PA (I;B)
c) Ectopic origin of the **right coronary artery** (opposite sinus) coursing between the Ao and the PA with documented ischemia (I;B)
d) Ectopic origin of the **LAD** coursing between the Ao and the PA (IIb;C)

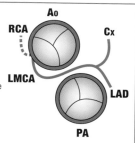

### ALCAPA SYNDROME

Anomalous left coronary artery arising from the pulmonary artery

**CLINICAL FEATURES:** ischemia; LV dysfunction; MI; ventricular arrhythmia; sudden death; may be well tolerated in the presence of collaterals of the RCA

**INDICATIONS FOR SURGERY** (coronary reimplantation)
> All patients with **ALCAPA syndrome** (I;C)

## CORONARY ARTERIOVENOUS FISTULA

Communication between a coronary artery and a heart chamber (RA; RV) or a vein (coronary sinus; vena cava; pulmonary vein) or sometimes the PA

**CLINICAL FEATURES:** continuous left parasternal murmur

**COMPLICATIONS**

a) Dilatation of the nutrient coronary artery
b) Rupture - dissection
c) Myocardial ischemia distal to the fistula
d) Endarteritis
e) Left heart failure

**INDICATIONS FOR SURGERY** (percutaneous closure by embolization or surgical closure)

a) Large fistula - Qp:Qs > 1.5 : 1 (I;C)
b) Small to moderate fistula with: ischemia or arrhythmia or LV dysfunction or LV dilatation or endarteritis (I;C)

## CONGENITAL SINUS OF VALSALVA ANEURYSM

**RUPTURE:** Sudden chest pain and dyspnea; continuous AV shunt with possible left and right heart failure; bounding pulse; continuous murmur ± thrill

a) Ruptured aneurysm of the right sinus of Valsalva: Ao - RVOT fistula
b) Ruptured aneurysm of the non-coronary sinus: Ao - RA fistula
c) Ruptured aneurysm of the left sinus of Valsalva: Ao - LA fistula

**DDX:** Infectious (endocarditis); Inflammatory - Vasculitis; Marfan; Iatrogenic

## MYOCARDIAL BRIDGE ("MILKING")

**Intramyocardial coronary segment** (usually LAD)

Compression of the coronary segment with each systole

**CONSEQUENCES:** usually none; sometimes ischemia - angina - LV dysfunction - arrhythmia / VT - sudden death

**MANAGEMENT:** BB; CCB; PCI or CABG if severe refractory ischemia

# 7.20/ VASCULAR RING

Malformation of the aortic arch associated with **compression of the esophagus and/or trachea** (dysphagia, respiratory symptoms, stridor)

a) Double aortic arch
b) Right aortic arch; associated with Kommerell's diverticulum compressing the trachea (diverticulum at the junction of the left subclavian artery and the descending aorta)
c) Aberrant origin of the right subclavian artery (posterior to the esophagus)
d) Retroesophageal descending aorta (compression of the trachea)

Adult congenital heart disease & heart disease in pregnant women

## 7.21/ COR TRIATRIATUM

Fibromuscular diaphragm dividing the LA into two chambers

Severity varies according to the degree of stenosis; nonobstructive form (benign) versus obstructive form (leads to PHT)

Management similar to that of MS

## 7.22/ HEART DISEASE IN PREGNANT WOMEN

### HEMODYNAMIC CHANGES DURING PREGNANCY

| HEMODYNAMIC CHANGES | CONSEQUENCES |
|---|---|
| ↗ 40-50% of plasma volume | Risk of congestion |
| ↗ 10-20% of HR | Poorly tolerated MS |
| ↗ 30-50% of cardiac output | |
| ↘ Peripheral resistance (especially ↘ DBP) | Tolerated poorly stenotic lesions (increased gradient) |
| ↗ Venous pressure in legs | Risk of stasis / DVT |
| Hypercoagulability | Increased thromboembolic risk |

### NORMAL PHYSICAL EXAMINATION OF THE PREGNANT WOMAN

↗ HR; normal or slightly ↗ CVP; Hyperdynamic state (pulse; apex); Apex may be broadened and slightly lateralized; leg edema is frequent

Accentuated S1 - accentuated splitting; S2 may appear to be constantly split at the end of pregnancy; S3 is frequent; left parasternal ejection murmur ≤ 3/6; continuous murmur (cervical venous "hum" or breast murmur)

### MATERNAL RISK OF CARDIAC EVENTS

**STRESS TEST**: high-risk pregnancy if < 70% of predicted functional capacity

**CARPREG SCORE** (1 point each):

| | |
|---|---|
| 1) History of heart failure - TIA - Stroke - Arrhythmia<br>2) NYHA ≥ III or cyanosis<br>3) Mitral valve area < 2 cm² or Aortic valve area < 1.5 cm² or LVOT gradient > 30 mmHg<br>4) Systemic ventricle systolic function < 40% | Risk of cardiac event during pregnancy:<br>• 0 point: 5 %<br>• 1 point: 27 %<br>• ≥ 2 points: 75 % |

\* Does not take PHT - mechanical valve - aortopathy into account

*Siu SC, Sermer M, Colman JM, et al. Circulation 2001; 104:515–521.*

### STAGE I: LOW-RISK PREGNANCY

- Uncomplicated, small or mild PS or patent ductus arteriosus or MVP
- Successfully repaired simple lesions (ASD; VSD; patent ductus arteriosus; anomalous pulmonary venous drainage)
- Isolated APC and PVC

### STAGE II: MILD-TO-MODERATE RISK PREGNANCY

- Unrepaired ASD or VSD
- Repaired TOF
- Most arrhythmias

*Stage II or III, depending on severity*
- Mild LV dysfunction
- HCM
- Valvular heart disease not considered to be WHO stage I or IV
- Marfan syndrome without Ao dilatation
- Bicuspid aortic valve with Ao < 45 mm
- Repaired CoA

### STAGE III: HIGH-RISK PREGNANCY (EXPERT FOLLOW-UP RECOMMENDED)

- Mechanical valve
- Systemic RV
- Fontan
- Cyanotic heart disease
- Complex congenital heart disease
- Marfan: Ao 40-45 mm
- Bicuspid aortic valve: Ao 45-50 mm

### STAGE IV: PREGNANCY CONTRAINDICATED

- **Severe pulmonary arterial hypertension**
- **Severe LV dysfunction (LVEF < 30% - NYHA III or IV)**
- **Previous peripartum cardiomyopathy with residual impairment of LV function**
- **Severe MS or severe AS**
- **Marfan: Ao > 45 mm**
- **Bicuspid aortic valve: Ao > 50 mm**
- **Unrepaired CoA**

## BICUSPID AORTIC VALVE STENOSIS

**Pregnancy contraindicated if ascending Ao > 50 mm (or > 25 mm/m²)**

> In the presence of Ao dilatation: TTE every 4-8 weeks; BB

**SEVERE AORTIC STENOSIS**: avoid pregnancy (particularly if symptoms or LV dysfunction or abnormal stress test); risk of hemodynamic instability during delivery; percutaneous valvuloplasty PRN in the presence of severe symptoms

## MITRAL STENOSIS

Moderate-to-severe MS is poorly tolerated; deterioration due to tachycardia and ↗ cardiac output; risk of pulmonary congestion and PHT

BB (Metoprolol); valvuloplasty PRN if refractory NYHA III-IV

## MITRAL REGURGITATION AND AORTIC REGURGITATION

Generally well tolerated if moderate regurgitation / NYHA ≤ II / normal LV function and dimensions

Diuretics and vasoactive agents PRN; Surgery if refractory NYHA III-IV

## PROSTHETIC VALVE

**Follow-up by an experienced multidisciplinary team**

**MECHANICAL VALVE**: significant maternal and fetal risks
> Thromboembolic risk (hypercoagulability of pregnancy)
> Risk associated with anticoagulation (fetal loss; placental hemorrhage; insufficient anticoagulation; embryopathy; management during delivery)

**UNFRACTIONATED HEPARIN (IV OR SC)**: less effective than warfarin; adjusted according to aPTT 6h post-injection (> 2 x normal)

**LMWH**: bid; dose according to **anti-Xa level 4 h post-injection (target: 0.8-1.2 IU/mL)**; review once a week; replace by unfractionated heparin > 36 h before delivery

**WARFARIN**: risk of embryopathy during the first trimester (4-10%); **lower risk with Warfarin ≤ 5 mg daily**

---

**WARFARIN DOSE ≤ 5 MG QD**: **continue Warfarin; replace by unfractionated heparin at the end of pregnancy prior to planned delivery**

**WARFARIN DOSE > 5 MG QD**: **LMWH or IV Heparin during first trimester; replace by Warfarin for 2nd and 3rd trimesters; then replace by unfractionated heparin prior to planned delivery**

---

## CYANOTIC HEART DISEASE

**Pregnancy contraindicated if SaO$_2$ < 85 %**

R→L shunt increased by ↘ peripheral resistance

Maternal hypoxia alters fetal growth and survival

## PULMONARY HYPERTENSION

Pregnancy contraindicated in the presence of severe pulmonary hypertension

**EISENMENGER: maternal mortality as high as 50%**                    +

## DILATED CARDIOMYOPATHY

**Avoid pregnancy if LVEF < 40%**

## PERIPARTUM CARDIOMYOPATHY

**DEFINITION**: "Idiopathic" cardiomyopathy with LV systolic dysfunction occurring around the last month of pregnancy or during the first 5 months post-partum

> Diagnosis of exclusion

**RISK FACTORS:** twin pregnancy, African American mother, advanced age, pre-eclampsia, smoking

**MANAGEMENT: A)** Hydralazine / Nitrates; **B)** BB (avoid Atenolol and Carvedilol; prefer beta-1 selective BB; Metoprolol is the best studied BB during lactation); **C)** Digoxin; **D)** Diuretics; **E)** Anticoagulate if intracardiac thrombus or LVEF < 35% or concomitant Bromocriptine

> ACE inhibitors (Captopril; Enalapril) are safe while breastfeeding

> Possible benefit of post-partum Bromocriptine (2-5 mg/day)

> Continue therapy with standard HF medications for ≥ 12 months

**Normalization of LVEF in 50% of women** (2 to 6 months)

Avoid subsequent pregnancy **(30% recurrence rate)**

## HYPERTROPHIC CARDIOMYOPATHY

Autosomal dominant; variable penetrance

High-risk pregnancy if symptoms at baseline or significant baseline LVOT gradient

## HYPERTENSION

**PRE-EXISTING HTN:** before pregnancy or < 20 weeks; rule out CoA

**GESTATIONAL HYPERTENSION:** *de novo* HTN (> 20 weeks after start of pregnancy); BP > 140/90 on 2 occasions; absence of proteinuria; returns to normal during the first 12 weeks postpartum

> **Management:** Labetalol; Methyldopa; Nifedipine

**PRE-ECLAMPSIA:** gestational HTN with the presence of proteinuria **(> 300 mg/24 h or > 30 mg/mmol on urine spot test)**

> **Risk factors:** primiparous; twin pregnancy; ≥ 40 years; BMI ≥ 35 kg/m²; family history of preeclampsia

> **Clinical features:** headache, blurred vision, abdominal pain, thrombocytopenia, abnormal LFTs, hemolysis, hyperreflexia - clonus, seizures, acute pulmonary edema, stroke

> **Management:** rest; sodium restriction; magnesium sulphate; delivery; IV Labetalol; Methyldopa; Nifedipine; IV Nitroglycerin; target SBP 140 to 160 mmHg and DBP 90 to 105 mmHg

## ATRIAL FIBRILLATION

Anticoagulant according to embolic risk

**CONTROL HR:** Digoxin; BB (Metoprolol); CCB (Verapamil)

**CONTROL RHYTHM:** ECV; CCV (Procainamide); Flecainide / Sotalol

Continuous fetal monitoring during intervention / AAD

## SUPRAVENTRICULAR TACHYCARDIA

**ACUTE:** Vagal maneuver or Adenosine or ECV; Metoprolol PRN; IV Procainamide; Continuous fetal monitoring during intervention

**PROPHYLAXIS:** Metoprolol or Digoxin; Flecainide / Sotalol PRN; Verapamil or ablation as 3rd line

## CONTRACEPTION

Avoid estrogens in women with cyanotic heart disease, AF or flutter, mechanical prosthetic valve, Fontan, thromboembolic history or LVEF < 40%

- Bonow RO, Mann DL, Zipes DP, Libby P. *Braunwald's Heart Disease. A textbook of cardiovascular medicine.* Saunders Elsevier. 2012. 1961 p.
- Marelli A, Beauchesne L, Mital S et al. Canadian cardiovascular society 2009 consensus conference on the management of adults with congenital heart disease: Introduction. *CJC*; 2010; *26:* e65-e69.
- Silversides CK, Dore A, Poirier N et al. Canadian cardiovascular society 2009 consensus conference on the management of adults with congenital heart disease: Shunt lesions. *CJC*; 2010; *26:* e70-e79.
- Silversides CK, Kiess M, Beauchesne L et al. Canadian cardiovascular society 2009 consensus conference on the management of adults with congenital heart disease: Outflow tract obstruction, coarctation of the aorta, tetralogy of Fallot, Ebstein anomaly and Marfan's syndrome. *CJC*; 2010; *26:* e80-e97.
- Silversides CK, Salehian O, Oechslin E et al. Canadian cardiovascular society 2009 consensus conference on the management of adults with congenital heart disease: Complex congenital cardiac lesions. *CJC*; 2010; *52:* e80-e97.
- ACC/AHA 2008 Guidelines for the Management of Adults With Congenital Heart Disease; *JACC* 2008; *52;* e143-e264
- 2008 Focused Update Incorporated Into the ACC/AHA 2006 Guidelines for the Management of Patients With Valvular Heart Disease. *JACC;* 2008; *52;* e1-e142.
- ESC Guidelines for the management of grown-up congenital heart disease (new version 2010). *EHJ.* 2010; *31:* 2915-57.
- Tobis J., Shenoda M. Percutaneous Treatment of Patent Foramen Ovale and Atrial Septal Defects. *JACC* 2012; *60;* 1722-32
- ESC Guidelines on the management of cardiovascular diseases during pregnancy. *EHJ.* 2011; *32;* 3147-97
- Khairy P, Van Hare GF, Balaji S et al. PACES/HRS Expert Consensus Statement on the Recognition and Management of Arrhythmias in Adult Congenital Heart Disease. *CJC* 2014; *30;* e1-e64.
- Congenital heart disease in the older adult: a scientific statement from the AHA. *Circulation* 2015; *131;* 1884-1931.
- Elkayam U. Clinical Characteristics of Peripartum Cardiomyopathy in the United States. *JACC* 2011; *58:* 659-670
- Otto, CM. *Textbook of clinical echocardiography.* Saunders Elsevier. 2009. 519 p.
- Johnston, SC. Patent Foramen Ovale Closure - Closing the Door Except for Trials. *NEJM* 2012; *366:* 1048-1050.
- UpToDate 2015

# Peripheral Vascular Disease

## 08

| 8.1/ | Aneurysm of the thoracic aorta | 276 |
| 8.2/ | Acute aortic syndrome | 279 |
| 8.3/ | Abdominal aortic aneurysm (AAA) | 282 |
| 8.4/ | Other aortic diseases | 283 |
| 8.5/ | Peripheral artery disease (PAD) | 285 |
| 8.6/ | Atherosclerotic renovascular disease | 289 |
| 8.7/ | Cerebrovascular disease | 290 |
| 8.8/ | Pulmonary embolism | 295 |
| 8.9/ | Heparin-induced thrombocytopenia (HIT) | 300 |
| 8.10/ | Pulmonary hypertension | 301 |

## 8.1/ ANEURYSM OF THE THORACIC AORTA

**ANEURYSM:** permanent and localized dilatation of an artery; **diameter > 150 %** of normal  +
diameter (for age / gender / BSA)
> **Ectasia**: arterial dilatation < 150% of normal diameter
> **Pseudo-aneurysm (false aneurysm)**: **rupture** of arterial wall contained by hematoma  +
and adjacent tissues

NORMAL DIMENSIONS

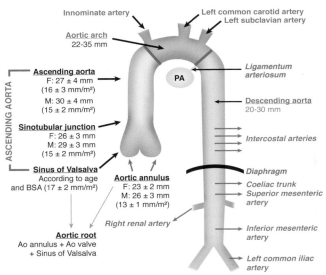

Innominate artery

Left common carotid artery
Left subclavian artery

Aortic arch
22-35 mm

PA

Ligamentum
arteriosum

**Ascending aorta**
F: 27 ± 4 mm
(16 ± 3 mm/m²)
M: 30 ± 4 mm
(15 ± 2 mm/m²)

Descending aorta
20-30 mm

ASCENDING AORTA

**Sinotubular junction**
F: 26 ± 3 mm
M: 29 ± 3 mm
(15 ± 2 mm/m²)

Intercostal arteries

**Sinus of Valsalva**
According to age
and BSA (17 ± 2 mm/m²)

**Aortic annulus**
F: 23 ± 2 mm
M: 26 ± 3 mm
(13 ± 1 mm/m²)

Diaphragm
Coeliac trunk
Superior mesenteric
artery

Right renal artery

**Aortic root**
Ao annulus + Ao valve
+ Sinus of Valsalva

Inferior mesenteric
artery

Left common iliac
artery

### RISK FACTORS

> **Atherosclerotic / Degenerative** (media degeneration): HTN; smoking; COPD; family history
> **Congenital**: Bicuspid aortic valve; Tetralogy of Fallot; CoA; VSD; Transposition of great arteries
> **Genetic**: Marfan; Ehlers-Danlos type IV; Turner; Loeys-Dietz; Noonan; Familial thoracic aortic aneurysm syndrome
> **Inflammatory**: Takayasu; Giant cell arteritis; Behçet; Ankylosing spondylitis; Spondyloarthropathies; SLE; Sarcoidosis
> **Infectious**: Syphilis; Salmonella; Staphylococcus; HIV

**PRESENTATION:** Asymptomatic; Aortic dissection; Aortic rupture; AR; Infectious aortitis; Compressive symptoms (recurrent laryngeal nerve; trachea; esophagus; SVC syndrome); Pain (neck; jaw; back; interscapular); Embolism (thrombus or cholesterol crystals); Fistula (aortoesophageal; aortobronchial)

**ECHOCARDIOGRAPHY:** diameter at end-diastole using the leading-edge of the anterior  +
wall to the leading of the posterior wall

**CT SCAN AND MRI:** measurement of outer diameter  +

**CXR:** large mediastinum; prominent aortic knob; trachea deviated to the right

# MANAGEMENT

**RISK FACTOR CONTROL:** HTN; Lipids; Smoking

**BB AND ACE INHIBITORS / ARB**

**AVOID ISOMETRIC EXERCISES**

| INDICATIONS FOR SURGERY – ASCENDING AORTIC ANEURYSM | |
|---|---|
| Degenerative ascending aortic aneurysm | ≥ 55 mm |
| Progressing aneurysm | > 5 mm / year |
| Symptomatic aneurysm | Compressive symptoms; Pain |
| Ao valve or CABG surgery | > 45 mm |
| Bicuspid aortic valve | > 55 mm (or > 50 mm with family history of dissection or progression ≥ 5 mm / year) |
| Marfan | 40-50 mm (▶▶| Genetic aortic syndromes) |
| Marfan or Genetic Syndrome or Bicuspid aortic valve | Maximum Ao area (cm²) / Patient's height (m) > 10 |
| Lœys-Dietz | ≥ 42 mm (TEE) or ≥ 44 mm (CT or MRI) |
| Turner | > 25 mm/m² |

| SURVEILLANCE – ASCENDING AORTIC ANEURYSM | |
|---|---|
| Aneurysm 35 - 44 mm | • Ensure stability with follow-up assessment 6 months after diagnosis<br>• Stable → Imaging every 1-3 years **(progression ≈ 1 - 2 mm / year)** |
| Aneurysm 45 - 54 mm | Imaging after 3-6 months (stability) then every 6-12 months |
| Pregnancy | Imaging every 6-8 weeks (until 3 months postpartum) |

# ANEURYSM OF AORTIC ARCH

**SURGERY:** requires profound hypothermia and circulatory arrest; temporary cerebral perfusion via the right axillary artery

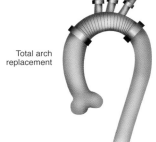

Total arch replacement

SURGICAL OPTIONS: Resection of the proximal hemi-arch; Total arch replacement; Stent with reimplantation of innominate arteries...

> **Elephant trunk procedure**: aneurysm of the aortic arch and descending aorta; allows subsequent stenting of the descending aorta

| MANAGEMENT – ANEURYSM OF THE AORTIC ARCH | |
|---|---|
| Isolated aneurysm of the aortic arch > 55 mm or compressive symptoms | Surgery (if acceptable surgical risk) |
| Aneurysm of the aortic arch < 40 mm | Imaging every 1-2 years |
| Aneurysm of the aortic arch > 40 mm | Imaging every 6-12 months |

---

# ANEURYSM OF THE DESCENDING THORACIC AORTA

| MANAGEMENT – ANEURYSM OF THE DESCENDING THORACIC AORTA | |
|---|---|
| Degenerative or traumatic aneurysm > 55 mm | TEVAR (when technically feasible) |
| Chronic dissection + [refractory symptoms or aneurysm > 55 mm or progression of diameter > 4 mm/year] | TEVAR (open surgery when TEVAR is contraindicated) |

SURGICAL PROCEDURE: CPB with retrograde femoral perfusion

> Risk of spinal cord ischemia

THORACIC ENDOVASCULAR AORTIC REPAIR (TEVAR): **stent deployment requires a normal aortic segment > 20 mm above and below the aneurysm (with diameter < 40 mm) and adequate vascular access**

> **Contraindications**: Severe Ao atherosclerosis (risk of atheroembolism); severe PAD (limiting femoral access)
> **Regular long-term surveillance following TEVAR**: CTscan or MRI after 1, 6 and 12 months and then yearly (or every 2 years if stable course)
> **Complications**: Stroke; Atheroembolism; Spinal cord ischemia; Paraplegia; MI; Ventricular arrhythmia; ARF; Transformation from type B to type A dissection; Stent fracture; Stent migration; Infection; Occlusion of arterial branches (subclavian; mesenteric; celiac trunk; renal)
>   • **Endoleak**: persistence of blood flow outside of the stent lumen towards the aneurysm sac

| TYPE I ENDOLEAK | Reperfusion and filling of the aneurysm sac via a leak in the proximal or distal portion of the stent (requires treatment) |
|---|---|
| TYPE II ENDOLEAK | Retrograde flow in the aneurysm sac via a branch artery (intercostal; lumbar; mesenteric) (observation) |
| TYPE III ENDOLEAK | Separation of stent components (fracture; separation) (requires treatment) |

### AORTIC DISSECTION

Tear of the media with bleeding inside the media and along the arterial wall

**Acute aortic syndrome**

Ao
dissection

Intramural
hematoma

Penetrating
atherosclerotic ulcer

| STANFORD CLASSIFICATION | |
|---|---|
| **Type A** | Involves the ascending Ao |
| **Type B** | No involvement of the ascending Ao |
| **DEBAKEY CLASSIFICATION** | |
| **Type I** | Ascending Ao → extends at least to the aortic arch (± descending Ao) |
| **Type II** | Confined to the ascending Ao |
| **Type III** | Confined to the descending Ao |

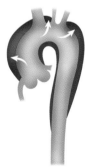

**Type A Ao dissection**
Involvement of the ascending Ao
(Surgical management)

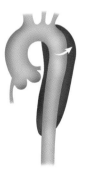

**Type B Ao dissection**
No involvement of the ascending Ao
(Initially medical treatment)

| ↗ AORTIC STRESS | DEGENERATION OF THE MEDIA |
|---|---|
| • Aortic aneurysm<br>• Aortic valve disease<br>• HTN<br>• CoA<br>• Recent aortic intervention<br>• Trauma / Deceleration<br>• Pheochromocytoma<br>• Cocaine<br>• Weightlifting<br>• Penetrating ulcer<br>• Infectious aortitis | ↗ metalloproteinases;<br>↘ elastic fibers; ↗ proteoglycans<br><br>• **Degenerative / Atherosclerotic**<br>• **Genetic**: Marfan; Ehlers-Danlos type IV; Bicuspid aortic valve; Turner; Loeys-Dietz; Familial thoracic aortic aneurysm and dissection<br>• **Vasculitis**: Takayasu; Giant cell arteritis; Behçet<br>• **Other**: Pregnancy; Polycystic kidneys; Chronic corticosteroid therapy |

PRESENTATION: Acute - severe - tearing pain; Retrosternal pain (type A) or back pain (type B)

> **Target organ ischemia:** Myocardial infarction; Stroke - TIA; Spinal cord ischemia (paraplegia / paraparesis) or mesenteric or renal or lower limbs; Ischemic neuropathy

> **Hemorrhagic**: Tamponade; Hemothorax; Hemomediastinum; Aortopulmonary or aorto-enteric or aorto-esophageal fistula

> **Aortic regurgitation**: Mechanisms: **A)** Aortic root dilatation (malcoaptation); **B)** Dissection involving a leaflet implantation site (leaflet prolapse); **C)** Transvalvular prolapse of the dissection flap; **D)** Underlying AR (bicuspid aortic valve)

CLINICAL FEATURES: Hypotension or Normotension or Hypertension (**measure BP in both arms**); Absent pulses (evaluate pulses in all extremities); **AR murmur**; Signs of tamponade; Neurological deficits; Abdominal signs

TEE: Dissection flap separating the true lumen and the false lumen (with independent movement); two flows on either side of the dissection flap on color Doppler; thrombus in the false lumen; look for the entry site and/or exit site of the dissection; pericardial effusion; myocardial ischemia (RWMA); AR; coronary ostia

| | TRUE LUMEN | FALSE LUMEN |
|---|---|---|
| **Size** | True < False | False > True |
| **Pulsation** | Systolic expansion | Systolic compression |
| **Direction of flow** | Anterograde (systolic) | Retrograde or<br>↘ Anterograde systolic flow |
| **Thrombus** | Rare | Common |
| **Contrast agent** | Rapid opacification | Delayed opacification |

a) **Aortic shadow** abnormal and enlarged
b) **Large mediastinum**: AP CXR → **> 8 cm at the carina**
c) **Calcium sign**: separation between calcification of the aortic intima and the lateral wall of the aortic knob **> 10 mm**
d) **Pleural effusion** (inflammatory reaction or hemothorax)
e) **Deviation of the trachea** towards the right (or deviation of the esophagus - NGT)
f) **Pulmonary edema** (AR)

**PREOPERATIVE CORONARY ANGIOGRAPHY**: it is reasonable not to perform coronary angiography in acute aortic syndrome, which constitutes a surgical emergency (class IIa recommendation)

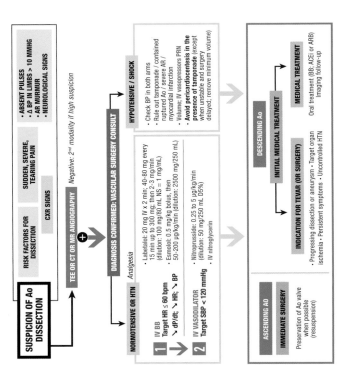

POSTOPERATIVE COMPLICATIONS: Aneurysm formation (at the site of dissection or at the site of anastomosis or elsewhere); Recurrent dissection; Graft dehiscence; Pseudoaneurysm; AR; Infection; Progression of false lumen

FOLLOW-UP BY CT ANGIOGRAPHY OR MR ANGIOGRAPHY: 1-3-6-12-18-24 months; then annually   **+**

> **Tybe B aortic dissection:** TEVAR or surgical repair if aneurysm > 55-60 mm or > 4 mm/year growth or target organ ischemia or recurrent pain

AVOID ISOMETRIC EXERCISES; CONTROL BP

## SPONTANEOUS INTRAMURAL HEMATOMA

Medial tear with bleeding inside the media, but absence of communication with the aortic lumen (absence of false lumen)

> Can propagate in an anterograde or retrograde fashion
> **May have an identical clinical presentation to that of aortic dissection**

IMAGING: Intramural thrombus; Enlarged wall **> 5 mm** (crescent-shaped or circular); Absence   **+** of flow (contrast) in wall

COURSE: Resolution or stabilization or aneurysm formation or progression to aortic dissection or aortic rupture

MANAGEMENT: Similar to aortic dissection (for corresponding segment)

a) **Ascending Ao →** urgent surgery
b) **Descending Ao →** initial medical treatment; Indication for TEVAR (or surgery) according to aortic diameter or persistent symptoms or progression or compromise of branches (with ischemia)

## PENETRATING ATHEROSCLEROTIC ULCER

Penetration of the aortic wall by an atherosclerotic ulcer (± secondary intramural hematoma); descending aorta in the majority of cases

COMPLICATIONS: Aortic dissection; Aortic rupture; Distal embolism (thrombus or cholesterol crystals); Aneurysm

MANAGEMENT

a) **Ascending Ao →** Surgery should be considered
b) **Descending Ao →** Initial medical treatment; Indication for TEVAR (or surgery) according to aortic diameter or persistent symptoms or progression or deteriorating associated intramural hematoma

# 8.3/ ABDOMINAL AORTIC ANEURYSM (AAA)

ANEURYSM: **Abdominal Ao diameter > 30 mm**

> Predominantly occurs in the infrarenal aorta
> Degeneration of the media ( ↗ metalloproteinases)
> **Risk factors**: Smoking; Family history; Age; Male gender; COPD; dyslipidemia; HTN

PRESENTATION: Asymptomatic; Embolism; Rapid expansion; Pain; Compression or erosion of adjacent structures; Rupture

ABDOMINAL ULTRASOUND: High sensitivity and specificity

> **Screening**: Male, 65 to 74 years with history of smoking; Male ≥ 60 years with family history of AAA

MANAGEMENT: Smoking cessation; treatment of HTN - dyslipidemia - DM; Surveillance of AAA

AAA REPAIR: Surgical or Percutaneous (EVAR) in a patient with **life expectancy > 2 years** +

| MANAGEMENT – ABDOMINAL AORTIC ANEURYSM | |
|---|---|
| Indication for aneurysm repair (EVAR or open surgery) | • ≥ 55 mm or<br>• Symptoms (pain) or<br>• Progression > 10 mm per year (> 5 mm over 6 months) or<br>• Infectious or inflammatory |
| AAA 30-39 mm | Surveillance every 3 years (progression ≈ 3 mm per year) |
| AAA 40-44 mm | Surveillance every 2 years |
| AAA > 45 mm | Surveillance every year |

EVAR: endovascular AAA repair (for infra-renal AAA); anatomical suitability → proximal aortic neck (segment between the lowest renal artery and the proximal extent of the aneurysm) > 10-15 mm of length (and < 32 mm in diameter); adequate vascular access required

★ EVAR and ★ DREAM: surgical versus endovascular AAA repair; ↘ operative mortality with EVAR; **similar long term mortality; ↗ reintervention with EVAR** +

SURGICAL AAA REPAIR SHOULD BE PREFERRED: anatomical criteria for EVAR not met or when regular long-term surveillance is impossible

> **Regular long-term surveillance following EVAR:** CT angiography or MR angiography at 1 month - 6 months - then annually; look for endoleakage, stent position, stability and exclusion of the aneurysm sac, stent fracture
> **Late complications of surgery**: para-anastomotic aneurysm; graft infection; graft-enteric fistula; imaging every 5 years

PATIENTS NOT CANDIDATES FOR SURGERY: **significant comorbidities → no benefit of EVAR on long term survival (★EVAR 2)**

# 8.4/ OTHER AORTIC DISEASES

## AORTIC ATHEROSCLEROTIC PLAQUE

COMPLEX PLAQUE: **Plaque thickness ≥ 4 mm or mobile / pedunculated debris (= thrombus) or ulceration** +

> ↗ embolic risk
> **Site**: particularly in the distal aortic arch and descending aorta

EMBOLISM: spontaneous or iatrogenic (post-intervention)

> **Thrombus (thromboembolism)**: thrombus forms on an unstable plaque then embolizes to a medium-to-large artery (stroke; TIA; leg ischemia; renal or splenic infarction; mesenteric ischemia)
>   • Consider anticoagulation if complex plaque in aortic arch with stroke / TIA (class IIb)
> **Cholesterol crystals (atheroembolism)**: crystal emboli to small arterioles ("blue toe"; retinal ischemia / Hollenhorst plaques; TIA; Confusion; ARF; HTN; *Livedo reticularis*; Petechiae; Purpura; Intestinal ischemia; Pancreatitis)
>   • **Hypocomplementemia; Eosinophilia**
>   • **Consider endarterectomy or stent** in the presence of an identified source of embolism and recurrent atheroembolism

MANAGEMENT: Secondary prevention; ASA - Statin - control HTN / DM; smoking cessation

| SYNDROME | DETAILS | FOLLOW-UP | MANAGEMENT |
|---|---|---|---|
| Marfan | • FBN1 mutation<br>• Dilatation of aortic root **(annulo-aortic ectasia)** and ascending Ao; **Type A dissection**<br>• Ghent diagnostic criteria ▶▶| - Chapter 7 | • TTE at diagnosis and after 6 months (stability) then every 6-12 months<br>• Follow-up by imaging of the entire aorta following repair of the ascending Ao | • BB; Losartan<br>• **Surgery: A)** > 50 mm; **B)** Progression > 5 mm/y; **C)** Family history of dissection < 50 mm;<br>**D)** Significant AR<br>• **Desire for pregnancy**: surgery if ≥ 40 mm |
| Lœys-Dietz | • Autosomal dominant<br>• TGFBR1 or 2 mutation<br>• Tortuosities / aneurysms / artery dissection<br>• Hypertelorism; Cleft palate or bifid uvula<br>• **Aneurysm of the aortic root; Aortic dissection** | • Imaging of the entire aorta at diagnosis and after 6 months (stability)<br>• **Annual MRI of the cerebrovascular circulation and as far as the pelvis** | • **Surgery if ascending Ao ≥ 42 mm (TEE; inner diameter) or ≥ 44 mm (CT or MRI; outer diameter)** |
| Ehlers-Danlos Type IV | • Autosomal dominant (COL3A1)<br>• **Risk of artery rupture** (including thoracic and abdominal aorta)<br>• **Risk of rupture of the uterus / intestine** | | • Role of prophylactic repair remains uncertain (friable tissues)<br>• Follow-up by imaging |
| Turner | • 45, X<br>• Small stature; Ovarian insufficiency<br>• **Bicuspid aortic valve (20%); CoA (10%); Ao aneurysm; Ao dissection** | • Look for risk factors of aortic dissection (bicuspid aortic valve / CoA / dilatation of thoracic Ao / HTN)<br>• **In the presence of risk factors:** annual TTE<br>• **Otherwise:** TTE every 3-5 years | • Surgery if maximum Ao area (cm²) / patient's height (m) > 10<br>• Surgery if diameter > 25 mm/m² |
| Non-syndromic familial thoracic aortic aneurysm and dissection | • Non-syndromic<br>• Autosomal dominant<br>• Variable penetrance<br>• **Genes identified:** TGFBR1 and 2; ACTA2; MYH11; MYLK; PRKG1 | • **Family screening:** 1st degree relatives of patients with unexplained dissection or aneurysm<br>• **Genetic testing** if several family members are affected | • TGFBR mutation: similar management to that of Loeys-Dietz |

# VASCULITIS WITH AORTIC INVOLVEMENT

Destruction of vessels (inflammation; ↗ metalloproteinases; granulomas)

| | |
|---|---|
| **Takayasu** | • **Vasculitis of the aorta and its branches (stenosis and/or aneurysm)**<br>• **Diagnostic criteria**: < 40 years; Claudication (upper limbs or lower limbs); ↘ Brachial pulse; Aortic or subclavian murmur; sBP Difference > 10 mmHg arms; Stenosis of the Ao or its branches (CT angiography or MR angiography)<br>• **Treatment**: Prednisone 50 mg; MTX; Azathioprine; Anti-TNFalpha |
| **Giant cell arteritis (temporal arteritis)** | • **Vasculitis of the aorta and its branches**<br>• **Diagnostic criteria**: > 50 years; de novo headache; tenderness over temporal artery (or ↘ pulse); ↗ ESR (> 50 mm/h); Positive biopsy<br>• Constitutional symptoms; Claudication of the jaw; Claudication of upper limbs; Visual symptoms; PMR; Aortic aneurysm / dissection<br>• **Treatment**: Prednisone 50 mg |
| **Behçet** | • **Diagnostic criteria**: Mouth ulcers; Genital ulcers; Uveitis or retinal vasculitis; Erythema nodosum; Pseudofolliculitis; Pathergy<br>• **Arterial involvement**: destruction of the media; aneurysm ± rupture (any artery can be affected) |
| **Ankylosing spondylitis** | • HLAB27+<br>• **Diagnostic criteria**: < 40 years; Low back pain; Morning stiffness; Slow progression; Improvement with exercise<br>• AR; Dilatation of the aortic root |

# TRAUMATIC AORTIC RUPTURE

Predominantly involves the **aortic isthmus** (deceleration injury)

BP in arms > BP in legs; radiofemoral delay; interscapular murmur

CXR: widened mediastinum; displaced nasogastric tube (hematoma); Dilatation of the aortic arch / descending aorta; pleural effusion

MANAGEMENT: TEVAR if suitable anatomy (or open surgery)

# INFECTIOUS AORTITIS

Contiguous invasion or septic embolism (endocarditis) or hematogenous spread

SITE: on a pre-existing aortic lesion (aneurysm; atherosclerotic plaque; site of iatrogenic injury); predominantly involves the infrarenal aorta

MICROORGANISMS: S. aureus; Salmonella; Streptocoque; E. coli; Neisseria; Fungi; TB; Syphilitic aortitis (10-25 years post-infection)

COMPLICATIONS: saccular aneurysm; fistula; pseudo-aneurysm; rupture

# 8.5/ PERIPHERAL ARTERY DISEASE

PAD: **cardiovascular risk equivalent to that of CAD**
> **5-year mortality**: 10-15% (75% from cardiovascular causes)

RISK FACTORS: Smoking; DM; HTN; Dyslipidemia; Age; CRF; Chronic inflammation

**PRESENTATION:** Asymptomatic; Intermittent claudication; Critical limb ischemia

**CLINICAL FEATURES:** ↘ pulse; murmur; pallor on elevation; ↗ erythema of limb in dependent position; coldness; muscle atrophy; hair loss; onychodystrophy; skin fissures; ulcers; devitalization - gangrene

| FONTAINE CLASSIFICATION | |
|---|---|
| I | Asymptomatic |
| II | Intermittent claudication |
| IIa | Claudication > 200 m |
| IIb | Claudication < 200 m |
| III | Rest pain / night pain |
| IV | Ulcer / Gangrene |

**DDX:** vasculitis (thromboangiitis obliterans; Takayasu; giant cell arteritis); CoA; fibromuscular dysplasia; external compression; radiotherapy; neurogenic claudication (lumbosacral radiculopathy); arthritis; myositis; venous insufficiency; popliteal artery entrapment syndrome

## ANKLE-BRACHIAL INDEX

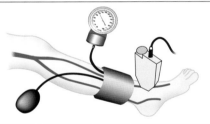

| ABI ≤ 0.90 | ABI 0.91 - 0.99 | ABI 1.0 - 1.4 | ABI > 1.4 |
|---|---|---|---|
| **Abnormal** | **Gray zone** | **Normal** | **Calcified noncompressible artery** |
| • Mild: 0.8-0.9<br>• Moderate: 0.5-0.8<br>• Severe: < 0.5 | ABI on exercise if persistent suspicion of PAD: diagnosis of vascular claudication if ABI ↘ by > 20-25 % | | DM / CRF / Age → Use toe-brachial index (diagnostic if < 0.7) |

**ABI:** ratio of sBP in ankle (posterior tibial artery or dorsalis pedis artery) / brachial artery

**INDICATION FOR ABI:** suspicion of PAD in the leg with:

> Suspected claudication; Poor wound healing; ≥ 50 years + [DM or Smoking]; ≥ 65 years; intermediate Framingham score

**OTHER EXAMINATIONS:** segmental BP measurements; Doppler US; MR angiography; CT angiography; Angiography

**MANAGEMENT OF RISK FACTORS:** Smoking cessation; Statin; Treatment of DM (HbA1c < 7%); Control of BP; ACE inhibitors (★ HOPE)

**ASA:** ↘ mortality - stroke - myocardial infarction (★ Antithrombotic Trialists' Collaboration)

> **Indications**
>   a) Symptomatic patient (claudication; critical limb ischemia; history of revascularization; history of amputation) (class I recommendation)
>   b) Asymptomatic patient with ABI ≤ 0.90 (class IIa recommendation); limited evidence
> **Clopidogrel as alternative treatment**: superior to ASA in ★ CAPRIE; marginal benefit of ASA and Clopidogrel combination in ★ CHARISMA

**SUPERVISED EXERCISE PROGRAM:** 30-45 min; 3 x / week; > 12 weeks; ↗ exercise capacity

**CILOSTAZOL (100 MG PO BID):** phosphodiesterase-3 inhibitor; ↘ platelet aggregation; direct arterial vasodilator; contraindicated in the presence of heart failure; beware of drug interactions

**PENTOXIFYLLINE (400 MG PO TID):** phosphodiesterase inhibitor; ↘ blood viscosity; ↗ erythrocyte deformability; marginal efficacy

**REVASCULARIZATION:** Indications → **A)** Symptoms refractory to medical treatment with impaired quality of life; **B)** Critical limb ischemia

| | | |
|---|---|---|
| **Aorto-iliac** | • First-line endovascular revascularization (with stent) (TASC II type A - B - C)<br>• Surgical revascularization: aortofemoral bypass graft with Dacron or PTFE prosthesis; femorofemoral bypass graft; axillofemoral bypass graft | |
| **Femoro-popliteal** | • First-line endovascular revascularization (TASC II type A - B - C)<br>• Stenting for intermediate length (TASC type II B)<br>• Surgical revascularization: femoropopliteal bypass graft preferably with autologous venous conduit (or PTFE prosthesis) | |
| **Infra-popliteal (below the knee)** | • Revascularization in the presence of persistent critical limb ischemia despite proximal revascularization<br>• First-line endovascular revascularization<br>• Stenting if suboptimal result<br>• Surgical revascularization: femorotibial or femoroperoneal bypass graft (autologous venous conduit) | |

Labels: Aorta; Iliac; Common femoral; Deep femoral; Superficial femoral; Popliteal; Anterior tibial; Peroneal; Posterior tibial; Dorsalis pedis

> **Mode of revascularization**: first-line endovascular treatment in most cases; decision by multidisciplinary team according to anatomy / durability / comorbidities / local expertise / patient preference
>   • **Percutaneous revascularization**: medium- and long-term patency decreased in the presence of a distal lesion / lesion > 10 cm / multiple lesions / poor distal runoff / DM / CRF

08

Peripheral Vascular Disease

- **Surgical revascularization:** preferred in the case of disseminated disease or technically difficult endovascular revascularization or TASC II type D (± type C)
> **Regular surveillance**: for all patients post-revascularization; history - ABI - physical examination; ± Doppler US (vein graft)
> **Antithrombotic therapy:** ASA for all patients; Clopidogrel 1 to 3 months post-stenting; consider Warfarin after bypass graft with vein graft

## CRITICAL LIMB ISCHEMIA

**08**

DEFINITION: **A)** Ischemic pain at rest; **B)** Ischemic lesion (ulcer; gangrene)
> **sBP at ankle**: < 50 mmHg (rest pain) or < 70 mmHg (ischemic lesion)

ONE-YEAR MORTALITY: **25 %**

MANAGEMENT: **A)** Analgesia; **B)** Urgent revascularization if tissues are still viable (endovascular if technically feasible); **C)** Amputation if tissues are devitalized; **D)** Secondary prevention - wound care - adjusted shoes - treatment of infectious complications

> ★ **BASIL**: revascularization by infrainguinal venous bypass graft similar to endovascular revascularization; ↘ reintervention with bypass graft; ↘ **mortality with bypass graft in patients surviving > 2 years**

## ACUTE LIMB ISCHEMIA

MECHANISM: embolism (cardiac; Ao; peripheral arteries); thrombosis *in situ*; thromboembolism from a popliteal artery aneurysm (repair of aneurysm as primary prevention if > 20 mm); thrombosis of infrainguinal bypass graft; trauma; dissection; thrombophilia - hyperviscosity; *phlegmasia cerulea dolens*; iatrogenic (endovascular procedure; IABP; extracorporeal cardiac mechanical support)

PRESENTATION: Pain; Coldness; Pallor; Loss of pulse (Doppler PRN); Paresthesia / Sensory deficit; Weakness / Paralysis

MANAGEMENT: Medical emergency; **A)** IV Heparin; **B)** Percutaneous thromboembolectomy and/or direct intraarterial thrombolysis (first-line); **C)** Surgical revascularization (second-line)

## ATHEROSCLEROSIS OF THE ARMS

Innominate / subclavian artery stenosis

SUBCLAVIAN STEAL SYNDROME: claudication of the arm; reversal of flow of the vertebral artery (vertigo; syncope; diplopia; dysarthria; ataxia) or of a mammary bypass graft (angina) to perfuse the arm

DETECTION: BP difference in arms ≥ 10 mmHg

TREATMENT: endovascular or surgical revascularization

# 8.6/ ATHEROSCLEROTIC RENOVASCULAR DISEASE

↘ Renal perfusion → activation of renin-angiotensin-aldosterone system → peripheral vasoconstriction + salt and water retention → HTN

BILATERAL RENAL ARTERY STENOSIS (OR FUNCTIONAL SOLITARY KIDNEY): ↗ BP + (renin-angiotensin-aldosterone system) with salt and water retention in the absence of compensatory sodium excretion → flash pulmonary edema

CONSEQUENCES: Asymptomatic; HTN; Flash pulmonary edema - Diastolic dysfunction; Progressive deterioration of renal function (ischemic nephropathy; hypertensive nephropathy in contralateral kidney + proteinuria)

MANAGEMENT

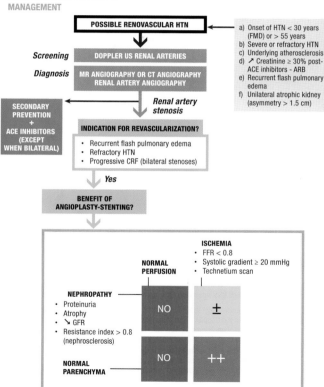

**POSSIBLE RENOVASCULAR HTN**

a) Onset of HTN < 30 years (FMD) or > 55 years
b) Severe or refractory HTN
c) Underlying atherosclerosis
d) ↗ Creatinine ≥ 30% post-ACE inhibitors - ARB
e) Recurrent flash pulmonary edema
f) Unilateral atrophic kidney (asymmetry > 1.5 cm)

*Screening*  DOPPLER US RENAL ARTERIES

*Diagnosis*  MR ANGIOGRAPHY OR CT ANGIOGRAPHY RENAL ARTERY ANGIOGRAPHY

*Renal artery stenosis*

SECONDARY PREVENTION + ACE INHIBITORS (EXCEPT WHEN BILATERAL)

**INDICATION FOR REVASCULARIZATION?**

· Recurrent flash pulmonary edema
· Refractory HTN
· Progressive CRF (bilateral stenoses)

*Yes*

**BENEFIT OF ANGIOPLASTY-STENTING?**

|  | NORMAL PERFUSION | ISCHEMIA<br>· FFR < 0.8<br>· Systolic gradient ≥ 20 mmHg<br>· Technetium scan |
|---|---|---|
| **NEPHROPATHY**<br>· Proteinuria<br>· Atrophy<br>· ↘ GFR<br>· Resistance index > 0.8 (nephrosclerosis) | NO | ± |
| **NORMAL PARENCHYMA** | NO | ++ |

STUDY: no benefit with stenting in ★ CORAL

# 8.7/ CEREBROVASCULAR DISEASE

## ETIOLOGIES – MECHANISMS

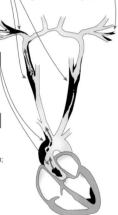

### HEMORRHAGIC STROKE (20%)

#### INTRACEREBRAL HEMORRHAGE

**RISK FACTORS**: HTN; Trauma; Bleeding diathesis; Amyloid angiopathy; Vascular malformation; Tumor; Drugs

#### SUBARACHNOID HEMORRHAGE

- Ruptured aneurysm
- Explosive headache
- Blood in CSF

### ISCHEMIC STROKE (80%)

#### ATHEROTHROMBOTIC (LARGE VESSELS)

- Intracranial or extracranial vessels
- Thrombosis *in situ* or Artery → artery embolism or Hypoperfusion
- ± Preceded by TIA in the same territory

#### CARDIOEMBOLIC

- Sudden onset
- Maximum deficit at onset
- Multiple territories

#### OTHER

Dissection; Thrombophilia; Hyperviscosity; Sickle-cell anemia; Systemic hypoperfusion; Arteritis; Vasospasm; Drugs; Cerebral venous thrombosis

### LACUNAR (SMALL PENETRATING VESSELS)

- Lipohyalinosis (HTN; DM)
- Pure motor; Pure sensory; Hemiparesis / Ataxia; Dysarthria / Clumsy hand

---

## TRANSIENT ISCHEMIC ATTACK (TIA)

TIA: transient episode (often < 1 h) of neurological dysfunction (focal cerebral or retinal or spinal ischemia) **in the absence of CNS infarction / permanent CNS injury**

ASSESSMENT: MRI (diffusion-weighted images - DWI) or brain CT scan; noninvasive imaging of head and neck vessels (carotid Doppler; CT angiography; MR angiography); ECG; TTE; ± TEE (cryptogenic TIA; suspicion of cardioembolic TIA); Holter; ± Evaluation of intracranial arteries (CT angiography or MR angiography or angiography or transcranial Doppler)

> **Evaluation of hereditary thrombophilia**: thrombophilia associated with venous >>> arterial thromboses; consider in the presence of cryptogenic TIA or suspected antiphospholipid syndrome (miscarriages; venous thrombosis; *livedo reticularis*) or personal or family history of systemic thrombosis
>> • **Look for**: protein C or S or antithrombin III deficiency; Leiden factor V; prothrombin mutation G20210A; lupus anticoagulant; anticardiolipin antibody

| ABCD² SCORE | | |
|---|---|---|
| ≥ 60 years | 1 point | 48-hour stroke risk |
| BP ≥ 140/90 | 1 point | 0-1: 0 % |
| Dysphasia without weakness or | 1 point | 2-3: 1 % |
| Unilateral weakness | 2 points | 4-5: 4 % |
| Diabetes | 1 point | 6-7: 8 % |
| Duration 0-59 min | 1 point | |
| Duration ≥ 60 min | 2 points | |

*Rothwell OM, Giles MF, Flossmann E, et al. Lancet. 2005; 366: 29-36.*
*Johnston SC, Rothwell PM, Nguyen-Huynh MN, et al. Lancet. 2007; 369: 283-92.*

# CARDIOEMBOLIC SOURCE

ASSESSMENT: ECG; 24-hour monitor / Holter; TTE; TEE

> **Additional ambulatory electrocardiographic monitoring** beyond 24-hour for subclinical AF detection if cardioembolic TIA suspected (★ EMBRACE; ★ CRYSTAL-AF)

| HIGH CARDIOEMBOLIC RISK | POTENTIAL CARDIOEMBOLIC RISK |
|---|---|
| • LA (LAA) or LV thrombus<br>• AF - Flutter<br>• Recent MI (< 1 month)<br>• Rheumatic MS<br>• Prosthetic valve<br>• Severe LV dysfunction<br>• Infective endocarditis<br>• Noninfective endocarditis (Libman-Sacks; Antiphospholipid syndrome; Nonbacterial thrombotic endocarditis)<br>• Myxoma - Fibroelastoma<br>• ASD or VSD | • Complex atherosclerosis of the aorta<br>• Aortic valve disease<br>• Mitral annular calcification<br>• MVP<br>• PFO<br>• Atrial septal aneurysm<br>• LV aneurysm without thrombus<br>• Spontaneous echo contrast in LA<br>• Regional wall motion abnormality<br>• HCM<br>• LV noncompaction |

# ISCHEMIC STROKE

| NIH STROKE SCALE (NIHSS): QUANTIFICATION OF NEUROLOGICAL IMPAIRMENT | |
|---|---|
| Level of consciousness | 0 - Alert;  1 - Drowsy;  2 - Stuporous;  3 - Comatose |
| Orientation (2 questions) | 0 - 2/2;  1 - 1/2;  2 - 0/2 |
| Response to 2 commands | 0 - 2/2;  1 - 1/2;  2 - 0/2 |
| Gaze | 0 - Normal lateral eye movements<br>1 - Partial gaze palsy<br>2 - Complete palsy |
| Visual fields | 0 - No visual loss<br>1 - Partial hemianopia<br>2 - Complete hemianopia<br>3 - Bilateral hemianopia |

Peripheral Vascular Disease

08

| Facial palsy | 0 - Normal<br>1 - Minor paralysis<br>2 - Partial paralysis<br>3 - Complete paralysis |
|---|---|
| A) Motor function - left arm<br>B) Motor function - right arm | 0 - No drift<br>1 - Drift in 5 s<br>2 - Some effort against gravity; limb falls in 10 s<br>3 - No effort against gravity<br>4 - No movement |
| A) Motor function - left leg<br>B) Motor function - right leg | 0 - No drift<br>1 - Drift in 5 s<br>2 - Some effort against gravity; limb falls in 10 s<br>3 - No effort against gravity<br>4 - No movement |
| Ataxia | 0 - Absent<br>1 - Present in one limb<br>2 - Present in two limbs |
| Sensory | 0 - Normal<br>1 - Mild-to-moderate sensory loss<br>2 - Severe to total sensory loss |
| Language | 0 - No aphasia; normal<br>1 - Mild-to-moderate aphasia<br>2 - Severe aphasia<br>3 - Mute, global aphasia |
| Dysarthria | 0 - Normal<br>1 - Mild-to-moderate dysarthria<br>2 - Severe dysarthria |
| Extinction and Neglect | 0 - No abnormality<br>1 - Visual, tactile, auditory, spatial, or personal inattention or extinction (1 sensory modality)<br>2 - Profound hemi-inattention or extinction to more than one modality |

**IMMEDIATE MANAGEMENT**: ABC; Cardiac monitor (> 24 h); IV line; O2 (if SaO$_2$ < 94%); Blood glucose; NPO

**EXAMINATIONS**: Unenhanced brain CT scan; Blood glucose; ECG; Electrolytes; Renal function; CBC; PT-aPTT; Troponin; ± Lumbar puncture (if suspicion of SAH and in the absence of bleeding on CT scan); ± EEG (rule out seizures)

**DDX**: Conversion; Hypertensive encephalopathy; Hypoglycemia; Complicated migraine; Seizures; Poisoning

**INTRAVENOUS THROMBOLYSIS**: **rtPA 0.9 mg/kg IV (max 90 mg) over 60 min** (10% of dose as a bolus over 1 min)

> ★ **NINDS rtPA Stroke Study**: < 3 h after onset of symptoms; improvement of neurological recovery at 3 months; similar mortality to that with placebo; cerebral hemorrhage in 6% of patients
> • **3 to 4.5 h of symptoms**: ★ ECASS-3; improvement of neurological recovery at 3 months

> **Post-thrombolysis**: intensive care; monitoring of neurological signs every 15-30 min for 6 h, then hourly for 24 h; Brain CT scan STAT if suspicion of intracranial hemorrhage; BP every 15-30 min for 6 h then hourly for 24 h; target BP < 180/105; repeat CT scan after 24 h

| CANDIDATES FOR INTRAVENOUS THROMBOLYSIS | |
|---|---|
| **< 3 h after onset of symptoms** | **3 to 4.5 h after onset of symptoms** |
| A) Ischemic stroke with measurable neurological deficit (not minor); <br> B) Absence of improvement of neurological deficit; <br> C) Caution in the presence of major neurological deficit (risk of hemorrhagic transformation); <br> D) Absence of SAH; <br> E) Absence of head injury or stroke < 3 months; <br> F) Absence of myocardial infarction < 3 months (risk of myocardial rupture; relative contraindication); <br> G) Absence of GI or urinary bleeding < 21 days; <br> H) Absence of major surgery < 14 days; <br> I) Absence of noncompressible arterial puncture < 7 days; <br> J) Absence of history of intracranial hemorrhage; <br> K) Absence of CNS neoplasm / AVM / intracranial aneurysm; <br> L) Absence of recent intracranial or spinal surgery; <br> M) BP < 185/110; <br> N) Absence of active internal bleeding; <br> O) INR < 1.7; <br> P) DOAC: normal sensitive detection test or last dose > 48 h (with normal renal function); <br> Q) Normal aPTT if heparin received < 48 h; <br> R) Platelet count > 100,000 mm3; <br> S) Blood glucose > 2.7 mmol/L; <br> T) Absence of seizures with residual neurological impairment; <br> U) Brain CT scan: absence of multilobar infarction (1/3 of a cerebral hemisphere) | Same criteria as for thrombolysis < 3 h of symptoms <br><br>  <br><br> **Exclusion criteria:** <br> a) > 80 years <br> b) Oral anticoagulants <br> c) NIHSS > 25 <br> d) History of stroke + DM <br> e) Ischemic lesion > 1/3 of the middle cerebral artery territory |

**INTRAARTERIAL REVASCULARIZATION**

> ★ **MR CLEAN**: stroke < 6 h + proximal occlusion in the anterior cerebral circulation; 89% treated with IV tPA before randomization; intraarterial thrombolysis and/or mechanical thrombectomy versus usual care; benefit on the functional outcomes
> ★ **ESCAPE**: stroke < 12 h + proximal intracranial occlusion in the anterior circulation; early thrombectomy associated with improved functional outcome and ↘ mortality

**MANAGEMENT OF BP**

> **BP > 220/120 mmHg**: 10-15% ↘ BP for 24 h (Nicardipine; Labetalol)
> **Thrombolysis considered**: target BP < 185/110
>   • Labetalol 10-20 mg IV x 1-2 min (can be repeated once)
>   • Nicardipine: 5 mg/h (titrate every 5-10 min up to 15 mg/h; when target BP has been achieved → 3 mg/h infusion)
> **Post-thrombolysis**: Labetalol 10 mg IV x 1-2 min (then every 10-20 min; max 300 mg) or Labetalol 10 mg IV then 2-8 mg/min infusion or Nicardipine (as above)
> **Post-stroke (long-term)**: target BP < 140/90 (ACE inhibitors and/or diuretics); resume antihypertensives 24 h after stroke

**ASA: 325 mg in < 48 h** (> 24 h in the case of thrombolysed stroke); benefit on the morbidity - mortality

**OTHER TREATMENTS: A)** Thromboprophylaxis / sequential compression device; **B)** Detection of dysphagia (water swallow test); **C)** Target normothermia and normoxemia; **D)** Nutritional support; **E)** Insulin if blood glucose > 10.3 mmol/L (avoid hypoglycemia); **F)** Rehabilitation

# SECONDARY PREVENTION

**RISK FACTORS:** ►►| Chapter 9; Treatment of HTN (from 24 h); Smoking cessation; Treatment of dyslipidemia (★ SPARCL); Treatment of DM; Moderate alcohol intake; Regular moderate physical exercise; Healthy weight; Balanced diet; Treat OSAHS

**ANTIPLATELET THERAPY:** indicated in a context of noncardioembolic TIA or ischemic stroke; ASA (50 to 325 mg daily) or ASA 25 mg / Dipyridamole 200 mg bid or Clopidogrel 75 mg daily

> **Evidence:** similar outcomes with Clopidogrel versus ASA / Dipyridamole (★ PRoFESS); no benefit of long-term combination of Clopidogrel and ASA (★ MATCH); ➘ adverse events with ASA / Dipyridamole versus ASA (★ ESPS-2; ★ ESPRIT)

**ATRIAL FIBRILLATION:** Warfarin (★ EAFT) or DOAC for secondary prevention

> **Initiation of A/C in acute stroke:** according to the severity of the stroke (risk of hemorrhagic transformation); anticoagulant therapy initiated < 14 days in ★ EAFT; wait 72 h for small stroke or 1 week for moderate stroke or 2 weeks for large stroke; no benefit of Heparin bridge
> **WATCHMAN:** LAA occlusion device; ★ PROTECT AF (noninferior to warfarin); consider when anticoagulation is contraindicated

**LVEF ≤ 35 %:** no evidence in support of warfarin for secondary prevention; Warfarin or ASA or Clopidogrel or ASA / Dipyridamole

**RHEUMATIC MITRAL STENOSIS:** Warfarin

**NONRHEUMATIC VALVULAR HEART DISEASE:** Aortic or mitral valve disease or mitral annular calcification or MVP; Antiplatelet therapy (IIb; C)

**PFO:** controversial subject; ►►| Chapter 7 - Congenital heart disease

**THROMBOPHILIA:** associated with venous >>> arterial thromboses; anticoagulation if concomitant DVT; Antiplatelet therapy or anticoagulation in the absence of DVT or an identifiable cause of stroke

> **Antiphospholipid syndrome:** anticoagulation indicated

# CAROTID ARTERY REVASCULARIZATION

**SYMPTOMATIC CAROTID ARTERY STENOSIS: benefit of surgical revascularization compared to medical treatment** (★ NASCET; ★ ECST; ★ VACS); NNT = 6

**ASYMPTOMATIC CAROTID ARTERY STENOSIS: benefit of surgical revascularization** in selected patients (★ ACAS and ★ ACST; studies conducted prior to the introduction of modern medical treatment); NNT = 33

**ANGIOPLASTY-STENTING VERSUS ENDARTERECTOMY: comparable long-term outcomes** (★ CREST; ★ SAPPHIRE)

> **Angioplasty-Stenting:** increased risk of periprocedural stroke compared to endarterectomy (particularly in patients > 70 years)
> **Prefer angioplasty-stenting:** anatomical / technical considerations (post-radiation; post-surgical; obesity; hostile neck; stenosis at different level); high operative risk - severe comoborbidities
> **Dual antiplatelet therapy:** 4 weeks

**REVASCULARIZATION IN THE PRESENCE OF MULTIPLE COMORBIDITIES: little evidence in favor of surgical or endovascular revascularization** (NYHA III-IV; CCS III-IV; CAD ≥ 2 vessels or LMCA; LVEF ≤ 30%; recent myocardial infarction; severe lung disease; advanced CRF)

| | SYMPTOMATIC (< 6 MONTHS) | | ASYMPTOMATIC |
|---|---|---|---|
| | **Carotid artery stenosis: 50-69% (angiography)** | **Carotid artery stenosis: 70-99% (noninvasive imaging)** | **Carotid artery stenosis > 70%** |
| **Endarterec-tomy** | I; B | I; A | IIa; A |
| | To be performed within 14 days of the neurological event unless contraindicated (IIa; B) | | Mortality - perioperative stroke < 3% |
| | Mortality - perioperative stroke < 6% Life expectancy > 5 years | | Life expectancy > 5 years |
| **Angioplasty-Stenting** | Alternative to surgery: I; B | Alternative to surgery: I; B | IIb; B (controversial) |
| | Mortality - perioperative stroke < 5% | | |

## INTRACRANIAL HEMORRHAGE

**MANAGEMENT:** Intensive care; Neurosurgical assessment; Target normothermia; Target blood glucose < 10.3 mmol/L; Thromboprophylaxis (sequential compression device; IVC filter PRN); Phenytoin in the presence of seizures; ± Continuous EEG monitoring

**ANTICOAGULATION:** Discontinue anticoagulation and antiplatelet therapy for more than 1-2 weeks and subsequently reassess the indication; weigh up the thromboembolic risk against the bleeding risk (high in cortical stroke secondary to amyloid angiopathy)

> **Reverse Warfarin: prothrombin complex concentrate** (Octaplex; Beriplex; Cofact; Proplex); complex of factors II - VII - IX - X; Target INR < 1.4
> - **Vitamin K:** 10 mg IV (max 1 mg/min)
> - **Fresh frozen plasma:** 8 units when prothrombin complex concentrate is not available

**BLOOD PRESSURE:** treat if sBP > 180 mmHg in the absence of intracranial hypertension; target BP < 160/90 (labetalol; nicardipine; esmolol; enalapril; hydralazine; nitroprusside; TNT)

**CONTROL OF INTRACRANIAL HYPERTENSION: target cerebral perfusion pressure > 60 mmHg (MAP - ICP) and ICP < 20-25 mmHg;** raise head of bed by 30°; analgesia; control of BP (target SBP < 180 mmHg and MAP < 130 mmHg, while maintaining adequate cerebral perfusion pressure); ventriculostomy (external CSF drainage); IV mannitol (target plasma osmolality: 300-310 mOsmol/kg); sedation; hyperventilation ($PaCO_2$: 30-35 mmHg); neuromuscular blockade; surgical evacuation of hematoma; barbiturate-induced coma

# 8.8/ PULMONARY EMBOLISM

**RISK FACTORS:** Age; Personal or family history of pulmonary embolism; Cancer; Trauma; Surgery; Immobilization; Pregnancy; Hormonal therapy; Oral contraceptive; Nephrotic syndrome; Chemotherapy

> **Thrombophilia:** Homozygous factor V Leiden; Homozygous prothrombin G20210A; Protein C deficiency; Protein S deficiency; Antiphospholipid syndrome / Lupus anticoagulant

**PRESENTATION:** Dyspnea; Pleuritic pain; Retrosternal chest pain; Cough; Hemoptysis; Paradoxical embolism; Syncope; Sudden death - Pulseless electrical activity

**CLINICAL FEATURES:** Tachypnea; Tachycardia; ± Shock; ± Cyanosis (R→ L shunt via PFO); ↘ SaO₂; Low-grade fever; JVD; Left parasternal heave; ↗ P2; TR murmur; right S3 or S4; Pleural friction rub (pulmonary infarction); signs of DVT in leg (edema; erythema; heat; pain; difference between legs)

**D-DIMERS: very sensitive but not specific**

**ECG:** Sinus tachycardia; S1Q3T3; *de novo* RBBB; T wave inversion (V1 to V4; inferior leads); Q in III and aVF; Qr in V1; ST depression or ST elevation in V1-V4; right axis deviation; AF / Flutter

**CXR:** PA dilatation; Atelectasis; Elevation of the diaphragm; Pleural effusion

> **Westermark sign:** Segmental oligemia secondary to proximal arterial occlusion
> **Hampton hump:** Triangular hyperdensity adherent to the pleura secondary to pulmonary infarction (consolidation with hemorrhage)

**TTE:** RV dilatation (↗ acute afterload); RV hypokinesia; PHT (non-preconditioned RV is unable to genereate a mPAP > 40 mmHg); TR; shunt via PFO; thrombus-in-transit visible in right chambers / PA; septal curvature towards the LV; dilated and noncompliant IVC

> **McConnell's sign:** hypokinesis of basal / mid RV free wall (preserved apex contractility) ✚

**LEG ULTRASOUND:** look for ↘ vein compressibility

## CONSEQUENCES OF PULMONARY EMBOLISM

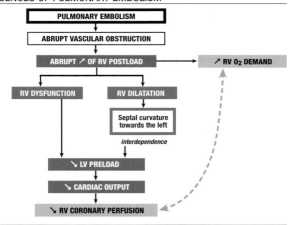

## ASSESSMENT

| WELLS CRITERIA – PRETEST PROBABILITY – DEEP VEIN THROMBOSIS | | |
|---|---|---|
| Active cancer | 1 point | |
| Paralysis or recent cast immobilization | 1 point | • **0 point:** low pretest probability |
| Bedridden > 3 days or surgery < 4 weeks | 1 point | • **1-2 points:** moderate pretest probability |
| Local vein tenderness | 1 point | • **1-2 points:** moderate pretest probability |
| Swelling of entire leg | 1 point | • **≥ 3 points:** high pretest probability |
| Difference between calves > 3 cm | 1 point | • **≥ 3 points:** high pretest probability |
| Pitting edema | 1 point | |
| Superficial collateral vein | 1 point | |
| Alternative diagnosis at least as likely | - 2 points | |

| WELLS CRITERIA – PRETEST PROBABILITY – PULMONARY EMBOLISM | | |
|---|---|---|
| Signs or symptoms of DVT | 3 points | • **0-1 point**: low pretest probability (10%)<br>• **2-6 points**: moderate pretest probability (30%)<br>• **≥ 7 points**: high pretest probability (65%) |
| Alternative diagnosis is less likely | 3 points | |
| HR > 100 bpm | 1.5 points | |
| Immobilization or surgery < 4 weeks | 1.5 points | |
| History of DVT or pulmonary embolism | 1.5 points | |
| Hemoptysis | 1 point | |
| Cancer (< 6 months or metastasis) | 1 point | |

*Wells PS, Anderson DR, Bormanis J, et al, Lancet 1997; 350:1795*
*van Belle A, et al. JAMA 2006; 295:172*

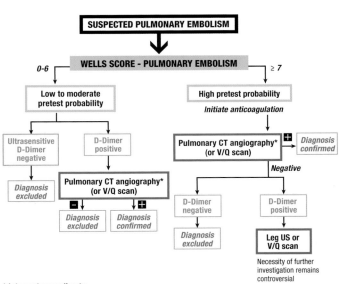

**\* Interpret according to:**

A) Pretest probability

B) Site of thrombus (main PA or lobar or segmental versus subsegmental PA)

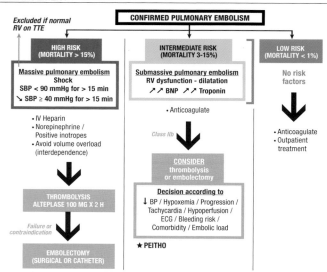

★ **PEITHO**: PE with RV dysfunction and ↗ Troponin; Tenecteplase + Heparin vs Heparin;
↘ Haemodynamic decompensation; similar all-cause 7-day mortality; ↗ intracranial bleeding;
↗ major hemorrhage

| Unfractionated heparin | · IV bolus: 80 IU/kg<br>· IV infusion: 18 IU/kg/h (target aPTT 1.5-2.5 x control or 60-80 s) | |
|---|---|---|
| Enoxaparin | · 1 mg/kg SC bid or 1.5 mg/kg qd | **LMWH** |
| Dalteparin | · 100 IU/kg SC bid or 200 IU/kg qd | · Better bioavailability<br>· More predictable effect<br>· Avoid if GFR < 30 mL/min |
| Tinzaparin | · 175 IU/kg SC bid | |
| Fondaparinux | · < 50 kg: 5 mg SC qd<br>· 50-100 kg: 7.5 mg SC qd<br>· > 100 kg: 10 mg SC qd | · Indirect Xa inhibitor<br>· Avoid if GFR < 30 mL/min |
| History of HIT | Argatroban or Bivalirudin or Lepirudin or Danaparoid | |

**WARFARIN: anticoagulant effect in 5 days**

> **Initially procoagulant effect: due to ↘ proteins C and S**                     +

> **Overlapping of warfarin with Heparin ≥ 5 days (and ≥ 24 h with INR ≥ 2.0)**

| Provoked pulmonary embolism or proximal DVT (secondary to surgery; trauma; pregnancy; hormonal therapy) | Thromboembolism and active cancer | Idiopathic or recurrent pulmonary embolism (or proximal DVT) |
|---|---|---|
| Anticoagulation x 3 months | LMWH (★ CLOT) Continue in the presence of active cancer (warfarin as alternative) | Anticoagulation x ≥ 3 months and consider long-term treatment (according to balance between the risks of recurrence and bleeding) |

**DOAC IN ACUTE PHASE OF THROMBOEMBOLIC DISEASE:** ★ EINSTEIN (Rivaroxaban 15 mg bid x 3 weeks then 20 mg qd); ★ AMPLIFY (Apixaban 10 mg bid x 7 days then 5 mg bid)

**SECONDARY PREVENTION** (after acute phase): Options → **A)** Warfarin; **B)** Rivaroxaban 20 mg qd (★ EINSTEIN-extension); **C)** Apixaban 2.5 mg bid (★ AMPLIFY-extension); **D)** Dabigatran 150 mg bid (★ RE-SONATE and ★ RE-MEDY); **E)** ASA 100 mg qd (★ ASPIRE and ★ WARFASA)

**IVC FILTER:** Indications → **A)** Bleeding / Contraindication to anticoagulation; **B)** Recurrent pulmonary embolism despite treatment (in the presence of a proximal thrombosis)
> ↘ Pulmonary embolism recurrence rate; ↗ DVT recurrence rate
> **Complications:** access site complication; recurrent DVT; IVC thrombosis; IVC perforation; migration; post-thrombotic syndrome
> Resume anticoagulation and **remove** the filter as soon as possible

**INTRAVENOUS THROMBOLYSIS:** ↘ mortality in massive pulmonary embolism
> **Alteplase 100 mg IV x 2 h** (without heparin); resume heparin without bolus at the end of thrombolysis if aPTT ≤ 80 s

**CATHETER-ASSISTED THROMBUS REMOVAL**
> **Indications:** Hemodynamic instability with → **A)** Contraindication to thrombolysis or **B)** Failure of thrombolysis (rescue)
> • **Consider surgery** in the presence of mobile thrombus-in-transit in right chambers or thrombus-in-transit in PFO

**LOCAL CATHETER THROMBOLYSIS FOR DVT: A)** Extensive ilio-femoral thrombosis with low bleeding risk (including *phlegmasia cerulea dolens*); **B)** Progression of thrombus despite treatment; **C)** Extensive upper extremity DVT (subclavian and axillary veins)
> **Benefit:** ↘ risk of postthrombotic syndrome
> **Pharmacomechanical approach:** local thrombolysis combined with catheter thrombectomy ± balloon venoplasty (± stent)

**UPPER EXTREMITY DVT:** Risk factors → central catheter; pacemaker; thoracic outlet syndrome (Paget-Schroetter disease); Cancer
> Risk of complications in the case of proximal DVT (starting at axillary vein)
> **Risk of PE:** 10 %
> **Anticoagulation:** ≥ 3 months
> • It is acceptable to observe upper extremity DVT **distal to the axillary vein**

**POSTTHROMBOTIC SYNDROME:** varicosities; hyperpigmentation; ulcers
> **Compression stockings:** 30-40 mmHg
> Consider angioplasty ± stenting in the presence of iliac vein obstruction

**THROMBOPROPHYLAXIS IN MEDICALLY HOSPITALIZED PATIENTS**
> **Unfractionated heparin:** 5000 IU SC bid or tid
> **LMWH:** Enoxaparin 40 mg SC qd or Dalteparin 5000 U SC qd
> **Fondaparinux:** 2.5 mg SC qd (useful in patients with a history of HIT)
> **Intermittent pneumatic compression:** contraindication to anticoagulants or multiple risk factors (with anticoagulant)

**TYPE 1 HIT:** Benign form

## TYPE 2 HEPARIN-INDUCED THROMBOCYTOPENIA

Immune form (IgG)

**PATHOPHYSIOLOGY:** Antibody directed against neoantigens on protein PF4 (protein released by activated platelets)

> Neoantigens are exposed following binding of PF4 with heparin → IgG binds simultaneously to the heparin-PF4 complex and to platelet Fc receptors → platelet activation with release of prothrombotic molecules → platelet consumption + intense thrombin production → multiple thromboses (venous or arterial)

**5-10 days post-exposure to heparin** (or earlier in the case of re-exposure < 3 months)

↘ **> 50% of platelets (compared to baseline count) or thrombosis beginning 5-10 days after the start of heparin** +

| 4 T SCORE | | | |
|---|---|---|---|
| | **2 POINTS** | **1 POINT** | **0 POINT** |
| **Thrombo-cytopenia** | > 50% decrease in platelet count and nadir ≥ 20,000/μL and no surgery in past 3 days | • > 50% decrease in platelet count and surgery in past 3 days or • 30-50% decrease in platelet count or • Nadir 10,000-20,000/μL | • < 30% decrease in platelet count or • Nadir < 10,000/μL |
| **"Timing" (post-exposure)** | Day 5 to Day 10 (or ≤ 1 day if prior heparin exposure within 30 days) | Uncertain interval (but probably between Day 5 and Day 10) or after Day 10 (or ≤ 1 day if prior heparin exposure within 30-100 days) | Decrease in platelet count ≤ Day 4 (no other heparin therapy during past 100 days) |
| **Thrombosis** | Confirmed new thrombosis; Skin necrosis at injection site; Anaphylactoid reaction to IV heparin bolus | Recurrent venous thrombosis while on anticoagulant therapy or suspected thrombosis or nonnecrotic skin lesions at injection site | None |
| **oTher causes** | No alternative cause to explain thrombocytopenia | Possible alternative cause | Probable alternative cause (recent surgery; bacteremia; chemotherapy; drugs…) |
| **6-8 points:** high probability (34%) **4-5 points:** intermediate probability (11%) **0-3 points:** low probability (0.9%) | | | |

*Lo GK, Warkentin TE, Sigouin CS et al. J Thromb Haemost. 2006; 4: 759-65.*

DIAGNOSTIC WORK-UP: to be performed in the case of intermediate to high probability (4 T score)

> **ELISA assay of anti-PF4 antibodies** (excellent NPV but low PPV)
> **Serotonin-release assay** (platelets containing labeled serotonin placed in contact with the patient's plasma and heparin); gold standard diagnostic test

PREVENTION: CBC every 2-3 days (starting on Day 5 of heparin therapy)

## MANAGEMENT OF TYPE 2 HIT

1) Stop all forms of heparin
2) Argatroban or Bivalirudin or Fondaparinux or Danaparoid
3) Initiate Warfarin **once the thrombocytopenia has resolved** (with IV co-administration of a direct thrombin inhibitor; overlapping for ≥ 5 days; discontinue after achieving therapeutic INR for 2 days); anticoagulation ≥ 3 months if confirmed thrombosis

> If the patient is treated with Warfarin at the time of HIT: reverse with vitamin K

# 8.10/ PULMONARY HYPERTENSION

| PHT | GROUP 1–3–4–5 PHT | POSTCAPILLARY (GROUP 2) |
|---|---|---|
| mPAP ≥ 25 mmHg | mPAP ≥ 25 mmHg Wedge ≤ 15 mmHg | mPAP ≥ 25 mmHg and Wedge > 15 mmHg |
| | | **Isolated postcapillary:** dPAP - Mean Wedge < 7 mmHg and/or PVR ≤ 3 WU |
| | | **With precapillary component:** dPAP - Mean Wedge ≥ 7 mmHg and/or PVR > 3 WU |

## ETIOLOGIES

| | mPAP ≥ 25 mmHg; Wedge ≤ 15 mmHg; PVR ≥ 3 WU |
|---|---|
| **Group 1: Pulmonary arterial hypertension (PAH)** | • **Idiopathic PAH**<br>• **Heritable PAH**<br>  - BMPR2; ALK1; Endoglin; SMAD9; CAV1; KCNK3 mutation<br>  - Hereditary hemorrhagic telangiectasia (Osler-Weber-Rendu)<br>• **PAH secondary to drugs - toxins** (Anorectics; Cocaine; Amphetamines)<br>• **PAH associated with**<br>  - **Collagen diseases**<br>    > Scleroderma - CREST; SLE; Mixed connective tissue disease; RA; Sjögren; Dermatomyositis<br>  - **HIV**<br>  - **Portal hypertension** (Cirrhosis)<br>    > Liver transplantation contraindicated if mPAP ≥ 35 mmHg or PVR > 250 dyn x s / cm$^5$<br>  - **Congenital heart disease** (Shunt)<br>    > VSD; Patent ductus arteriosus; ASD; Anomalous pulmonary venous return; AV canal defect; Complex congenital heart disease<br>  - **Schistosomiasis** |

| Group 1* | • **Pulmonary veno-occlusive disease and pulmonary capillary hemangiomatosis**<br> - Similar presentation to that of PAH<br> - Suspect in the presence of pulmonary edema following administration of pulmonary artery vasodilators<br> - Characteristic changes on pulmonary HDCT (subpleural thickened septal lines; centrilobular ground-glass opacities; lymphadenopathy) |
|---|---|
| **Group 2: PHT secondary to left heart disease** | **mPAP ≥ 25 mmHg; Wedge > 15 mmHg**<br> • LV systolic dysfunction<br> • LV diastolic dysfunction<br> • Left-sided valvular heart disease • Pulmonary veins stenosis |
| **Group 3: Pulmonary hypertension secondary to lung disease** | • COPD • Interstitial lung disease<br> • Mixed lung disease • Sleep-disordered breathing<br> • Alveolar hypoventilation • High altitude |
| **Group 4** | • Thromboembolic pulmonary hypertension |
| **Group 5: Uncertain mechanism** | • **Hematological disease:** Myeloproliferative disease (Polycythemia vera; Essential thrombocytosis; CML); Splenectomy; Chronic hemolytic anemia (Sickle-cell anemia; Hereditary spherocytosis; Homozygous beta-thalassemia)<br> • **Systemic disease:** Sarcoidosis; Langerhans cell histiocytosis; Lymphangioleiomyomatosis; Neurofibromatosis; Vasculitis<br> • **Metabolic disease**: Glycogen storage disease; Gaucher; Thyroid disease<br> • **Other:** Neoplastic obstruction; Fibrosing mediastinitis; Dialysis |

**Reversible causes of PHT secondary to ↗ transpulmonary blood flow**
Exercise; Anemia; Pregnancy; Sepsis; Hyperthyroidism; Volume overload

## ASSESSMENT

PRESENTATION: Dyspnea on exertion; Fatigue; Retrosternal chest pain; Syncope; Palpitations; Leg edema; Ortner's syndrome (recurrent laryngeal nerve compression by dilated PA); Hemoptysis

CLINICAL FEATURES: Hypotension; Cold extremities; ± Cyanosis; JVD (↗ A wave; ↗ V wave); left parasternal heave; Pulmonary artery palpable in left second intercostal space; ↗ P2; Ejection click / Systolic ejection murmur at pulmonary site; Holosystolic murmur (TR; ↗ on inspiration); PR murmur (Graham-Steel); Right S3 and/or S4; Pulsatile liver; Anasarca
> Look for signs of collagen disease (sclerodactyly; arthritis; telangiectasias; Raynaud; rash) and liver disease (spider naevi; testicular atrophy; palmar erythema); look for clubbing

ASSESSMENTS: HIV; ANA; RF; LFTs (± liver US); BNP; TSH; Thrombophilia screening (group 4)

ECG: RAH; RVH; R axis deviation; T wave inversion in R precordial leads; RBBB; Atrial arrhythmias

CXR: central PA dilatation; RA-RV dilatation; pruning (loss) of the peripheral blood vessels (oligemia)

TTE: ↗ PAP; RA and RV dilatation (RV / LV basal diameter ratio > 1.0); PA dilatation (> 25 mm); RVH; RV dysfunction (RIMP - S' - TAPSE - Strain); Curvature of the septum towards LV; Small left chambers; TR; Pericardial effusion; Look for shunt; Look for cause of PHT due to heart disease
> **Screening: A)** Scleroderma: annually (+ DLCO / biomarkers); **B)** Sickle-cell anemia: annually

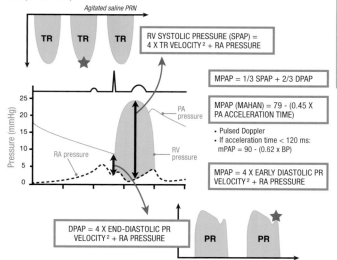

*Agitated saline PRN*

| TR | TR | TR |

RV SYSTOLIC PRESSURE (SPAP) =
4 X TR VELOCITY² + RA PRESSURE

MPAP = 1/3 SPAP + 2/3 DPAP

MPAP (MAHAN) = 79 - (0.45 X
PA ACCELERATION TIME)

- Pulsed Doppler
- If acceleration time < 120 ms:
  mPAP = 90 - (0.62 x BP)

MPAP = 4 X EARLY DIASTOLIC PR
VELOCITY² + RA PRESSURE

DPAP = 4 X END-DIASTOLIC PR
VELOCITY² + RA PRESSURE

| PR | PR |

PA pressure
RA pressure
RV pressure

**CARDIAC MRI:** More favorable prognostic factors → Ejection volume > 25 mL/m² or RV end-diastolic volume < 84 mL/m² or LV end-diastolic volume > 40 mL/m²

**PULMONARY ASSESSMENT:** CXR; PFTs; Pulmonary high-resolution CT; Arterial blood gases; V/Q scan (± CT angiography / pulmonary angiography); Nocturnal saturometry / Polysomnography
> **PFTs:** PAH associated with mild-to-moderate ↘ lung volumes and ↘ DLCO (40 to 80% of predicted)
> **Rule out thromboembolic PHT (Group 4) in all patients by V/Q scan**     +

**RIGHT/LEFT CATHETERIZATION**
> **Look for a shunt** (oximetry run)
> **Wedge pressure** (end of expiration) ± LVEDP; 500 mL bolus PRN to reveal diastolic dysfunction
> **Cardiac output:** Thermodilution (in the absence of significant TR or low output state or shunt) or Fick
> **PVR (WU)** = mPAP - Wedge / Cardiac output
> **Diastolic pressure gradient** = dPAP - Mean Wedge
> **Vasoreactivity test** (Idiopathic PAH; Heritable PAH; Drug-induced PAH)
> · **Positive: absolute** ↘ **of mPAP ≥ 10 mmHg (to mPAP < 40 mmHg) in the absence**     +
>   **of** ↘ **cardiac output**

| INHALED NO (FIRST LINE) | IV EPOPROSTENOL | IV ADENOSINE |
|---|---|---|
| 10 to 20 ppm | 2 - 12 ng/kg/min | 50 to 350 µg/kg/min |

> **Hepatic venous pressure gradient** = Wedged hepatic venous pressure - IVC pressure; normal value between 1-5 mmHg (≥ 10 mmHg → portal hypertension / cirrhosis)

**MONITORING OF FUNCTIONAL CAPACITY:** WHO functional class (equivalent to NYHA); 6MWT; Stress test; Cardiopulmonary test / VO₂ max

# MANAGEMENT

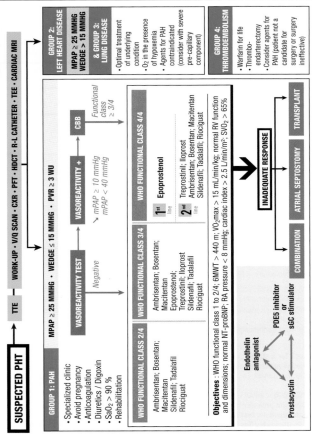

**SUSPECTED PHT** → TTE → **WORK-UP** · V/Q SCAN · CXR · PFT · HDCT · R-L CATHETER · TEE · CARDIAC MRI

MPAP ≥ 25 MMHG · WEDGE ≤ 15 MMHG · PVR ≥ 3 WU

**GROUP 1: PAH**
- Specialized clinic
- Avoid pregnancy
- Anticoagulation
- Diuretics / Digoxin
- SaO$_2$ > 90 %
- Rehabilitation

**VASOREACTIVITY TEST**

*Negative* → 

**VASOREACTIVITY +**
↘ mPAP ≥ 10 mmHg
mPAP < 40 mmHg

→ **CCB** — *Functional class ≥ 3/4*

**WHO FUNCTIONAL CLASS 2/4**
Ambrisentan; Bosentan; Macitentan
Sildenafil; Tadalafil
Riociguat

**WHO FUNCTIONAL CLASS 3/4**
Ambrisentan; Bosentan; Macitentan
Epoprostenol;
Treprostinil; Iloprost
Sildenafil; Tadalafil
Riociguat

**WHO FUNCTIONAL CLASS 4/4**

1st line — **Epoprostenol**

2nd line — Treprostinil; Iloprost
Ambrisentan; Bosentan; Macitentan
Sildenafil; Tadalafil; Riociguat

**INADEQUATE RESPONSE** →

COMBINATION     ATRIAL SEPTOSTOMY     TRANSPLANT

Endothelin antagonist
PDE5 inhibitor or sGC stimulator
Prostacyclin

**Objectives :** WHO functional class 1 to 2/4; 6MWT > 440 m; VO$_2$max > 15 mL/min/kg; normal RV function and dimensions; normal NT-proBNP; RA pressure < 8 mmHg; cardiac index > 2.5 L/min/m$^2$; SvO$_2$ > 65%

**GROUP 2: LEFT HEART DISEASE**
MPAP ≥ 25 MMHG
WEDGE > 15 MMHG
- Optimal treatment of underlying condition

**& GROUP 3: LUNG DISEASE**
- O$_2$ in the presence of hypoxemia
- Agents for PAH contraindicated (consider with severe pre-capillary component)

**GROUP 4: THROMBOEMBOLISM**
- Warfarin for life
- Thrombo-endarterectomy
- Consider agents for PAH (patient not a candidate for surgery or surgery ineffective)

O$_2$ (target: SaO$_2$ > 90% and PaO$_2$ > 60 mmHg)

AVOID PREGNANCY

REHABILITATION / AEROBIC EXERCISE PROGRAM

AVOID HIGH ALTITUDE; O$_2$ in plane when SaO$_2$ < 92% (or PaO$_2$ < 60 mmHg)

VACCINATION (Influenza - Pneumococcus)

SODIUM RESTRICTION (< 2.4 g/day) in the presence of volume overload

DIURETICS for volume overload

DIGOXIN (right heart failure or atrial tachyarrhythmias)

| DRUG THERAPY FOR GROUP 1 PAH | | |
|---|---|---|
| **Anticoagulation** | **Warfarin**<br>Target INR: 2.0 to 2.5 | Consider in idiopathic PAH or Heritable PAH or PAH due to anorexigens (class IIb recommendation) |
| **Calcium channel blocking agents** | **Nifedipine** (120 - 240 mg)<br>**Diltiazem** (720 - 960 mg)<br>**Amlodipine** (20 - 30 mg PO) | In patients with idiopathic PAH, Heritable PAH or drug induced PAH and positive vasoreactivity test<br>Continue if WHO functional class 1 to 2/4 with marked hemodynamic improvement |
| **Prostanoids (prostacyclins)**<br><br>**Vasodilators Antiproliferative agents** | **Epoprostenol**<br>2 ng/kg/min (target 25 - 40 ng/kg/min) | **Only agent demonstrated to ↘ mortality in IPAH** (★ Primary Pulmonary Hypertension Study Group)<br>Need for intravenous administration (risk of local infection and catheter obstruction / sepsis) |
| | **Treprostinil** (SC or IV or inhaled)<br>• s/c: 1-2 to 20 - 80 ng/kg/min<br>• Inhaled: 30 - 45 μg qid | Associated with infusion site pain |
| | **Iloprost aerosol**<br>2.5 - 5 μg (6-9 per day) | Associated with flushing and jaw pain |
| **Prostacyclin IP receptor agonist** | **Selexipag**<br>200-1600 μg PO bid | Headache; Diarrhea; Nausea; Flushing |
| **Endothelin receptor antagonist**<br><br>**Vasodilator** | **Ambrisentan**<br>2.5 - 5 - 10 mg PO qd | Adverse effects: liver function test abnormalities; edema |
| | **Bosentan**<br>125 mg PO bid | Monitor liver function monthly |
| | **Macitentan**<br>3 or 10 mg PO qd | Can cause anemia |
| **Phospho-diesterase-5 inhibitor**<br>↗ NO | **Sildenafil**<br>20 mg PO tid | Associated with headache, flushing, epistaxis<br>**Do not combine with soluble guanylatecyclase stimulator** |
| | **Tadalafil**<br>2.5 - 10 - 20 - 40 mg PO qd | |
| **Soluble guanylate cyclase stimulator**<br>↗ NO | **Riociguat**<br>2.5 mg PO tid | Approved for group 1 PAH (★ PATENT) and thromboembolic PHT (★ CHEST)<br>Risk of syncope<br>**Do not combine with PDE–5 inhibitor** |

**BALLOON ATRIAL SEPTOSTOMY FOR RA-RV DECOMPRESSION:** creation of a R → L shunt; ↘ RV filling pressures; improvement of LV filling; ↗ cardiac output (**at the cost of hypoxemia**)

> **Indications:** Severe PAH with treatment-refractory right heart failure (including inotropes) or recurrent syncope or bridge to transplant

**LUNG TRANSPLANT:** Progressive treatment-refractory PAH; WHO functional class 3-4/4

> **5-year survival:** 52-75%; risk of bronchiolitis obliterans - rejection - opportunistic infections

**GROUP 2 PHT:** left heart disease causing **venous PHT with passive retrograde transmission of increased pressure**

> **Wedge > 15 mmHg;   Diastolic pressure gradient < 7 mmHg (dPAP - Mean Wedge)**   +
> May be associated with pulmonary hemosiderosis (leakage of RBC from capillaries) with formation of fibrosis
> **Pulmonary artery vasodilators: risk of pulmonary edema in the presence of ↗ LV**   + **filling pressures**
> - **PAH-approved therapies are not recommended in group 2 PHT**
> - **PDE-5 inhibitors / Macitentan**: awaiting the results of the ★ Sil-HF and ★ MELODY-1

> **Postcapillary PHT with precapillary component**: development of arterial PHT with ↗ PVR as mechanism of adaptation to pulmonary edema
> - **Active component**: ↗ pulmonary artery vasomotor tone and/or fixed obstructive arterial structural remodeling
> - **Diastolic pressure gradient ≥ 7 mmHg (dPAP - Mean Wedge)**   +
> - **Consider pulmonary artery vasodilators** on an individual basis by the expert PH centre

**GROUP 4 PHT:** organized thrombus associated with the arterial wall with lobar or segmental or subsegmental perfusion abnormality

> Pulmonary arteriopathy superimposed (similar to idiopathic PAH)
> **V/Q scan:** screening test of choice
> - CT pulmonary angiography / Conventional pulmonary angiography for confirmation
> **Thromboendarterectomy:** treatment of choice (deep hypothermia circulatory arrest)
> - Consider balloon pulmonary angioplasty if technically non-operable
> **Anticoagulation** for life
> **Consider pulmonary artery vasodilators** when thromboendarterectomy is impossible or gives mixed results; prefer Riociguat (beneficial in ★ CHEST)

**PAH ASSOCIATED WITH CONGENITAL HEART DISEASE (SHUNT)**

| EINSENMENGER | PAH WITH L→R SHUNT | PAH WITH SMALL SEPTAL DEFECT | POST-CORRECTION PAH |
|---|---|---|---|
| • Large defect<br>• Severely ↗ PRV<br>• Reversed shunt (or bidirectional)<br>• Cyanosis; Erythrocytosis; multisystem features | • Moderate-to-large defect<br>• No cyanosis at rest<br>• Do not operate if PVR > 4.6 WU (or indexed PVR > 8 WU/m²) | • VSD < 1 cm<br>• ASD < 2 cm<br>• ↗ PVR disproportional to congenital anomaly<br>• Similar profile to idiopathic PAH | • PAH despite absence of a residual defect |

> **Shunt distal to the tricuspid valve** (VSD; patent ductus arteriosus; truncus arteriosus) subjects pulmonary arteries to much higher pressure stress than pre-tricuspid shunt

- Bonow RO, Mann DL, Zipes DP, Libby P. *Braunwald's Heart Disease. A textbook of cardiovascular medicine.* Elsevier. 2012. 1961 p.
- 2014 ESC Guidelines on the diagnosis and treatment of aortic diseases. *EHJ* 2014; *41*; 2873-2926.
- 2010 ACCF /AHA /AATS /ACR /ASA /SCA /SCAI /SIR /STS /SVM Guidelines for the Diagnosis and Management of Patients With Thoracic Aortic Disease. *JACC* 2010; *55*; e27-e129.
- Patel HJ, Deeb M. Ascending and Arch Aorta Pathology, Natural History, and Treatment. *Circulation* 2008; *118*: 188-195.
- Echocardiography in aortic diseases: EAE recommendations for clinical practice. *EJE* 2010; *11*; 645-658
- Otto, CM. *Textbook of clinical echocardiography.* Saunders Elsevier. 2009. 519 p.
- Kent KC. Abdominal Aortic Aneurysms. *NEJM* 2014; *371*; 2101-2108.
- 2011 ACCF/AHA Focused Update of the Guideline for the Management of Patients With Peripheral Artery Disease. *JACC* 2011; *58*; 2020-2045
- ESC Guidelines on the diagnosis and treatment of peripheral artery diseases. *EHJ.* 2011; *32*: 2851-2906
- ACC/AHA 2005 Guidelines for the Management of Patients With Peripheral Arterial Disease (Lower Extremity, Renal, Mesenteric, and Abdominal Aortic): Executive Summary. *JACC* 2006; *47*; 1239-1312.
- Inter-Society Consensus for the Management of Peripheral Arterial Disease (TASC II). *J Vasc Surg.* 2007; *45*; S5-67
- Antithrombotic Therapy in Peripheral Artery Disease Antithrombotic Therapy and Prevention of Thrombosis, 9th ed: American College of Chest Physicians Evidence-Based Clinical Practice Guidelines. *CHEST* 2012; *141:* e669S-e690S
- Seddon M, Saw J. Atherosclerotic renal artery stenosis: Review of pathophysiology, clinical trial evidence, and management strategies. *CJC* 2011; *27*; 468-480.
- Definition and Evaluation of Transient Ischemic Attack. *Stroke.* 2009; *40:* 2276-2293
- Guidelines for the Early Management of Adults With Ischemic Stroke. *Stroke.* 2007; *38:* 1655-1711
- 2010 American Heart Association Guidelines for Cardiopulmonary Resuscitation and Emergency Cardiovascular Care. Part 11: Adult Stroke. *Circulation* 2010; *122;* S818-S828
- Expansion of the Time Window for Treatment of Acute Ischemic Stroke With Intravenous Tissue Plasminogen Activator. *Stroke.* 2009; *40:* 2945-2948.
- Goldman ME. Croft LB. Echocardiography in Search of a Cardioembolic Source. *Curr Probl Cardiol* 2002; *27:* 342-358.
- Guidelines for the Prevention of Stroke in Patients With Stroke or Transient Ischemic Attack. *Stroke.* 2011; *42:* 227-276
- 2011 ASA / ACCF / AHA / AANN / AANS / ACR / ASNR / CNS / SAIP /SCAI /SIR / SNIS / SVM / SVS Guideline on the Management of Patients With Extracranial Carotid and Vertebral Artery Disease. *JACC* 2011; *57;* e16-e94.
- Guidelines for the Management of Spontaneous Intracerebral Hemorrhage. *Stroke.* 2010; *41:* 2108-2129
- Guidelines for the Primary Prevention of Stroke. *Stroke.* 2011; *42:* 517-584
- Hamon M, Baron J-C, Viader F et al. Periprocedural Stroke and Cardiac Catheterization. *Circulation.* 2008; *118:* 678-683
- 2014 ESC Guidelines on the diagnosis and management of acute pulmonary embolism. *EHJ* 2014; *35;* 3033-3073.
- Management of Massive and Submassive Pulmonary Embolism, Iliofemoral Deep Vein Thrombosis, and Chronic Thromboembolic Pulmonary Hypertension. A Scientific Statement From the America Heart Association. *Circulation* 2011; *123;* 1788-1830.

08

Peripheral Vascular Disease

- Diagnosis of DVT Antithrombotic Therapy and Prevention of Thrombosis, 9th ed: American College of Chest Physicians Evidence-Based Clinical Practice Guidelines. *CHEST* 2012; *141;* e351-418.
- Antithrombotic Therapy for VTE Disease. Antithrombotic Therapy and Prevention of Thrombosis, 9th ed: American College of Chest Physicians Evidence-Based Clinical Practice Guidelines. *CHEST* 2012; *141;* e419-e494.
- Treatment and Prevention of Heparin-Induced Thrombocytopenia. Antithrombotic Therapy and Prevention of Thrombosis, 9th ed: American College of Chest Physicians Evidence-Based Clinical Practice Guidelines. *CHEST* 2012; *141;* e495s-e530s.
- Greinacher A. Heparin-induced thrombocytopenia. *NEJM* 2015; *373;* 252-261.
- ACCF/AHA 2009 Expert Consensus Document on Pulmonary Hypertension. *JACC* 2009; *53;* 1573-1619.
- 2015 Guidelines for the diagnosis and treatment of pulmonary hypertension. *EHJ* 2016; *37;* 67-119.
- Simonneau G, Gatzoulis M, Adatia A. Updated Clinical Classification of Pulmonary Hypertension. *JACC* 2013; *62;* D34-D41.
- Hoeper M, Bogaard H, Condliffe R. Definitions and Diagnosis of Pulmonary Hypertension. *JACC* 2013; *62;* D42-D50.
- Galiè N, Corris P, Frost A. Updated Treatment Algorithm of Pulmonary Arterial Hypertension. *JACC* 2013; *62;* D60-D72.
- McLaughlin V, Gain SP, Howard L. Treatment Goald of Pulmonary Hypertension. *JACC* 2013; *62;* D73-D81.
- Kim N, Delcroix M, Jenkins D. Chronic Thromboembolic Pulmonary Hypertension. *JACC* 2013; *62;* D92-D99.
- Vachiéry JL, Adir Y, Barberà JA. Pulmonary Hypertension Due to Left Heart Diseases. *JACC* 2013; *62;* D100-D108.
- Haïat R, Leroy G. *Prescription guidelines in cardiology,* 5th edition. Éditions Frison-Roche. 2015. 350 p.
- UpToDate 2015

# Miscellaneous

**09**

| | | |
|---|---|---|
| 9.1/ | Preoperative assessment (noncardiac surgery) | 310 |
| 9.2/ | Primary & Secondary prevention of cardiovascular disease | 314 |
| 9.3/ | Smoking cessation | 315 |
| 9.4/ | Dyslipidemia | 316 |
| 9.5/ | Hypertension | 323 |
| 9.6/ | Diabetes | 329 |
| 9.7/ | Physical activity | 333 |
| 9.8/ | Weight & Diet | 336 |
| 9.9/ | Obstructive sleep apnea syndrome | 338 |
| 9.10/ | Driving & Air travel | 339 |
| 9.11/ | Cardiovascular complications of systemic diseases | 341 |
| 9.12/ | Cardiovascular complications of trauma | 343 |
| 9.13/ | Poisoning | 344 |
| 9.14/ | Swan-Ganz catheter placement | 346 |
| 9.15/ | Cardiopulmonary resuscitation | 347 |

# 9.1/ PREOPERATIVE ASSESSMENT (noncardiac surgery)

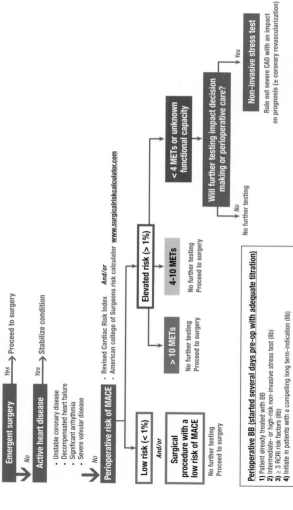

**PREOPERATIVE ASSESSMENT - NON-CARDIAC SURGERY**

**Emergent surgery** → *Yes* → Proceed to surgery

*No*

**Active heart disease** → *Yes* → Stabilize condition
- Unstable coronary disease
- Decompensated heart failure
- Significant arrhythmia
- Severe valvular disease

*No*

**Perioperative risk of MACE** · Revised Cardiac Risk Index    ***And/or***
· American college of Surgeons risk calculator www.surgicalriskcalculator.com

***And/or***

**Low risk (< 1%)**

**Surgical procedure with a low risk of MACE**

No further testing
Proceed to surgery

**Elevated risk (> 1%)**

**> 10 METs**
No further testing
Proceed to surgery

**4-10 METs**
No further testing
Proceed to surgery

**< 4 METs or unknown functional capacity**

**Will further testing impact decision making or perioperative care?**

*No* → No further testing

*Yes* →

**Non-invasive stress test**
Rule out severe CAD with an impact on prognosis (± coronary revascularization)

**Perioperative BB (started several days pre-op with adequate titration)**
1) Patient already treated with BB
2) Intermediate- or high-risk non-invasive stress test (IIb)
3) ≥ 3 RCRI risk factors (IIb)
4) Initiate in patients with a compelling long term-indication (IIb)

## EVALUATION OF FUNCTIONAL CAPACITY

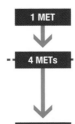

**1 MET**
- Eating; dressing; going to the toilet
- Walking indoors
- Walking 1-2 blocks (3.2-4.8 kph)
- Light housework (washing dishes; dusting)

**4 METs**
- Climbing one flight of stairs
- Walking at 6.4 kph
- Running a short distance
- Heavy housework (scrubbing floors; moving furniture)
- Golf - Bowling - Dancing - Doubles tennis - Playing ball
- Swimming - Singles tennis - Skiing - Basketball

**10 METs**

## REVISED CARDIAC RISK INDEX (RCRI) DURING NONCARDIAC SURGERY

| | |
|---|---|
| 1) History of CAD<br>2) History of heart failure<br>3) History of cerebrovascular disease<br>4) Insulin-treated DM<br>5) Pre-op Creatinine > 2 mg/dL (> 176 mmol/L)<br>6) Intrathoracic or intraperitoneal or vascular surgery | **Risk of cardiac events** (MI; pulmonary edema; VF; cardiac arrest; complete heart block)<br><br>0 point = low risk (0.5%)<br>1 point = moderate risk (1.3%)<br>2 points = moderate risk (3.6%)<br>≥ 3 points = high risk (9.1%) |

*Lee TH, Marcantonio ER, Mangione CM. Circulation 1999; 100; 1043-1049*

## CARDIAC RISK ASSOCIATED WITH SURGERY

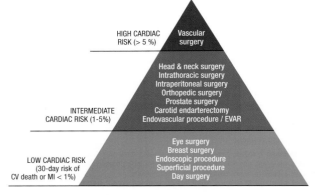

HIGH CARDIAC RISK (> 5 %) — Vascular surgery

INTERMEDIATE CARDIAC RISK (1-5%) — Head & neck surgery / Intrathoracic surgery / Intraperitoneal surgery / Orthopedic surgery / Prostate surgery / Carotid endarterectomy / Endovascular procedure / EVAR

LOW CARDIAC RISK (30-day risk of CV death or MI < 1%) — Eye surgery / Breast surgery / Endoscopic procedure / Superficial procedure / Day surgery

## NONINVASIVE STRATIFICATION

**OBJECTIVE**: to exclude the presence of severe CAD with an impact on prognosis and which would require revascularization, regardless of the type of surgery

**PREOPERATIVE REVASCULARIZATION: no benefit on perioperative events,** even in the presence of significant ischemia on noninvasive stratification (★ CARP; ★ DECREASE-V)

**INDICATIONS FOR PREOPERATIVE REVASCULARIZATION: identical to stable CAD or unstable angina or NSTEMI or STEMI** (▶▶| Chapter 2 - CAD)    **+**

## PERIOPERATIVE BETA-BLOCKERS AND STATINS

**BB - INDICATIONS**: **1)** Patient already treated with BB (Class I recommendation); **2)** Intermediate- or high-risk non-invasive stress test (IIb); **3)** ≥ 3 RCRI risk factors (IIb); **4)** Initiate in patients with a compelling long term indication (IIb)

**BB - MODALITY OF USE**: Start BB therapy several days preoperatively; titrate the dose targeting a resting HR of 60-80 bpm; avoid hypotension

> ★ **POISE**: High-dose Metroprolol succinate started **2-4 h preoperatively** versus placebo; ↘ primary outcomes (cardiovascular mortality; MI) but ↗ all-cause mortality and ↗ stroke

**STATINS - INDICATIONS:** **1)** Patient already on statin (I); **2)** Initiate if undergoing vascular surgery (IIa); **3)** Initiate in patients with clinical indications who are undergoing elevated-risk procedures (IIb)

## PERIOPERATIVE ECG AND TROPONIN

**ECG: Preoperative** → CAD, arrhythmia, PAD, cerebrovascular disease or structural heart disease (except for low-risk procedures); **Post-operative** → **A)** Signs or symptoms suggestive of ischemia / MI / arrhythmia; **B)** Usefulness of routine screening in asymptomatic patient is uncertain

**POSTOPERATIVE TROPONIN**: Indications → **A)** Signs or symptoms suggestive of ischemia or MI; **B)** Usefulness of routine screening in asymptomatic patient is uncertain (IIb)

**DIAGNOSIS OF PERIOPERATIVE MYOCARDIAL INFARCTION**: ▶▶| Chapter 2 (Definition of MI)

> **Consider type 1 myocardial infarction (rupture of fragile plaque) or type 2 (O_2 supply/ demand mismatch); Type 1 MI causes < 5% of troponin elevation postoperatively**    **+**

## PERMANENT PACEMAKER AND DEFIBRILLATOR

**PACEMAKER-DEPENDENT PATIENT: Reprogram in VOO or DOO mode** or apply a magnet during the operation (asynchronous stimulation)

**DEFIBRILLATOR**: **Temporarily** deactivate tachyarrhythmia therapies or apply a magnet during the operation

> **N.B.**: a magnet applied to a defibrillator deactivates tachyarrhythmia therapies, **but does not change the pacing mode to VOO or DOO**; risk of inappropriate inhibition of pacing

## SPECIFIC ENTITIES

**HCM**: avoid dehydration / vasodilators / hypotension / beta-agonists

**SEVERE AORTIC STENOSIS**

> **Asymptomatic**: complete preoperative clinical reassessment with stress test; consider AVR before elective high-risk non-cardiac surgery; monitor intravascular volume; avoid tachycardia; avoid intraoperative hypotension (treat with phenylephrine)
> **Patient refusing AVR or not a candidate or requiring urgent surgery**: operative mortality ≥ 10%; consider TAVI or balloon valvuloplasty if hemodynamically unstable

**POST-PCI SURGERY AND DUAL ANTIPLATELET THERAPY**

> **Post-PTCA**: wait **2-4 weeks** (then operate under ASA)
> **Post-BMS**: dual antiplatelet therapy for a minimum of **2-4 weeks** (then operate under ASA)
>  • Discontinue Clopidogrel 5-7 days preoperatively
> **Post-DES**: dual antiplatelet therapy for a **strict minimum of 3 to 6 months** with new
>  generation stents (consider bridging with IV tirofiban / eptifibatide / cangrelor if surgery required
>  before this time) then operate under ASA

| | MECHANICAL VALVE PROSTHESIS | ATRIAL FIBRILLATION | THROMBOEMBOLIC DISEASE |
|---|---|---|---|
| **High thrombo-embolic risk (annual risk > 10%)** | • Mitral valve prosthesis<br>• Old generation aortic valve prosthesis (cagedball; tilting-disk)<br>• Stroke or TIA < 6 months | • CHADS 5 or 6<br>• Stroke or TIA < 3 months<br>• Rheumatic disease | • Thromboembolism < 3 months<br>• Severe thrombophilia (protein C or S or antithrombin deficiency; antiphospholipid antibodies; multiple anomalies) |
| | • Stop Warfarin 5 days pre-op + Bridge with IV heparin or LMWH<br>  - **Prosthetic Valve or AF →** Enoxaparin 1 mg/kg bid or Dalteparin 100 IU/kg bid; **Venous thromboembolism →** Enoxaparin 1.5 mg/kg qd or Dalteparin 200 IU/kg qd<br>• INR on the day before surgery (vitamin K 1 mg PO if INR > 1.5)<br>• Stop IV Heparin 4-6 h pre-op; Last dose of LMWH 24 h pre-op (Enoxaparin 1 mg/kg or Dalteparin 100 IU/kg administered 24 h pre-op)<br>• Resume Warfarin 12-24 h post-op if adequate hemostasis<br>• Resume Heparin (without bolus) or LMWH 48-72 h post-op depending on hemostasis<br>• Consider IVC filter in the presence of venous thromboembolism < 4 weeks | | |
| **Moderate thromboembolic risk (annual risk 5-10%)** | **Bileaflet aortic valve prosthesis with ≥ 1 risk factor:**<br>AF • History of stroke or TIA • HTN • DM • Heart failure • > 75 years | CHADS 3 or 4<br><br>(no benefit in ★BRIDGE; mean CHADS = 2.3) | • Thromboembolism 3-12 months<br>• Nonsevere thrombophilia: Leiden factor V or prothrombin mutation (heterozygous)<br>• Active neoplasia |
| | • Case-by-case decision for heparin bridge (thromboembolic risk versus perioperative bleeding risk) | | |
| **Low thromboembolic risk (annual risk < 5%)** | Bileaflet aortic valve prosthesis with no other risk factor | CHADS 0 to 2 (with no history of stroke or TIA) | Thromboembolism > 12 months (with no other risk factor) |
| | • Heparin bridge not recommended | | |

**MINOR PROCEDURES**: do not discontinue Warfarin for superficial skin or ophthalmic (cataract) or dental procedures (use tranexamic acid)

**PERIOPERATIVE DOAC: ►►I** Chapter 6

# 9.2/ PRIMARY & SECONDARY PREVENTION OF CARDIOVASCULAR DISEASE

## EVALUATION OF THE RISK OF ADVERSE CARDIOVASCULAR EVENTS

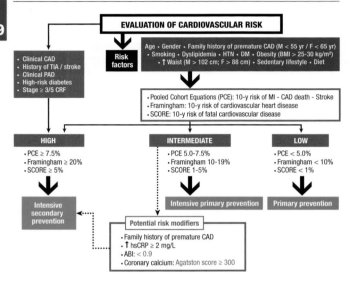

## CARDIOVASCULAR DISEASE - PRIMARY PREVENTION

**CONTROL OF CONVENTIONAL RISK FACTORS:** ▶▶| Smoking cessation; ▶▶| Dyslipidemia; ▶▶| HTN; ▶▶| DM; ▶▶| Weight & Diet; ▶▶| Physical exercise

**ASA**: not recommended as part of routine primary prevention     +

> ★ **Antithrombotic Trialists' Collaboration**: marginal benefit of ASA for primary   +
> prevention (high NNT); bleeding risk
> **Consider ASA for primary prevention**: in the presence of a low bleeding risk but high cardiovascular risk (subclinical atherosclerosis; multiple risk factors; family history of premature cardiovascular disease) (Class IIb recommendation; C)

## CARDIOVASCULAR DISEASE - SECONDARY PREVENTION

| Smoking | Complete cessation |
|---|---|
| Dyslipidemia | High dose statin; Target → ≥ 50% ↘ LDL |
| HTN | Target BP < 140/90 (< 140/85 in the presence of DM) |

| Antiplatelet therapy | ASA: for life (★ Antithrombotic Trialists')<br>• Clopidogrel as alternative (★ CAPRIE)<br>• No benefit of ASA + Clopidogrel combination (★ CHARISMA) |
|---|---|
| ACE inhibitors | As secondary prevention for all patients<br>(especially when LVEF ≤ 40% or HTN or DM or CRF) |
| BB | • LVEF ≤ 40%: Long term<br>• Normal LVEF: can be stop 3 years after ACS<br>• Antianginal: Long term |
| DM | HbA1c < 7% |
| Physical exercise | > 30 min moderate exercise 5 x per week |
| Obesity | • BMI: 18.5 - 24.9 kg/m² • Waist: M < 102 cm and F < 88 cm |
| Healthy diet | Healthy and balanced diet |
| Influenza vaccine | Annually |
| Hormonal therapy; NSAID | Avoid |

# 9.3/ SMOKING CESSATION

**30% of deaths related to CAD can be attributed to smoking**

**BENEFITS**: reduction of cardiovascular risk to achieve a similar level to that of nonsmokers after 5 years of smoking cessation

**INTERVENTION**

1) Confirm that the patient is a smoker; 2) Strongly recommend smoking cessation; 3) Ask the patient whether he/she wants to stop smoking (if the patient refuses, suggest reducing consumption ± nicotine replacement therapy); 4) Establish a plan and a date for complete cessation; 5) Inform the patient's friends and relatives; 6) Remove all objects related to smoking; 7) Cease all activities related to smoking; 8) Have a plan in the case of temptation / relapse; 9) Propose drug therapy; 10) Propose support by a smoking cessation center; 11) **www.smokefree.gov** ; 12) Ensure regular follow-up

**DRUG THERAPY**

| Nicotine gum | **Initially 1 gum every 1–2 h then decrease (maximum: 24 gums per day)**<br>• ≤ 24 cigarettes / day: 2 mg gum<br>• ≥ 25 cigarettes / day: 4 mg gum | • 6-month abstinence rate: 19%<br>• **Adverse effects**: Nausea; Oropharyngeal irritation |
|---|---|---|
| Transdermal nicotine patch | • < 10 cigarettes / day: 14 mg patch for 6 weeks then 7 mg patch for 4 weeks then stop<br>• > 10 cigarettes / day: 21 mg patch for 6 weeks then 14 mg patch for 2 weeks then 7 mg patch for 2 weeks | • 6-month abstinence rate: 23%<br>• **Adverse effects**: Local skin reaction; Nausea; Insomnia |
| Bupropion SR | • Inhibits dopamine and norepinephrine reuptake<br>• Bupropion SR 150 mg PO daily for 3 days then bid for 12 weeks then stop<br>• Start 10 days before smoking cessation<br>• Can be combined with nicotine replacement therapy | • 6-month abstinence rate: 24%<br>• **Adverse effects**: Decreased seizure threshold; Insomnia; Xerostomia; Nightmares |

| Varenicline | • Partial agonist of acetylcholine nicotinic receptor<br>• Varenicline 0.5 mg PO daily for 3 days then bid for 3 days then 1 mg bid for 11 weeks then stop<br>• Start 1 to 2 weeks before smoking cessation<br>• Can be combined with nicotine replacement therapy | Contraindicated in the case of pregnancy or breastfeeding or CRF or mental illness |
|---|---|---|

# 9.4/ DYSLIPIDEMIA

**DIET:** source of triglycerides (glycerol bound to 3 fatty acid chains) and dietary Cholesterol

**LIPOPROTEINS:** transport TG and cholesterol in the blood

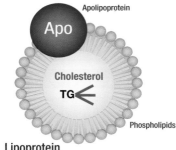

Lipoprotein

**CHYLOMICRONS:** large nonatherogenic lipoproteins transporting TG from the gastrointestinal tract; apoB48

**VLDL:** large nonatherogenic lipoproteins transporting TG from the liver; apoB100

**LDL: atherogenic lipoproteins responsible for atherosclerosis; mainly contain cholesterol; apoB100**  +

> **Calculated LDL (mmol/L) = TC - HDL - (0.45 x TG) (valid if TG < 4.5 mmol/L)**
> **Calculated LDL (mg/dL) = TC - HDL - (TG / 5) (valid if TG < 400 mg/dL)**

**NON-HDL CHOLESTEROL (= TC - HDL):** cholesterol contained in LDL - VLDL - IDL - Lp(a); predictive of cardiovascular risk

> **ApoB:** comprises LDL - VLDL - IDL - Lp(a)

**HDL:** antiatherogenic properties; contains apolipoprotein **ApoA1**

**HYPERTRIGLYCERIDEMIA: TG-enriched LDL → formation of smaller and denser LDL (due to modification by hepatic lipase) → dense, atherogenic LDL**  +

> **HyperTG:** TG-enriched HDL (CTEP) → ↗ recovery of HDL by the liver → ↘ HDL  +
> **HyperTG:** associated with metabolic syndrome (↗ TG; ↘ HDL; dense, atherogenic LDL)  +
> **HyperTG: risk of pancreatitis** (especially if TG > 10 mmol/L or > 885 mg/dL)

**LP(a):** apolipoprotein(a) bound to a molecule of LDL; associated with an increased risk of cardiovascular events; plasma concentration is genetically determined

# SCREENING FOR DYSLIPIDEMIA

- Male ≥ 40 years
- Female ≥ 50 years (or postmenopausal)
- DM
- HTN
- Smoking
- BMI > 27 kg/m²
- CRF - CrCl < 60 mL/min
- Atherosclerosis

- Family history of premature CAD (M < 55 years; F < 65 years)
- Family history of dyslipidemia
- SLE - RA - Psoriatic arthritis - Ankylosing spondylitis - Inflammatory bowel disease
- COPD
- Erectile dysfunction
- HIV (treated with antiretroviral agents)
- Clinical features of familial dyslipidemia (xanthomas; xanthelasmas; arcus senilis)

# DYSLIPIDEMIA: UNDERLYING CAUSES

**HYPERCHOLESTEROLEMIA**: Hypothyroidism; Cholestasis; Nephrotic syndrome; CRF; Cushing; Corticosteroids; Anorexia; HIV protease inhibitors

**HYPERTRIGLYCERIDEMIA:** Obesity; DM; Alcohol; CRF; Hypothyroidism; Corticosteroids; Antipsychotics (Clozapine; Olanzapine); Nonselective BB; Thiazides; Cyclosporine; HIV protease inhibitors; Retinoic acid; Hormonal therapy; Sirolimus; Bile acid sequestrants

↘ **HDL**: Smoking; Obesity; Sedentary lifestyle; DM; CRF; HyperTG; Nonselective BB; Corticosteroids; Anabolic steroids; Cyclosporine

# GENETIC DISORDERS OF LIPOPROTEINS

| | | | |
|---|---|---|---|
| **Familial hyper-cholesterolemia** | ↗ LDL | - **LDL–R receptor mutation**<br>- 1,000 mutations identified<br>- Autosomal dominant | - Arcus senilis<br>- Xanthelasmas<br>- **Pathognomonic tendinous xanthomas** (extensor tendons; MCP; Achilles tendon)<br>- Premature CAD |
| **Defective Apo B100** | ↗ LDL | - ↘ Affinity for LDL-R receptor<br>- Autosomal dominant | - Similar presentation to familial hyper-cholesterolemia |
| **Familial LPL deficiency** | ↗ TG | - **Abnormal catabolism of chylomicrons** and VLDL | - **Pancreatitis**<br>- **Lipemia retinalis**<br>- **Eruptive xanthomas**<br>- **Lactescent serum** |
| **Familial Apo-C-II deficiency** | ↗ TG | - **Apo-CII is the LPL activator** | - Similar presentation to familial LPL deficiency |
| **Familial dysbeta-lipoproteinemia** | ↗ TC<br>↗ TG | - **Homozygote for ApoE2** (less effective binding to hepatic receptors)<br>- Accumulation of **remnant lipoproteins** (IDL; remnant chylomicrons) | - Premature CAD<br>- **Tuberous xanthomas** (elbows; knees)<br>- **Palmar xanthomas**<br>- **Consider diagnosis:** ApoB (g/L) / TC (mmol/L) ratio < 0.15 |

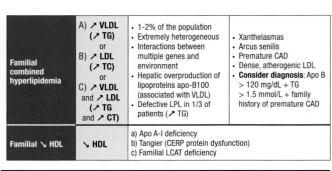

| | A) ↗ VLDL (↗ TG) or B) ↗ LDL (↗ TC) or C) ↗ VLDL and ↗ LDL (↗ TG and ↗ CT) | • 1-2% of the population<br>• Extremely heterogeneous<br>• Interactions between multiple genes and environment<br>• Hepatic overproduction of lipoproteins apo-B100 (associated with VLDL)<br>• Defective LPL in 1/3 of patients (↗ TG) | • Xanthelasmas<br>• Arcus senilis<br>• Premature CAD<br>• Dense, atherogenic LDL<br>• **Consider diagnosis**: Apo B > 120 mg/dL + TG > 1.5 mmol/L + family history of premature CAD |
|---|---|---|---|
| **Familial combined hyperlipidemia** | | | |
| **Familial ↘ HDL** | ↘ HDL | a) Apo A-I deficiency<br>b) Tangier (CERP protein dysfunction)<br>c) Familial LCAT deficiency | |

## MANAGEMENT - CANADIAN TARGETS

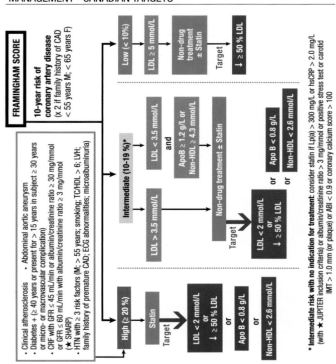

**FRAMINGHAM SCORE**

**10-year risk of coronary artery disease**
(x 2 if family history of CAD < 55 years M; < 65 years F)

• Clinical atherosclerosis  • Abdominal aortic aneurysm
• Diabetes (≥ 40 years or present for > 15 years in subject ≥ 30 years or micro- or macrovascular complication)
• CRF with GFR ≤ 45 mL/min or albumin/creatinine ratio ≥ 30 mg/mmol or GFR ≤ 60 mL/min with albumin/creatinine ratio ≥ 3 mg/mmol (★ SHARP)
• HTN with ≥ 3 risk factors (M: > 55 years; smoking; TC/HDL > 6; LVH; family history of premature CAD; ECG abnormalities; microalbuminuria)

**Low (< 10%)** → **LDL ≥ 5 mmol/L** → **Non-drug treatment ± Statin** → **Target ↓ ≥ 50 % LDL**

**Intermediate (10-19 %)\***

LDL < 3.5 mmol/L and ApoB ≥ 1.2 g/L or Non-HDL ≥ 4.3 mmol/L → **Non-drug treatment ± Statin** → **Apo B < 0.8 g/L** or **Non-HDL < 2.6 mmol/L**

LDL > 3.5 mmol/L → **Non-drug treatment ± Statin** → **Target LDL < 2 mmol/L** or **↓ ≥ 50 % LDL**

**High (≥ 20 %)** → **Statin** → **Target LDL < 2 mmol/L** or **↓ ≥ 50 % LDL** or **Apo B < 0.8 g/L** or **Non-HDL < 2.6 mmol/L**

**\* Intermediate risk with no indication for treatment:** consider statin if Lp(a) ≥ 300 mg/L or hsCRP > 2.0 mmol/L (with ★ JUPITER inclusion criteria) or albumin/creatinine ratio > 3 mg/mmol or positive stress test or carotid IMT > 1.0 mm (or plaque) or ABI < 0.9 or coronary calcium score > 100

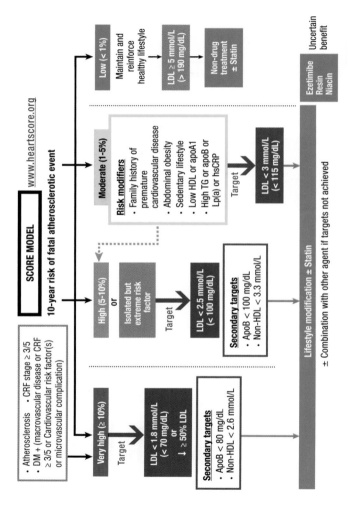

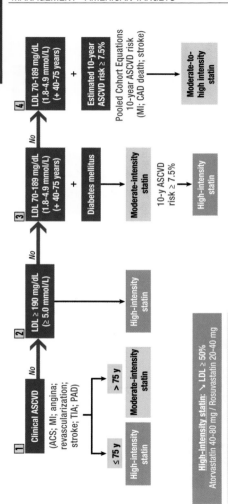

**1** Clinical ASCVD

(ACS; MI; angina; revascularization; stroke; TIA; PAD)

≤ 75 y → **High-intensity statin**

> 75 y → **Moderate-intensity statin**

**2** LDL ≥ 190 mg/dL (≥ 5.0 mmol/L) → **High-intensity statin**

*No*

**3** LDL 70-189 mg/dL (1.8-4.9 mmol/L) (+ 40-75 years)

Diabetes mellitus → **Moderate-intensity statin**

10-y ASCVD risk ≥ 7.5% → **High-intensity statin**

*No*

**4** LDL 70-189 mg/dL (1.8-4.9 mmol/L) (+ 40-75 years)

+

Estimated 10-year ASCVD risk ≥ 7.5%

Pooled Cohort Equations 10-year ASCVD risk (MI; CAD death; stroke) → **Moderate-to-high intensity statin**

**High-intensity statin:** ↘ LDL ≥ 50%
Atorvastatin 40-80 mg / Rosuvastatin 20-40 mg

**Moderate-intensity statin:** ↘ LDL 30-50%
Atorvastatin 10-20 mg / Rosuvastatin 5-10 mg /
Simvastatin 20-40 mg / Pravastatin 40-80 mg

Less evidence for statin therapy
in NYHA II-IV HF or Hemodialysis

**ASCVD:** Atherosclerotic cardiovascular disease

**Consider statin therapy**
· LDL ≥ 160 mg/dL (≥ 4.1 mmol/L)
· Evidence of genetic hyperlipidemia
· Family history of premature ASCVD (< 55 y M - < 65 y F)
· Hs-CRP ≥ 2 mg/L
· CAC ≥ 300 Agatston units
· ABI < 0.9

**NONDRUG TREATMENT**: healthy diet; diet rich in omega-3 fatty acids; target healthy weight (BMI 18.5 to 24.9 kg/m²); regular physical exercise; smoking cessation; moderate alcohol consumption (maximum: 2 glasses per day for M and 1 glass per day for F)

**DRUG TREATMENT**: First-line Statin

**HYPERTRIGLYCERIDEMIA**: avoid alcohol and secondary causes; ↘ carbohydrates; increase omega-3 consumption; exercise and weight loss; control of DM

> **TG > 10 mmol/L (> 885 mg/dL) → Fibrate for prevention of pancreatitis**
> **TG 5-10 mmol/L (440-885 mg/dL) → Consider Fibrate (undemonstrated benefit)**

↘ **HDL**: smoking cessation; weight loss; exercise; moderate alcohol consumption

> **Niacin**: no benefit in ★ AIM-HIGH and ★ HPS2-THRIVE studies

| STATINS (HMG–COA REDUCTASE INHIBITORS) | | |
|---|---|---|
| **Atorvastatin** | 10-80 mg | • ↘ **LDL (30-50%)**<br>• ↘TG (10-30 %); ↗ HDL (5-10 %)<br>• ↘ intracellular cholesterol synthesis → ↗ expression of LDL-R receptor<br>• **Pleiotropic effects**: stabilization of atherosclerotic plaque; antiinflammatory effect; antithrombotic effect; improves endothelial function<br>• **Adverse effects**: ↗ Transaminases; Myalgia / Myositis / Rhabdomyolysis; Drug interactions; ↗ risk of DM |
| **Fluvastatin** | 20-80 mg | |
| **Lovastatin** | 20-80 mg | |
| **Pravastatin** | 10-40 mg | |
| **Rosuvastatin** | 5-40 mg | |
| **Simvastatin** | 10-40 mg | |

| BILE ACID SEQUESTRANTS (RESINS) | | |
|---|---|---|
| **Colesevelam** | 4 to 6 tablets (in 1 or 2 daily doses) | • ↘ **LDL (15-30 %)**<br>• **Adverse effects:** GI symptoms (constipation; discomfort); ↘ absorption of medications; ↗ TG |
| **Colestipol** | 1 or 5 g / unit; 2-6 units / days (with meals) | |

| CHOLESTEROL ABSORPTION INHIBITOR | | |
|---|---|---|
| **Ezetimibe** | 10 mg | • ↘ **LDL (20 %)**<br>• Interferes with NPC1-L1 protein of intestinal epithelial cells<br>• ★ **IMPROVE-IT**: Ezetimibe + Simvastatin vs. Simvastatin post ACS; ↘ MI and Stroke |

| FIBRATES | | |
|---|---|---|
| **Fenofibrate** | 200 mg | • ↘ **TG (35-50 %)**<br>• ↗ HDL (5-10 %); ↘ LDL (10-20 %)<br>• ↗ LPL activity; ↘ Hepatic secretion of VLDL<br>• **No benefit in ★ ACCORD study**<br>• **Adverse effects**: ↗ Creatinine (adjust according to CrCl); Myotoxicity (avoid Gemfibrozil with statin); Rash; Drug interactions; ↗ Transaminases |
| **Bezafibrate** | 400 mg | |
| **Gemfibrozil** | 600 mg bid | |

| NICOTINIC ACID | | |
|---|---|---|
| Niacin | 1 g tid | • ↗ HDL (25 %); ↘ TG (30 %); ↘ LDL (20 %) |
| Slow-release niacin (Niaspan) | 1-2 g daily | • ↗ Hepatic production of apo A1<br>• ↘ HDL catabolism<br>• ↘ Hepatic production of VLDL<br>• **No benefit in ★ AIM-HIGH and ★ HPS2-THRIVE studies**<br>• **Adverse effects:** Flushing (↘ with ASA); Hyperuricemia; Hyperglycemia; Hepatotoxicity; Gastritis |

| CETP INHIBITORS |
|---|
| ↗ HDL; Anacetrapib; Dalcetrapib (no benefit in ★ dal–OUTCOMES); Evacetrapib |

| PCSK9 INHIBITORS |
|---|
| ↘ LDL |
| ★ **ODYSSEY long term:** ↘ LDL (62 %); ↘ MACE with Alirocumab vs. Placebo |
| ★ **OSLER:** ↘ LDL (61 %); ↘ cardiovascular events and MACE with Evolocumab vs. Placebo |

## STATINS

★ **CHOLESTEROL TREATMENT TRIALISTS':** each 1 mmol/L (40 mg/dL) ↘ of LDL → 20-25% ↘ RR of cardiovascular mortality or myocardial infarction     +

**PRIMARY PREVENTION:** ★ WOSCOPS (Pravastatin); ★ AFCAPS/TexCAPS (Lovastatin); ★ HPS (Simvastatin); ★ ASCOT (Atorvastatin); ★ JUPITER (Rosuvastatin)

**SECONDARY PREVENTION:** ★ 4S (Simvastatin); ★ CARE (Pravastatin); ★ LIPID (Pravastatin); ★ HPS (Simvastatin)
> **Intensive treatment:** ★ A-to-Z and ★ SEARCH (Simvastatin); ★ PROVE-IT, ★ TNT, ★ ALLIANCE, ★ IDEAL and ★ SPARCL (Atorvastatin)

**ADVANCED HEART FAILURE (LVEF < 30 %):** no benefit (★ CORONA; ★ GISSI-HF)

**RENAL FAILURE ON DIALYSIS:** no benefit (★4D; ★AURORA)

## MONITORING OF STATIN THERAPY

**LIPID PROFILE:** At 4 to 12 weeks; then annually when dose adjusted and targets achieved

**DECREASING DOSE: may be considered when LDL < 1.0 mmol/L (< 40 mg/dL)**     +

**MYALGIA:** Discontinue Statin then resume several weeks later to **prove toxicity** (+ monitoring of CK)
> **Proven toxicity:** A) Reintroduce the same statin at a lower dose; B) Fluvastatin; C) Rosuvastatin 5-10 mg daily (or every 2 days or once a week); D) Ezetimibe - Niacin - Fibrate
> **Consider other conditions:** Hypothyroidism; CRF; liver disease; PMR; steroid myopathy; vitamin D deficiency; primary muscle diseases

**MYOSITIS:** myalgia + ↗ CK > ULN

**RHABDOMYOLYSIS:** severe myalgia; CK > 10,000 IU/L; Myoglobinuria; ± ARF

**RISK FACTORS FOR MYOPATHY:** statin dose; drug interactions; > 75 years; CRF (prefer Atorvastatin); liver disease; alcohol; pre-existing myopathy

| AST – ALT | | CK | |
|---|---|---|---|
| **Baseline measurement and as necessary** | | **Assay as necessary in the presence of myalgia** | |
| ↗ < 3 x ULN | ↗ ≥ 3 x ULN | ↗ ≤ 5 x ULN | ↗ > 5 x ULN |
| • Continue treatment<br>• AST - ALT in 6 weeks<br>• If stable → stop monitoring AST - ALT | • Discontinue Statin<br>• Consider DDx (alcohol; drugs; NASH)<br>• Monitor AST - ALT until normalization<br><br>**Normalization**<br>a) Reintroduce at a lower dose<br>b) Different statin<br>c) Ezetimibe - Niacin - Fibrate | • Continue statin in the absence of symptoms<br>• Repeat CK in 6 weeks<br>• Discontinue Statin in the presence of symptoms or ↗ CK<br>• If stable and asymptomatic → stop monitoring CK | • Discontinue Statin<br>• Consider rhabdomyolysis (± hydration)<br>• Monitor CK until normalization<br>• Consider DDx<br><br>**Normalization**<br>a) Reintroduce at a lower dose<br>b) Different statin<br>c) Ezetimibe - Niacin - Fibrate |

**09**

Miscellaneous

# 9.5/ HYPERTENSION

## ASSESSMENT

| **DIAGNOSIS OF HYPERTENSION** | |
|---|---|
| **Office** | **1ˢᵗ VISIT:** SBP ≥ 140 and/or DBP ≥ 90 |
| | **SUBSEQUENT VISIT:**<br>• Diagnosis of HTN if **target organ damage or DM or GFR < 60 mL/min**<br>• Diagnosis of HTN if **SBP ≥ 180 and/or DBP ≥ 110**<br>• Otherwise<br>  › **Office**: diagnosis of HTN if **SBP ≥ 160 and/or DBP ≥100** x first 3 visits (mean)<br>  › **Office**: diagnosis of HTN if **SBP ≥ 140 and/or DBP ≥ 90** x first 5 visits (mean)<br>  › **ABPM or BP measured at home** |
| **ABPM (24 h)** | • Daytime SBP: ≥ 135 or<br>• 24-hour SBP: ≥ 130 or<br>• Night: SBP ≥ 120; ↘ < 10 % | • Daytime DBP: ≥ 85 or<br>• 24-hour DBP: ≥ 80 or<br>• Night: DBP ≥ 70; ↘ < 10 % |
| **BP at home** | Daytime SBP: ≥ 135 mmHg | Daytime DBP: ≥ 85 mmHg |
| | • ≥ 2 readings daily (on getting out of bed and at bedtime) for 7 days (mean of days 2 to 7)<br>• Recommended apparatus: www.hypertension.ca | |
| **Hypertensive emergency** | HTN diagnosed immediately | |

| **STAGE OF HTN** | | |
|---|---|---|
| **Grade 1**<br>140-159 and/or 90-99 | **Grade 2**<br>160-179 and/or 100-109 | **Grade 3**<br>≥ 180 and/or ≥ 110 |

## BLOOD PRESSURE MEASUREMENT TECHNIQUE

**a)** After resting for 5 min; no coffee or cigarettes for > 30 min; legs uncrossed; **b)** Patient seated in a chair with a back with the arms level with the heart; **c)** Inflatable cuff covers **> 80% of the arm circumference**; Cuff > 3 cm above the cubital fossa; **d)** Inflate to 30 mmHg above the level at which the radial pulse is lost; **e)** Deflate by 2 mmHg per beat; **f)** ≥ 3 measurements on the same arm (determine the mean of the last 2 measurements); **g)** Measure BP in both arms; **h)** Measure BP 1 min and 3 min after standing (rule out OH)

> › **First audible sound = SBP (Korotkoff phase I)**
> › **Last audible sound = DBP (Korotkoff phase V)**
>   • If sounds persist until 0 mmHg, use the point at which the sounds become softer to define DBP (phase IV)

**WORK-UP:** Electrolytes; Creat; Urinalysis; Albumin/creat ratio; Fasting glucose; Lipids; CBC; ECG

**ABPM (AMBULANT BLOOD PRESSURE MONITORING):** verify response to treatment; nocturnal HTN (insomnia; OSAHS; obesity; CRF; OH; dysautonomia); evaluate fluctuating BP

> › **White coat syndrome**: high BP in the doctor's office; home BP or daytime ABPM < 130-135/80-85 mmHg; no signs of target organ damage
> › **Masked HTN**: normal BP in the doctor's office; ↗ daytime BP (stress; work...)

## SEARCH FOR TARGET ORGAN DAMAGE

**HEART DISEASE:** CAD; Heart failure; LVH (ECG; TTE)

**CEREBROVASCULAR DISEASE:** stroke; TIA; Intracerebral hemorrhage; SAH; Vascular dementia; Carotid IMT ≥ 1 mm or plaques

**PERIPHERAL ARTERY DISEASE (PAD):** Aortic dissection; AAA; Claudication - Leg ischemia; ABI < 0.9

**RENAL DISEASE:** Hypertensive nephroangiosclerosis; CrCl < 60 mL/min; Microalbuminuria (30-300 mg/24 h or albumin/creatinine ratio 3.4-34 mg/mmol or 30-300 mg/g) or Macroalbuminuria

**HYPERTENSIVE RETINOPATHY:** Hemorrhages; microaneurysms; cotton wool spots or hard exudates; papilledema

## UNDERLYING CAUSES OF HYPERTENSION

**LOOK FOR AN UNDERLYING CAUSE IN THE PRESENCE OF:** severe HTN; sudden onset or sudden deterioration of HTH; treatment failure; target organ damage disproportionate to the duration of HTN

| Chronic renal disease | • Salt and water retention / Volume overload | • Urinalysis; Creatinine; Renal US; ± biopsy |
|---|---|---|
| Renovascular disease | • ►►| Chapter 8 (Peripheral vascular disease) | • Doppler renal arteries; MR angiography; CT angiography |
| CoA | • HTN in arms; ↘ Femoral pulses; Murmur between scapulae | • TTE; MR angiography; CT angiography; Cardiac cath |
| Primary hyper-aldosteronism | • Adenoma; Adrenal hyperplasia<br>• Hypokalemia (spontaneous or severe diuretic-induced); Refractory HTN; ± Hypernatremia; Muscle weakness | • ↗ Plasma Aldosterone / Renin ratio (high sensitivity)<br>• Suppression test with salt load (absence of ↘ of Aldosterone)<br>• Adrenal CT scan or MRI<br>• Adrenal vein catheterization |

| Cushing syndrome | • Truncal obesity; Violaceous striae; Thin skin; Muscle wasting; Osteoporosis; Buffalo hump | • Urinary cortisol<br>• Suppression test (1 mg dexamethasone)<br>• CT scan of adrenal glands |
|---|---|---|
| Pheochromo-cytoma | • Labile HTN; Headache; Profuse sweating; Palpitations<br>• Exacerbated by stress / anesthesia / BB / caffeine / manipulation of the tumor<br>• ± Dilated CM with HTN<br>• Associated with Von Hippel-Lindau syndrome; MEN; Neurofibromatosis | • Plasma metanephrines (sensitivity 99%)<br>• Urine metanephrines<br>• CT scan or MRI of adrenal glands |
| Medications – Drugs | NSAID; Corticosteroids; Cyclosporine; Tacrolimus; EPO; Ephedrine; Decongestants; Cocaine; Amphetamines; Oral contraceptive; MAO inhibitors - SSRI; Midodrine; Anabolic steroids | |

**Other:** Acromegaly; Hypothyroidism; Hyperparathyroidism; Pregnancy; Acute glomerulonephritis; Renal crisis (scleroderma); Rebound HTN (nonadherence to treatment); Smoking; Alcohol; Obesity; Sodium; OSAHS; Liquorice; Chronic pain; Intracranial neoplasm

## MANAGEMENT

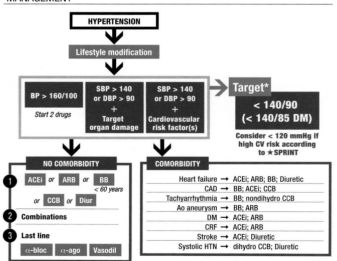

**\* AMERICAN TARGETS (JNC 8)**

• < 60 years (or DM or CRF) → < 140/90 mmHg   • > 60 years → < 150/90 mmHg

★ **SPRINT**: sBP ≥ 130 mmHg + ≥ 50 years old + increased CV risk (CV disease; GFR 20-60 ml/min; Framingham > 15% /10-year; ≥ 75 years) + no diabetes / no prior stroke; target → **sBP < 120 mmHg vs. < 140 mmHg**; study terminated prematurely; ↘ **MACCE**; ↘ **Mortality**

**NONDRUG TREATMENT**: healthy weight (BMI 18.5 to 24.9 kg/m2); waist < 102 cm (M) and < 88 cm (F); regular physical exercise; moderate alcohol consumption; sodium < 2.4 g daily; healthy diet (rich in fruit and vegetables; low-fat; DASH diet); smoking cessation; relaxation techniques

## DRUG TREATMENT

> ★ **ALLHAT**: Chlorthalidone and Lisinopril and Amlodipine are comparable
> ★ **ASCOT**: Hypertensive patients with ≥ 3 cardiovascular risk factors; Amlodipine + Perindopril superior to Atenolol + Thiazide (study terminated prematurely; ↘ stroke, ↘ mortality)
> ★ **ACCOMPLISH**: Hypertensive patients with CAD or high risk of CAD; **Benazepril + Amlodipine superior to Benazepril + HCTZ**

| ANGIOTENSIN–CONVERTING ENZYME (ACE) INHIBITORS | | |
|---|---|---|
| Benazepril | 5 mg to 40 mg qd | |
| Captopril | 6.25 mg tid to 50 mg tid | |
| Cilazapril | 1.25 mg to 10 mg qd | |
| Enalapril | 2.5 mg to 40 mg qd | |
| Fosinopril | 10 mg to 40 mg qd | • ↗ Bradykinin (cough; angioedema) |
| Lisinopril | 5 mg to 40 mg qd | • **Accept ↗ creatinine ≤ 30%** |
| Perindopril | 2.5 to 10 mg qd (2 to 8 mg in Canada) | • Deterioration of renal function with bilateral renal artery stenosis |
| Quinalapril | 5 mg to 40 mg qd | • Hyperkalemia |
| Ramipril | 1.25 mg to 10 mg qd | |
| Trandolapril | 0.5 mg to 4 mg qd | |
| ANGIOTENSIN II RECEPTOR BLOCKERS (ARB) | | |
| Candesartan | 8 mg to 32 mg qd | |
| Irbesartan | 75 mg to 300 mg qd | • ARF; Hyperkalemia; OH; Angioedema |
| Losartan | 25 to 100 mg qd | • Deterioration of renal function with bilateral renal artery stenosis |
| Olmesartan | 20 mg to 40 mg qd | • Do not add ARB to ACE inhibitors (harmful effect in ★ ONTARGET) |
| Telmisartan | 20 mg to 80 mg qd | |
| Valsartan | 40 mg to 320 mg qd | |
| DIRECT RENIN INHIBITORS | | |
| Aliskiren | 150 mg to 300 mg qd | Adverse effect of pro-renin? |
| CALCIUM CHANNEL BLOCKERS | | |
| Amlodipine | 5 mg to 10 mg qd | • Dihydropyridines (Amlodipine and Nifedipine): OH; leg edema; flushing; headache |
| Nifedipine | XL: 30 mg to 120 mg qd | |
| Verapamil | SR: 120 mg qd to 240 mg bid | • Non-dihydropyridines (Diltiazem and Verapamil): negative inotropic agent; negative chronotropic agent |
| Diltiazem | CD: 120 mg to 360 mg qd | |

| DIURETICS | | |
|---|---|---|
| Indapamide | 1.25-2.5 mg daily | |
| Chlorthalidone | 12.5-50 mg daily | |
| Hydrochlorothiazide | 6.25-50 mg daily | |
| Metolazone | 2.5-10 mg daily | • Avoid thiazides if CrCl < 30 mL/min |
| Bumetanide | 0.5-5 mg daily | • Adverse effects (thiazides): |
| Furosemide | 20-600 mg daily | hyponatremia; hypomagnesemia; |
| Torsemide | 2.5-10 mg daily | hypokalemia; OH; glucose intolerance; |
| Eplerenone | 25-100 mg daily | hypercalcemia; ARF; sulfonamide |
| Spironolactone | 25-100 mg daily | allergy; gout |
| Triamterene | 50-300 mg daily | |
| Amiloride | 5-10 mg daily | |

| BETA-BLOCKERS | | |
|---|---|---|
| Acebutolol | 100 mg bid to 400 mg bid | |
| Atenolol | 25 mg to 100 mg qd | |
| Bisoprolol | 2.5 mg to 10 mg qd | |
| Carvedilol | 3.125 mg bid to 50 mg bid | Bronchospasm; Bradycardia; Negative inotropic agent; Exacerbation of PAD; |
| Labetalol | 100 mg bid to 400 mg bid | Fatigue; Erectile dysfunction; Rebound effect on withdrawal; Unopposed alpha |
| Metoprolol | 25 mg bid to 100 mg bid | stimulation (pheochromocytoma); ↗ TG and ↘ HDL (nonselective); Masks |
| Nadolol | 40 mg to 240 mg qd | symptoms of hypoglycemia; glucose intolerance |
| Nebivolol | 2.5 mg to 20 mg qd | |
| Pindolol | 2.5 mg bid to 40 mg bid | |
| Propranolol | LA: 80 mg to 320 mg qd | |
| Timolol | 2.5 mg bid to 20 mg bid | |

| ALPHA-BLOCKERS | | |
|---|---|---|
| Doxazosin | 1 mg to 16 mg qd | • Not recommended as first-line |
| Prazosin | 0.5 mg tid to 5 mg tid | • OH; Fluid retention (risk of heart failure) |
| Terazosin | 1 mg to 20 mg qd | • Doxazosin used as third line in ★ ASCOT |

| CENTRAL ALPHA-ADRENERGIC AGONISTS (VASOMOTOR ACTIVITY CENTER) | | |
|---|---|---|
| Methyldopa | 250-3000 mg daily | Sedation; Dry mouth; Impotence; Galactorrhea; ANA+; Autoimmune anemia |
| Clonidine | 0.1 mg to 0.8 mg bid | Sedation; Dry mouth; Rebound effect on withdrawal |

| DIRECT VASODILATORS | | |
|---|---|---|
| Hydralazine | 10 mg to 50 mg qid | • Relaxation of precapillary arterioles<br>• Reflex sympathetic activation; Lupus |
| Nitroglycerin | Imdur: 60-240 mg / 24h<br>Nitrodur: 0.2 to 0.8 mg/h | Nausea; Headache; Hypotension; Tolerance |

## HYPERTENSION IN THE ELDERLY

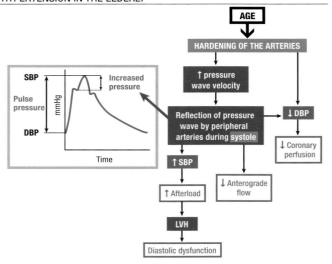

★ **HYVET**: > 80 years; SBP > 160 mmHG; Indapamide / Perindopril vs Placebo; Benefit of treatment (↘ all-cause mortality; ↘ adverse events)

**INITIATE TREATMENT IF SBP > 160 mmHG** (no RCT with SBP < 160 mmHg)

> **Target → SBP ≤ 150 mmHg**                                                                     +
  • Caution when DBP < 60 mmHg
  • Monitoring of adverse effects: BP supine-standing

**PSEUDOHYPERTENSION: HTN on sphygmomanometer, but normal BP on intraarterial**          +
**measurement**; secondary to rigid arteries that are not compressible by the cuff

> **Osler's maneuver**: radial pulse palpable when cuff inflated

## TREATMENT-RESISTANT HYPERTENSION

BP > 140/90 mmHg despite ≥ 3 medications at adequate doses (including a diuretic)

**ETIOLOGIES**: nonadherence; failure to comply with salt restriction; dehydration (↗ stimulation of renin and aldosterone); **insufficient dose of diuretic; HTN secondary to an underlying cause**; hyperaldosteronism; OSAHS

> **Pseudo-resistance**: **A)** White coat syndrome; **B)** Pseudohypertension in the elderly

**MANAGEMENT**: Combination of ≥ 3 medications; look for underlying cause; use a sufficient dose of diuretic; mineralocorticoid receptor antagonist; alpha-blocking agent (Doxazosin); percutaneous radiofrequency renal denervation (no benefit in ★ Simplicity HTN-3)

## HYPERTENSIVE CRISIS

### SBP ≥ 180 MMHG OR DBP ≥ 110 MMHG

**HYPERTENSIVE URGENCY**: absence of target organ damage

> Often associated with discontinuation of treatment, nonadherence to treatment and/or anxiety
> **Management:** gradual treatment (over 24-48 h); consider oral treatment (Captopril; Furosemide; Propranolol; Nifedipine); avoid target organ hypoperfusion

**HYPERTENSIVE EMERGENCY: target organ damage; immediate treatment required; invasive hemodynamic monitoring; target ↘ DBP by 10-15% x 30-60 min** ＋

> **Retinal damage:** hemorrhages; exudates; papilledema
> **CNS damage:** Hypertensive encephalopathy (headache; irritability; altered state of consciousness); thrombotic stroke; hemorrhagic stroke; SAH
  • **Cerebral autoregulation:** ↗ intracerebral blood pressure when DBP > 110-130 mmHg (autoregulatory mechanisms no longer effective); risk of cerebral edema
> **Cardiac damage:** Aortic dissection; acute heart failure; acute coronary syndrome
> **Renal damage:** ARF
> **Other:** Eclampsia / HELLP syndrome; Microangiopathic hemolytic anemia

| | | |
|---|---|---|
| **Nitroprusside** | IV infusion: 0.25-10 µg/kg/min (short duration) | Nausea; Vomiting; Cyanide toxicity; Avoid in the presence of CNS damage or ARF or liver failure |
| | Standard dilution: 50 mg/250 mL D5 % | |
| **IV Nitroglycerin** | Perfusion: 5-60 µg/min | Headache; Vomiting; Methemoglobinemia; Tolerance |
| | Standard dilution: 50 mg/250 mL D5 % | |
| **Labetalol** | • IV bolus: 20-80 mg every 10 min<br>• IV infusion: 2 mg/min (max 300 mg / 24 h) | Vomiting; Faintness; Nausea; Block; OH |
| | Standard dilution: 200 mg/160 mL NS (= 1 mg/mL) | |
| **Esmolol** | • Bolus: 0.25-0.5 mg/kg/min x 4 min<br>• IV infusion: 0.05-0.3 mg/kg/min | Hypotension; Nausea; Block |
| | Standard dilution: 2500 mg/250 mL | |
| **IV Nicardipine** | IV infusion: 5-15 mg/h | Headache; Nausea; Flushing; Tachycardia |

## 9.6/ DIABETES

**TYPE 1 DM:** autoimmune (or idiopathic) destruction of pancreatic beta cells

**TYPE 2 DM:** insulin resistance and/or abnormal insulin secretion

| DIAGNOSIS OF DIABETES | PREDIABETES | | |
|---|---|---|---|
| | **Abnormal fasting blood glucose** | **Glucose intolerance** | **Prediabetes** |
| · **Fasting blood glucose**: ≥ 7.0 mmol/L (≥ 126 mg/dL) or<br>· **Random blood glucose**: ≥ 11.1 mmol/L (≥ 200 mg/dL) or<br>· **Blood glucose 2 h after 75 g glucose load**: ≥ 11.1 mmol/L or<br>· **HbA1c**: ≥ 6.5 % | **Fasting blood glucose:** 6.1 - 6.9 mmol/L (110 - 124 mg/dL)<br>Rule out Glucose intolerance | **Blood glucose 2 h after 75 g glucose load:** 7.8 - 11.0 mmol/L (140 - 200 mg/dL) | **HbA1c:** 6.0 - 6.4%<br>Rule out Glucose intolerance |
| | More intensive management of cardiovascular risk factors; consider Metformin or Acarbose | | |

## GLYCEMIC CONTROL - TYPE II DIABETES

### BENEFITS OF GLYCEMIC CONTROL

> **Reduction of microvascular complications**: retinopathy; nephropathy; neuropathy (★ DCCT - ★ UKPDS - ★ ADVANCE)
> **Little evidence concerning the benefit on macrovascular complications**: ★ ADVANCE and ★ VADT; ★ ACCORD demonstrated excess mortality for target HbA1c < 6%

| GLYCEMIC CONTROL TARGETS | | |
|---|---|---|
| **HbA1c** | **Fasting blood glucose & Preprandial blood glucose** | **2 h postprandial blood glucose** |
| **≤ 7 %**<br>every 3 months (every 6 months when target achieved) | **4.0 - 7.0 mmol/L (72 - 126 mg/dL)** | **5.0 - 10.0 mmol/L**<br>(5.0 - 8.0 when target HbA1c not achieved) |

1) **NONDRUG TREATMENT**: weight loss (< 5%); balanced diet / follow-up by a nutritionist; regular moderate aerobic physical exercise (30 min; 5 times a week)

> **Stress test prior to training program:** consider in patients at high-risk of cardiovascular disease (or with microvascular complication) in the case of training with an intensity greater than rapid walking

2) **FIRST-LINE DRUG TREATMENT:** Metformin

3) **SECOND-LINE DRUG TREATMENT:** in combination with Metformin

> Sulfonylurea (or Meglitinide) and/or Incretins
> Bedtime basal insulin therapy

4) **INSULIN THERAPY**: 3 approaches

   a) **Bedtime basal insulin therapy**: combined with oral antidiabetic; **starting dose of 10 units at bedtime**; increase by 1 unit per day, targeting a fasting blood glucose of 4.0-7.0 mmol/L (72 - 126 mg/dL); avoid nocturnal hypoglycemia

   b) **Premixed insulin: starting dose of 5-10 units bid** (before breakfast and before dinner); increase the morning dose by 1 unit, targeting evening blood glucose before dinner of 4.0 - 7.0 mmol/L (idem for the evening dose, targeting morning fasting blood glucose of 4.0 - 7.0 mmol/L)

   c) **Intensive insulin therapy**: total daily dose = 0.3 to 0.5 kg unit; 40% of the total dose as bedtime basal insulin therapy; 20% of the total dose as bolus doses tid with each meal

| | | | |
|---|---|---|---|
| **Biguanide** | Metformin: 250 mg bid to 850 mg tid | Decreases hepatic glucose synthesis | ↘ HbA1c by 0.8%<br><br>**Adverse effects:** Nausea; Diarrhea; Lactic acidosis (contraindicated if GFR < 30 mL/min)<br><br>Weight loss<br><br>Benefit on the risk of MI and mortality in obese patients in ★ UKPDS |
| **Sulfonylureas** | • Gliclazide: 60 mg qd to 120 mg qd<br>• Glimepiride: 1 to 8 mg qd<br>• Glyburide: 2.5 mg qd to 10 mg bid | Stimulates insulin secretion by the pancreas | ↘ HbA1c by 0.7%<br><br>**Adverse effects:** Hypoglycemia (prefer Gliclazide which is associated with the lowest risk of hypoglycemia); weight gain<br><br>Benefit on the risk of MI in ★ UKPDS |
| **Meglitinide** | Repaglinide: 0.5 mg tid to 4 mg qid | Stimulates insulin secretion by the pancreas | ↘ HbA1c by 1-1.5 %<br><br>Short duration of action (to be taken < 30 min before the meal)<br><br>**Adverse effects:** Hypoglycemia; Weight gain |
| **Incretin - GLP-1 analog ("glucagon-like peptide 1")** | • Exenatide: 5 to 10 µg SC bid<br>• Liraglutide: 0.6 to 1.8 mg SC daily | **GLP-1:**<br>↗ insulin secretion;<br>↘ glucagon secretion; delays gastric emptying | ↘ HbA1c by 1 %<br><br>**Weight loss**<br><br>**Adverse effects:** Nausea; Vomiting |
| **Incretin - DPP-4 inhibitors** | • Sitagliptin: 100 mg qd<br>• Linagliptin: 5 mg qd<br>• Saxagliptin: 5 mg qd | Inhibits the breakdown of GLP-1 | ↘ HbA1c by 0.7 %<br><br>Safe post-ACS (★EXAMINE; Alogliptin)<br><br>**Adverse effects:**<br>↗ hospitalization for heart failure with Saxagliptin in ★SAVOR but not with Sitagliptin in ★TECOS |
| **Alpha-glucosidase inhibitor** | Acarbose: 25 mg tid to 100 mg tid | Decreases intestinal absorption of carbohydrates | ↘ HbA1c by 0.6 %<br><br>**Adverse effects:** Bloating |
| **Thiazolidine-dione (TZD)** | Pioglitazone: 15 mg to 45 mg qd | Increases peripheral insulin sensitivity | ↘ HbA1c by 0.8 %<br><br>**Adverse effects:** Weight gain; Edema; contraindicated in heart failure (★ DREAM); bladder tumor; fracture |

| **SGLT2 inhibitors** | Canagliflozin Dapagliflozin Empagliflozin | ↘ glucose reabsorption by the renal proximal tubule | ↘ **All-cause mortality** with Empagliflozin in ★ EMPA-REG ↘ BP; Weight loss **Adverse effects:** urinary tract infections; candidiasis; ↗ LDL |
|---|---|---|---|
| **RAPID ACTING INSULIN** • Aspart (NovoRapid) • Lispro (Humalog) | | | • Onset of action: 10-15 min • Peak action: 1-2 h • Duration of action: 3-5 h |
| **REGULAR INSULIN** • Humulin-R • Novolin ge Toronto | | | • Onset of action: 30 min • Peak action: 2-3 h • Duration of action: 6.5 h |
| **INTERMEDIATE-ACTING INSULIN** • Humulin-N • Novolin ge NPH | | | • Onset of action: 1-3 h • Peak of action: 5-8 h • Duration of action: up to 17 h |
| **LONG-ACTING INSULIN** • Detemir (Levemir) • Glargine (Lantus) | | | • Onset of action: 90 min • Duration of action: up to 24 h |
| **PREMIXED INSULIN** Humulin 30/70; Novolin ge 30/70; Biphasic insulin aspart (NovoMix 30); Insulin lispro / lispro protamine (Humalog Mix25)… | | | |

# MANAGEMENT - TYPE II DIABETES

**CARDIOVASCULAR RISK:** 2- to 3-fold higher prevalence of coronary artery disease than in nondiabetic subjects; coronary artery disease occurs 10 years earlier

**CONTROL OF CARDIOVASCULAR RISK FACTORS:** healthy weight; waist < 102 cm (M) and < 88 cm (F); BMI 18.5 - 24.9 kg/m2; healthy diet; regular physical exercise; smoking cessation

**CONTROL BP:** target BP < 140/85 and prefer ACEi (or ARB) as first-line treatment

> ★ **ACCORD-BP**: no benefit of targeting SBP < 120 versus < 140 mmHg

**ANTIPLATELET THERAPY (ASA):**

> **Secondary prevention**: indicated for all patients
> **Primary prevention**: uncertain benefit (ongoing ★ ASCEND and ★ ACCEPT-D studies); not recommended routinely; consider if high 10-year risk of cardiovascular events in the absence of bleeding risk (class IIb recommendation); **decision based on clinical judgment**

**STATIN:** ★ CARDS and ★ HPS studies of primary prevention demonstrated a benefit

> **European guidelines - Indications: A)** Very high risk → DMI or DMII + (macrovascular disease or CRF ≥ 3/5 or cardiovascular risk factors or microvascular complication); **B)** High risk → DMII + (absence of cardiovascular risk factors and absence of target organ damage)
> **Canadian guidelines - Indications**: Diabetes + (≥ 40 years or present for > 15 years in a patient ≥ 30 years or macrovascular disease or microvascular complication)
> **American guidelines - Indications**: Diabetes + 40-75 years + LDL ≥ 70 mg/dL (≥ 1.8 mmol/L)

**ACEI: cardioprotective effect:** (★ HOPE, ★ EUROPA and ★ ADVANCE); indicated in the presence of HTN or clinical macrovascular disease or ≥ 55 years or in the presence of a microvascular complication

> **ARB: when ACEi are not tolerated;** ★ ONTARGET → Telmisartan non-inferior to Ramipril; ★ TRANSCEND → no benefit of Telmisartan versus placebo (patients intolerant to ACEi)

**NONINVASIVE ASSESSMENT OF CAD (PROGNOSTIC PURPOSES):** Indications → **A)** Symptoms (retrosternal chest pain; dyspnea); **B)** Baseline ECG abnormalities; **C)** Atherosclerosis (PAD - TIA - stroke - murmur)

> **Revascularization**: benefit of revascularization by bypass graft (versus PCI) on mortality and risk of MI (★ FREEDOM)                                                    +

**VACCINATION:** Influenza (annually); Pneumococcus

**OTHER:** self-monitoring of blood glucose; screening for retinopathy (every 1-2 years); screening for neuropathy (big toe; Semmes-Weinstein 10 g monofilament test or 128 Hz tuning fork); examination of feet; prevention of diabetic ulcer; PDE-5 inhibitor for erectile dysfunction

**HYPOGLYCEMIA:** Blood glucose < 4 mmol/L (72 mg/dL) + symptoms (tremor; palpitations; anxiety; profuse sweating; nausea; confusion; weakness); **treatment with 15 g of oral carbohydrate or 1 mg of Glucagon SC (or IM) or 1 ampoule of 50% dextrose IV**

## DIABETIC NEPHROPATHY

**CHRONIC NEPHROPATHY:** GFR < 60 mL/min and/or microalbuminuria or macroalbuminuria

**SCREENING:** albumin / creatinine ratio and serum creatinine (and GFR) every year

**MANAGEMENT:** optimal control of blood glucose and BP; ACEi or ARB; Nephrological follow-up if sustained deterioration or GFR < 30 mL/min or significant macroalbuminuria; aggressive treatment of cardiovascular risk factors (high risk of adverse events)

| ALBUMINURIA | | | NEPHROPATHY | | |
|---|---|---|---|---|---|
| | Albumin / creatinine ratio (mg/mmol) | Albumin mg / 24h | Stage | Renal damage | GFR (mL/min) |
| Normal | < 2.0 | < 30 | 1 | Minimal - Absent | ≥ 90 |
| Micro-albuminuria | 2.0 - 20.0 | 30 - 300 | 2 | Mild | 60 - 89 |
| Macro-albuminuria | > 20.0 | > 300 | 3 | Moderate | 30 - 59 |
| | | | 4 | Severe | 15 - 29 |
| | | | 5 | End-stage | < 15 |

# 9.7/ PHYSICAL ACTIVITY

## PHYSIOLOGY OF EXERCISE

1) ↗ **CARDIAC OUTPUT:** ↗ up to 4- to 6-fold
   a) ↗ **Stroke volume** (↗ venous return → Frank-Starling law; catecholamines → positive inotropes)
   b) ↗ **HR** (HRmax ≈ 220 - age)

2) **REDISTRIBUTION OF PERFUSION:** vasodilatation in muscles; vasoconstriction of other systems (except for CNS and heart)

3) ↗ **$O_2$ EXTRACTION BY MUSCLES**

4) ↗ **CORONARY PERFUSION:** ↗ up to fivefold; vasodilatation of coronary arterioles
   > **$MVO_2$:** myocardial $O_2$ consumption; determined by **HR / SBP / LV end-diastolic volume / wall thickness / contractility**                                        +

**BENEFITS OF EXERCISE ON CONVENTIONAL CARDIOVASCULAR RISK FACTORS**

> **HTN:** ↘ 3.4 / 2.4 mmHg
> **Dyslipidemia:** ↗ HDL 0.06 mmol/L (2.3 mg/dL); ↘ TG
> **Obesity:** ↘ 7 kg in 1 year (in combination with diet)
> **Diabetes:** ↘ HbA1c by 0.8%

**IMPROVEMENT OF OTHER PARAMETERS**: functional capacity; quality of life; mental health; endothelial function; inflammatory state; ischemic threshold

> **Physical activity**: ↘ **mortality and** ↘ **cardiovascular events in patients with CAD** (meta-analyses); ↘ mortality and hospitalizations in patients with LVEF < 35% (★ HF-ACTION; after adjustments)

**BENEFITS OF TRAINING**: ↗ VO$_2$ max; ↗ stroke volume; lower HR for the same level of exercise (same HRmax); ↗ arteriovenous O$_2$ difference; delayed ventilatory threshold; ↘ MVO$_2$ for the same level of exercise

**RISKS OF PHYSICAL EXERCISE**

a) **< 35 years**: sudden death / arrhythmia / genetic condition (HCM; congenital coronary artery anomalies; myocarditis; ARVD; Channelopathy; CAD; Acute aortic syndrome; Aortic stenosis; DCM; WPW; *commotio cordis*)

b) **> 35 years**: CAD / MI (especially in sedentary subject performing unusually strenuous exercise)

## INTENSITY OF PHYSICAL EXERCISE

**1 MET:** = O$_2$ consumption at rest while seated (3.5 mL O$_2$/kg/min)

| < 3 METs | 3 – 5 METs | 5 – 7 METs | 7 – 9 METs | > 9 METs |
|---|---|---|---|---|
| • Washing<br>• Shaving<br>• Dressing<br>• Washing the dishes<br>• Sewing<br>• Playing a musical instrument<br>• Golf (caddy)<br>• Walking (3.2 kph)<br>• Fishing<br>• Pool | • Washing the windows<br>• Electric lawnmower<br>• Making a bed<br>• Dancing<br>• Golf<br>• Sailing<br>• Tennis (doubles)<br>• Volleyball (6 players)<br>• Ping-pong<br>• Walking (6.4 kph) | • Manual lawnmower<br>• Climbing stairs (slowly)<br>• Badminton<br>• Tennis (singles)<br>• Basketball<br>• Walking (8 kph)<br>• Bike-riding (16 kph)<br>• Swimming (breaststroke) | • Shoveling snow<br>• Climbing stairs (moderate speed)<br>• Canoe<br>• Soccer<br>• Jogging (8 kph)<br>• Swimming (front crawl)<br>• Bike-riding (19 kph)<br>• Mountain-climbing | • Climbing stairs (rapidly)<br>• Shoveling heavy snow<br>• Handball<br>• Squash<br>• Running (> 10 kph)<br>• Bike-riding (> 21 kph) |

## EVALUATION OF THE RISK OF PHYSICAL EXERCISE

**PRE-TRAINING STRESS TEST**: **A)** DM; **B)** Symptoms or multiple cardiovascular risk factors or known heart disease; **C)** Strenuous physical exercise by a sedentary subject (M > 45 years and F > 55 years)

| CATEGORY | CHARACTERISTICS | MANAGEMENT |
|---|---|---|
| **Class A:**<br>**In good**<br>**health** | • M < 45 years or F < 55 years with no symptoms, no heart disease and no major cardiovascular risk factors<br>• M > 45 years or F > 55 years with no symptoms, no heart disease and ≤ 1 major cardiovascular risk factor<br>• M > 45 or F > 55 years with no symptoms, no heart disease with ≥ 2 major cardiovascular risk factors | • No restriction<br>• No supervision required<br>• Physical examination / Stress test as necessary (according to cardio-vascular risk factors / type of strenuous exercise) |
| **Class B:**<br>**Stable**<br>**heart**<br>**disease** | • Stable CAD<br>• Nonsevere valvular heart disease<br>• Stable congenital heart disease (according to 36th Bethesda conference)<br>• Stable cardiomyopathy (LVEF ≤ 30%)<br>• Abnormal stress test (no class C abnormalities)<br><br>**+**<br>**CLINICAL CHARACTERISTICS**<br>NYHA I or II; No decompensated heart failure; ≥ 6 METs; No ischemia < 6 METs; Normal BP response to exercise; No VT on effort - rest; Able to selfmonitor | • Individualized prescription **(50% of HR reserve then increase)**<br>• Medical supervision with monitoring during the initial phase (6-12 sessions)<br>• Nonmedical supervision thereafter until the patient is able to self-monitor |
| **Class C:**<br>**Moderate**<br>**to high**<br>**risk** | • CAD<br>• Nonsevere valvular heart disease<br>• Moderate congenital heart disease (36th Bethesda conference)<br>• Cardiomyopathy (LVEF ≤ 30%)<br>• Partially controlled ventricular arrhythmia<br><br>**+**<br>**CLINICAL CHARACTERISTICS**<br>NYHA III-IV; Stress test < 6 METs; Ischemia < 6 METs; Abnormal BP response to exercise; NSVT on exercise; History of cardiac arrest; Potentially dangerous medical condition | • Individualized prescription **(40% of HR reserve then increase)**<br>• Medical supervision with monitoring until safety is confirmed (> 12 sessions)<br>• Can be classified as class B when exercise is safe |
| **Class D:**<br>**Unstable**<br>**condition** | • Unstable ischemia<br>• Severe valvular heart disease / symptoms<br>• Severe congenital heart disease<br>• Decompensated heart failure<br>• Uncontrolled arrhythmia<br>• Other condition worsened by exercise | • Exercise contraindicated<br>• Target treatment of the disease |

*Fletcher GF, Balady GJ, Amsterdam EA. Exercise Standards for Testing and Training; A Statement for Healthcare Professionals From the American Heart Association. Circulation. 2001;104:1694-1740*

**COMPETITIVE SPORT:** according to the 36th Bethesda conference

## PRESCRIPTION OF AEROBIC (ISOTONIC) PHYSICAL EXERCISE

**FREQUENCY**: 5 times a week

**DURATION**: 30 min (in 10-min fractions if necessary)

**INTENSITY**: moderate
> **Target**: ideally 450 to 750 METs x min / week (1000 kcal / week)
> **Kcal/min**: = (METs x 3.5 x kg weight) / 200
> **Strenuous aerobic exercise**: 3 times a week; 20 min per session

| MODERATE AEROBIC EXERCISE | VIGOROUS AEROBIC EXERCISE |
|---|---|
| • **% VO$_2$ max**: 45-59 %<br>• **% HR reserve**: 45-59 %<br>• **% HRmax**: 55-69 % | • **% VO$_2$ max**: 60-85 %<br>• **% HR reserve**: 60-85 %<br>• **% HRmax**: 70-90 % |
| • **Borg scale**: 12-13 / 20<br>Comfortable while talking (≈ ventilatory threshold ≈ 50 % VO$_2$Max) | • **Borg scale**: 14-16 / 20<br>Conversation is difficult during exercise |
| • **METs**: 4 - 6 METs (middle-aged)<br>5 - 7 METs (young)<br>3 - 5 METs (elderly)<br>2 - 3 METs (very elderly) | • **METs**: 6 - 8.5 METs (middle-aged)<br>7 - 10 METs (young)<br>5 - 7 METs (elderly)<br>3 - 4 METs (very elderly) |
| • **Type of exercise**: rapid walking; bike-riding; swimming; dancing; pool aerobics; elliptic exercise machine | • **Type of exercise**: rapid walking uphill; jogging; rapid swimming; hockey; singles tennis; shoveling snow |

- **Target HR according to HR reserve**: = (prescribed % x HR reserve) + resting HR
- **HR reserve**: = HRmax on stress test - resting HR
- **HRmax**: = 220 - age
- **HRmax**: = HRmax on stress test limited by symptoms

- **Ischemia on stress test**: Target HR on exercise must be at least 10 bpm lower than ischemic threshold (or target HR = 70% of HR at the ischemic threshold)

## PRESCRIPTION OF RESISTANCE TRAINING (STATIC; ISOMETRIC)

**FREQUENCY:** twice a week

**CONTENT:** 1-3 series of 8 to 12 repetitions of the prescribed load (counterweight machine or dumbbells)

**8-10 MUSCLE GROUPS:** Biceps; Triceps; Shoulders; Pectorals; Back; Abdominal muscles; Leg muscles

**PRESCRIBED LOAD:** maximum load that can be lifted once → 35% of this maximum load for arms and 45% for legs

## 9.8/ WEIGHT & DIET

## WEIGHT CONTROL

**BMI**: = Mass (kg) / Height $^2$ (m$^2$)

| Underweight | BMI < 18.5 kg/m² |
| --- | --- |
| Healthy weight | BMI 18.5 - 24.9 kg/m² |
| Overweight | BMI 25.0 - 29.9 kg/m² |
| Obesity - Class I | BMI 30.0 - 34.9 kg/m² |
| Obesity - Class II | BMI 35.0 - 39.9 kg/m² |
| Obesity - Class III (morbid) | BMI ≥ 40 kg/m² |

**BENEFIT OF WEIGHT CONTROL ON CARDIOVASCULAR RISK FACTORS**: ↘ BP; improves lipid profile (↘ TG; ↘ atherogenic lipoproteins; ↗ HDL); ↘ DM; ↘ OSAHS; ↘ inflammatory state; improves endothelial function

## WEIGHT LOSS

| BMI | **Target 18.5 - 24.9 kg/m²** |
| --- | --- |
| WAIST (midpoint between superior iliac crest and costal margin) | **Target < 102 cm M and < 88 cm F** (ideally < 94 cm M and < 80 cm F) |

**1) LIFESTYLE MODIFICATION**: healthy diet; regular physical exercise; behavioral therapy (selfmonitoring; eat more slowly; eat smaller servings; nutritional education...)

> **Targets**: weight loss of 5% in 3-6 months (realistic target)
> **Measurements**: energy deficit of 500 kcal per day (loss of 1-2 pounds per week); Regular exercise program (30 min; 5 times a week)

**2) DRUG TREATMENT**: indicated after failure of nondrug treatment for 6 months with BMI > 30 kg/m² (or > 27 kg/m² with comorbidities)

| **Pancreatic lipase inhibitor** | Orlistat 120 mg tid + fat-soluble vitamin supplement | Inhibits digestion and absorption of dietary fat by 30% | Bloating; Steatorrhea; Abdominal cramps; Renal stones |
| --- | --- | --- | --- |
| **Selective serotonin agonist** | Lorcaserin | Early satiety | Faintness; Nausea; Headache; URTI; Uncertain long-term safety (valvular heart disease?) |

**3) BARIATRIC SURGERY**: indicated in the presence of class III obesity (or class II obesity with secondary comorbidities) and failure of other treatment modalities with an acceptable operative risk

> **Options**: Vertical gastroplasty with laparoscopic banding or laparoscopic Roux-en-Y gastric bypass

## HEALTHY DIET

DASH diet or Mediterranean diet or AHA diet; emphasize intake of vegetables, fruits, whole grains, nontropical vegetable oils, nuts, low-fat dairy products, fish, poultry; limit intake of sodium - sweets - sugar-sweetened beverages - red meats

**BENEFIT ON CONVENTIONAL CARDIOVASCULAR RISK FACTORS**: ↘ LDL; ↘ BP; ↘ Weight; ↘ DM

**MEDITERRANEAN DIET**: rich in olive oil / nuts / fruit and vegetables; ↘ cardiovascular mortality in secondary prevention (★ Lyon diet heart study) and ↘ cardiovascular events in primary prevention (★ PREDIMED)

| Total calories - Energy balance | Intake equal to energy expenditure<br>**Normal intake: 22 kcal/kg (± 20%)** |
|---|---|
| Fat | **< 35 % of total energy intake** |
| Mono- and polyunsaturated fatty acids (fish; vegetable oils; nuts) | • Increase intake<br>• **Omega-3 fatty acids → ↘ cardiovascular mortality**<br>(★ GISSI-Prevention) |
| Saturated fatty acids | < 7% of total energy intake<br>Avoid red meat - high-fat dairy products - tropical oils (palm; coconut) |
| Trans fatty acids / Hydrogenated oils | Limit to a minimum; < 1% of total energy intake;<br>↗ LDL and ↘ HDL |
| Dietary cholesterol | < 200-300 mg daily |
| Carbohydrates | **45 - 60% of total energy intake**<br>Prefer whole grain products - low-fat dairy products - fruit and vegetables<br>Avoid carbohydrates with a high glycemic index (potatoes; white bread; white rice; soft drinks) |
| Proteins | **15 - 20% of total energy intake** |
| Fibers (whole grains; fruit; vegetables; nuts) | Increase intake; 25 - 50 g daily |
| Fruit and vegetables | ≥ 8-10 servings per day |
| Fish | At least twice a week |
| Sodium | < 2.4 g per day |
| Alcohol | M: 20 g per day (2 glasses); F: 10 g per day (1 glass)<br>(caution in the presence of DM - HTN - Liver disease - History of alcohol abuse) |
| Red meat; High-fat dairy products | Limit to a minimum |

## METABOLIC SYNDROME

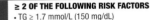

| **CENTRAL OBESITY (WAIST)**<br>USA - Canada:<br>    M: ≥ 102 cm; F: ≥ 88 cm<br>Europid: M: ≥ 94 cm; F: ≥ 80 cm | **+** | **≥ 2 OF THE FOLLOWING RISK FACTORS**<br>• TG ≥ 1.7 mmol/L (150 mg/dL)<br>• HDL: M < 1.03 and F < 1.3 mmol/L (40 - 50 mg/dL)<br>• BP ≥ 130/85 (or treated HTN)<br>• Fasting blood glucose ≥ 5.6 mmol/L (100 mg/dL) |
|---|---|---|

↗ risk of cardiovascular disease and DMII

**MANAGEMENT**: control of cardiovascular risk factor; regular exercise; weight loss

# 9.9/ OBSTRUCTIVE SLEEP APNEA SYNDROME

**OBSTRUCTIVE APNEA**: absence of airflow for ≥ 10 s despite active ventilatory efforts

**OBSTRUCTIVE HYPOPNEA**: ↘ airflow < 50% for ≥ 10 s with ↘ SaO₂ ≥ 4 %

**APNEA-HYPOPNEA INDEX (AHI): mean number of episodes of apnea and hypopnea per hour (mild if AHI ≥ 5; severe if AHI ≥ 30)**

**CLINICAL FEATURES:** snoring; daytime sleepiness; witnessed apnea during the night; morning headache; disorders of concentration

**HARMFUL EFFECTS:** sympathetic stimulation; transient hypoxemia; marked fluctuations of intrathoracic pressure (↗ afterload); nocturnal HTN; treatment-resistant HTN; diastolic dysfunction; nocturnal angina

**ASSOCIATIONS:** obesity; DM; metabolic syndrome; AF; CAD; stroke; heart failure; nonischemic dilated cardiomyopathy; PHT

**DIAGNOSIS:** Polysomnography (screening by nocturnal saturometry)

**TREATMENT:** Weight loss; CPAP; Oral device; Surgery

## 9.10/ DRIVING & AIR TRAVEL

|  | PRIVATE VEHICLE | COMMERCIAL VEHICLE |
|---|---|---|
| **STEMI** | 1 month | 3 months |
| **NSTEMI - Significant damage (RWMA)** | 1 month | 3 months |
| **Unstable angina or NSTEMI without RWMA** | 48 h post-PCI (7 days in the absence of PCI) | 7 days post-PCI (30 days in the absence of PCI) |
| **CAD - PCI** | 48 h post-PCI | 7 days post-PCI |
| **CABG** | 1 month | 3 months |
| **LMCA** | Disqualified if > 70% | Disqualified if > 50% |
| **VF - Absence of reversible cause** | 6 months | Disqualified |
| **Unstable VT** | 6 months | Disqualified |
| **VT or VF - Reversible cause (MI; Electrocution; Drugs)** | Disqualified until correction of reversible cause | |
| **Stable sustained VT - LVEF < 30%** | 3 months | Disqualified |
| **Stable sustained VT - LVEF ≥ 30%; without ICD** | 4 weeks | 3 months |
| **Symptomatic SSS** | Disqualified until treatment | |
| **LBBB or Bifascicular block or Mobitz I or Bifascicular block + 1st degree AV block** | No restriction in the absence of alteration of LOC | No restriction in the absence of alteration of LOC and in the absence of higher grade of AV block on annual Holter |
| **Mobitz II (infranodal)** | Disqualified | Disqualified |
| **Alternating RBBB and LBBB** | Disqualified | Disqualified |
| **3rd degree AV block** | Disqualified | Disqualified |

| Pacemaker | 1 week post-implantation (no alteration of LOC postimplantation; functioning pacemaker) | 1 month post-implantation (no alteration of LOC postimplantation; functioning pacemaker) |
|---|---|---|
| **ICD - Primary prevention (NYHA I to III)** | 4 weeks | Disqualified |
| **ICD - Secondary prevention (VF or VT with alteration of LOC)** | 6 months | |
| **ICD - Secondary prevention (stable VT; NYHA I to III)** | 1 week + interval associated with VT | |
| **Therapy (ATP or shock) with alteration of LOC** | 6 months | |
| **Brugada / Long QT / ARVD** | 6 months after episode with alteration of LOC | Disqualified |
| **EPS (without induced VT) or ablation procedure** | 48 h | 1 week |
| **SVT / AF / Flutter with alteration of LOC** | • Ablation: 48 h<br>• Medical treatment: 3 months | • Ablation: 1 week<br>• Medical treatment: 3 months |
| **Classical vasovagal syncope - 1st episode** | No restriction | No restriction |
| **Classical vasovagal syncope - Recurrence (< 12 months)** | 1 week | 12 months |
| **Syncope with treated cause (e.g.: pacemaker)** | 1 week | 1 months |
| **Situational syncope** | 1 week | 1 week |
| **Unexplained syncope - 1st episode** | 1 week | 12 months |
| **Unexplained syncope - Recurrence (< 12 months)** | 3 months | 12 months |
| **AS** | NYHA I or II; No alteration of LOC | Asymptomatic - NYHA I - Area ≥ 1 cm² - LVEF ≥ 35% |
| **AR - MS - MR** | NYHA I or II; No alteration of LOC | No alteration of LOC - NYHA I - LVEF ≥ 35% |
| **Mechanical valve or Bioprosthesis** | 6 weeks<br>Anticoagulation (if indicated)<br>No thromboembolic complication | 3 months<br>NYHA I and LVEF ≥ 35%<br>Anticoagulation (if indicated)<br>No thromboembolic complication |
| **NYHA I or II** | No restriction | LVEF ≥ 35% |
| **NYHA III** | No restriction | Disqualified |
| **NYHA IV** | Disqualified | Disqualified |

| Heart transplant | 6 week<br>NYHA I or II | 6 months<br>NYHA I; LVEF ≥ 35%<br>No ischemia on annual<br>noninvasive test |
| LVAD - continuous<br>flow ventricular assist<br>device | 2 months<br>NYHA I-III | Disqualified |
| HCM | No alteration of LOC | Wall thickness < 30 mm; No<br>syncope; No NSVT (annual<br>Holter); No family history of<br>sudden death; No ↘ BP on<br>exercise |

## AIR TRAVEL

**INDICATION FOR O₂: A)** PaO₂ < 70 mmHg; **B)** CCS III/IV angina; **C)** NYHA III/IV heart failure;
**D)** Cyanotic congenital heart disease; **E)** PHT - Right heart failure

| Stable angina / NYHA I - II - III | O₂ if NYHA III |
| Post-myocardial infarction / NYHA I | 6-8 weeks |
| Heart failure / NYHA I - II - III | O₂ if NYHA III |
| Valvular heart disease / NYHA I - II - III | O₂ if NYHA III or PHT |
| Congenital heart disease /<br>NYHA I - II - III | O₂ if NYHA III or PHT or PaO₂ < 70 mmHg |
| ICD / NYHA I - II | 1 month post-ICD therapy associated with<br>presyncope or syncope |

# 9.11/ CARDIOVASCULAR COMPLICATIONS OF SYSTEMIC DISEASES

## HIV

Heart failure - Dilated cardiomyopathy - Myocarditis; Pericardial effusion / Pericarditis; Infective and noninfective endocarditis (non-bacterial thrombotic endocarditis); PHT; Neoplasia → Kaposi sarcoma (epicardial) / NHL; Accelerated atherosclerosis / Endothelial dysfunction; Early-onset cerebrovascular disease; Protease inhibitors → lipodystrophy / ↗ TG - ↗ LDL - ↘ HDL / Glucose intolerance; Arrhythmias - ↗ QT; Dysautonomia; Vasculitis; Drug interactions

## VASCULITIS

**TAKAYASU - GIANT CELL ARTERITIS - BEHÇET: ▶▶|** Chapter 8

**KAWASAKI**: young children (< 5 years); fever; rash; conjunctivitis; lymphadenopathy; mucosal lesions; erythema of extremities then desquamation

> **Cardiac involvement**: pericardial effusion; myocarditis; MI; aortitis; AR; heart failure; arrhythmias; coronary arteritis
> **Coronary artery stenoses or aneurysms**: < 6 weeks after onset of the disease; proximal lesions; short-term, medium-term and long-term risk of thrombosis
> **Treatment**: ASA; IV Ig; consider anticoagulation if multiple aneurysms or thrombus

**CHURG & STRAUSS**: pericarditis; myocarditis; coronary arteritis; heart failure; mesenteric ischemia

**POLYARTERITIS NODOSA (MEDIUM VESSEL VASCULITIS):** HTN; heart failure; arteritis; coronary aneurysms; angina; myocardial infarction; pericarditis

## CONNECTIVE TISSUE DISEASES

**RHEUMATOID ARTHRITIS**: pericarditis; pericardial effusion; constriction; accelerated CAD; blocks (rheumatoid nodules); granulomatous valve lesions with regurgitation (mitral; aortic); rheumatoid aortitis; PHT (rheumatoid lung disease)

**HLA-B27-ASSOCIATED SPONDYLOARTHROPATHIES:** aortitis / aortic root dilatation; aortic valvulitis; AR; blocks; early CAD

**SYSTEMIC LUPUS ERYTHEMATOSUS**: pericarditis; pericardial effusion; constrictive pericarditis; coronary arteritis; accelerated CAD; nonbacterial endocarditis (Libman-Sacks; nonmobile vegetations); valvulitis (fibrosis; retraction; regurgitation); myocarditis; sinus tachycardia; congenital AV block; PHT; aortitis

> **Drug-induced lupus**: hydralazine; procaïnamide; quinidine
> **Antiphospholipid syndrome (antiphospholipid antibodies or lupus anticoagulant)**: arterial or venous thrombosis; myocardial infarction; stroke; intracardiac thrombus; PHT; nonbacterial endocarditis; valvulitis (fibrosis; regurgitation)

**SCLERODERMA**: Raynaud; renal crisis; pericarditis; pericardial effusion; microvascular ischemia; myocardial fibrosis; heart failure (diastolic > systolic); conduction disorders; PHT

**POLYMYOSITIS**: myocarditis / heart failure; blocks; PHT

## ENDOCRINE DISEASES

**ACROMEGALY**: HTN; LVH; heart failure; diastolic dysfunction; stroke; insulin resistance; aortic root dilatation; mitral regurgitation

**CUSHING'S DISEASE**: Accelerated CAD; hyperglycemia / insulin resistance; dyslipidemia; HTN; LVH; heart failure; dilated cardiomyopathy; stroke; PAD

**HYPERPARATHYROIDISM**: ↗ contractility; short QT; calcifications (valvular; aortic)

**HYPOCALCEMIA**: Prolonged QT; ↘ contractility

**HYPERTHYROIDISM**: high output; ↘ systemic resistance; systolic HTN (↗ pulse pressure); sinus tachycardia; ↗ plasma volume; angina (↗ O$_2$ demand); vasospasm; PHT; AF; heart failure

**HYPOTHYROIDISM**: low output state; ↗ systemic resistance; sinus bradycardia; diastolic HTN; ↗ LDL; hypertriglyceridemia; pericardial effusion; prolonged QT; low voltage; ↗ risk of CAD; diastolic dysfunction

**PHEOCHROMOCYTOMA**: HTN; tachycardia; concentric LVH; myocarditis; cardiomyopathy similar to Takotsubo

## MUSCULAR DYSTROPHIES

**PERMANENT PACEMAKER: A)** Third-degree or advanced second-degree AV block (class I recommendation); **B)** May be considered with any degree of AV block (including first degree) in patients with Steinert disease, Kearns-Sayre syndrome or limb-girdle muscular dystrophy (class IIb)

**BECKER DYSTROPHY AND DUCHENNE DYSTROPHY**: X-linked; ↗ CK; **progressive dilated cardiomyopathy**; MR; hypertrabeculations; arrhythmias; blocks

> **Duchenne**: prominent R wave in V1 (↗ R/S ratio); Q wave in left precordials; short PR; RVH

**MYOTONIC DYSTROPHY**: autosomal dominant; **predominantly affects conduction tissue**; blocks; arrhythmias (AF; flutter; VT; bundle branch reentry VT); systolic and/or diastolic dysfunction; LVH; MVP

> **Follow-up**: Annual ECG and Holter

**EMERY-DREIFUSS DYSTROPHY: DCM**; arrhythmias (AF; Flutter; atrial asystole with junctional rhythm; VT; VF); conduction disorders (including dystrophy secondary to **lamin A/C** mutation)

**LIMB-GIRDLE MUSCULAR DYSTROPHY: DCM**; prominent R wave in V1; blocks

## OTHER NEUROLOGICAL DISEASES

**FRIEDREICH'S ATAXIA**: autosomal recessive; **concentric HCM** (sometimes localized in the septum); LVOT obstruction; diffuse T wave inversion; possible progression to DCM

**MITOCHONDRIAL DISEASES**: HCM; DCM; blocks (Kearns-Sayre syndrome); preexcitation

**DESMIN-RELATED MYOPATHY**: autosomal dominant; conduction disorders; DCM; RCM

**GUILLAIN-BARRÉ SYNDROME**: HTN; OH; sinus tachycardia; ST abnormalities; tachyarrhythmias / bradyarrhythmias; asystole

**MYASTHENIA GRAVIS**: myocarditis; arrhythmias; blocks

**ACUTE CEREBROVASCULAR DISEASE:** ST elevation or depression; T wave inversion; Q waves; ↗ QT (with peaked T wave); neurogenic stunned myocardium; Takotsubo cardiomyopathy; systolic dysfunction; acute pulmonary edema; VT - VF; Torsade de pointes; bradyarrhythmias

## CHRONIC RENAL DISEASE

### INDEPENDENT CARDIOVASCULAR RISK FACTOR

Accelerated and aggressive CAD; cardiomyopathy; LVH; HTN; valvular heart disease (Ao sclerosis; MAC); vascular calcifications; toxicity of cardiovascular drugs; dyslipidemia (↘ HDL; ↗ TG - ↗ LDL); cardiorenal syndrome; arrhythmias; blocks; infective endocarditis; anemia associated with heart failure; risk of contrast nephropathy; inflammatory state

> To convert serum creatine level mg/dL to mmol/L, multiply by 88.4
> **High output heart failure (AV fistula)**: Nicoladoni - Branham sign → ↘ cardiac output (↘ LVOT VTI) after manual compression of the fistula; predictive improved cardiac output after fistula ligation

# 9.12/ CARDIOVASCULAR COMPLICATIONS OF TRAUMA

**PENETRATING INJURY**: knife; bullet

> Tamponade; Ischemia (coronary trauma); Complex lesion (valves; coronary arteries; intracardiac fistula)

**NONPENETRATING INJURY**: compression or deceleration or contusion; safety belt; airbag; steering wheel; fall; collision; rib fractures; CPR

> Contusion; systolic dysfunction; LV free wall rupture (tamponade or hemothorax); RA rupture; ventricular septal rupture; ruptured chordae tendineae or papillary muscle; ruptured valve leaflet (Ao > M > T); Ao rupture; rupture of pericardium (cardiac hernia); arrhythmias; blocks; myocardial infarction (thrombosis; dissection; coronary laceration); *commotio cordis*

**SEVERE BURN:** toxic myocardial depression for several days (in addition to significant hypovolemia)

**ELECTROCUTION:** cardiac arrest (VF; asystole); myocardial necrosis; ischemia; arrhythmias; conduction disorder; ECG abnormalities; dysautonomia

## MANAGEMENT

ABC; ACLS; Cardiac monitor; NS Bolus; Transfusion; Ultrasound (FAST); OR - Urgent left anterolateral thoracotomy in the case of structural damage

## 9.13/ POISONING

### COCAINE POISONING

**SYMPATHOMIMETIC AGENT**: inhibition of presynaptic reuptake of norepinephrine and dopamine

**CARDIOVASCULAR COMPLICATIONS**: sympathetic stimulation; HTN; LVH; ischemia; MI; DCM (excess catecholamines); myocarditis; heart failure (systolic and/or diastolic); arrhythmia; sudden death; endocarditis; aortic dissection; stroke - intracranial hemorrhage; Takotsubo; Brugada pattern on ECG; ↗ QT (effect on sodium and potassium channels)

**MYOCARDIAL INFARCTION**: ↗ $O_2$ demand; vasospasm; accelerated CAD; thrombosis (↗ platelet activation / aggregation); ↗ plaque rupture; coronary dissection

> **Treatment of myocardial infarction:** $O_2$; ASA; Benzodiazepines; Nitrates; CCB (Diltiazem 20 mg IV); Coronary angiography if persistent ST elevation (thrombolysis if coronary angiography not available and in the absence of contraindication); avoid BB (unopposed alpha-adrenergic stimulation)

### BETA-BLOCKER POISONING

**PRESENTATION**: Symptoms often appear within first 6 h after ingestion: bradycardia; hypotension; cardiogenic shock; altered LOC; seizures; hypoglycemia; bronchospasm

**ASSESSMENT**: ECG; Glucose; Electrolytes; $Ca^{2+}$; BUN; Creatinine; Acetaminophen - Salicylate; beta-HCG

> **ECG**: sinus bradycardia; ↗ PR interval; ↗ QRS interval (Propranolol or Acebutolol); bradyarrhythmia; asystole

**MANAGEMENT:** ABC; Monitor; Atropine (0.5-1 mg IV every 3-5 min up to 0.04 mg/kg); Bolus NS; IV Dextrose; Benzodiazepine if seizures; Activated charcoal (50 g) if patient presents 1-2 h postingestion; Poison Center

**IF NECESSARY (IN THE FOLLOWING ORDER)**

a) **Glucagon:** IV bolus 5 mg over 1 min (± 2nd bolus in 10 min); if improvement → start infusion (2-5 mg/h); target MAP 60 mmHg; Antinausea treatment (Ondansetron)

b) **IV Calcium:** Calcium chloride (1 g of 10% solution = 10 mL via central line up to a dose of 3 g if necessary) or Calcium gluconate (30 mL of a 10% solution via a central or peripheral line); Monitoring of serum calcium

c) **Vasopressors:** Epinephrine (1-10 μg/min; titrate to achieve MAP of 60 mmHg)

d) **High-dose insulin / Glucose (D5-10%) infusion;** ▶▶| CCB poisoning; $K^+$ - $Mg^{2+}$ supplement PRN

e) **IV fat emulsion** (parenteral nutrition)

f) **Sodium bicarbonate** (1-2 mEq/kg IV ± infusion) if ↗ QRS interval

g) **Endovenous pacemaker:** frequent capture failure; only slight hemodynamic improvement; consider if failure of drug treatment

h) **IABP / Ventricular assist device** if failure of drug treatment

i) **Consider hemodialysis** if failure of drug treatment (Atenolol; Nadolol; Sotalol; Acebutolol)

# CALCIUM CHANNEL BLOCKER POISONING

**DIHYDROPYRIDINE CCB**: arterial vasodilatation; reflex tachycardia; effects of nondihydropyridine CCB with high-dose ingestion

**NONDIHYDROPYRIDINE CCB**: peripheral vasodilatation; bradycardia; negative inotropic agent

**ASSESSMENT**: ECG; Glucose; Electrolytes; $Ca^{2+}$; BUN; Creatinine; Acetaminophen - Salicylate; beta-HCG

**MANAGEMENT**: ABC; Monitor; Bolus NS; Atropine (0.5-1 mg IV every 2-3 min up to 3 mg); activated charcoal (50 g) if patient presents in 1-2 h post-ingestion; Poison Center

**IV CALCIUM**: Calcium chloride (10-20 mL of solution 10% x 10 min via central line; repeat up to 4 x if necessary every 20 min) or Calcium gluconate (30 to 60 mL of a 10% solution via a central or peripheral line); Monitoring of serum calcium

> **Infusion**: Calcium chloride (0.2-0.4 mL/kg/h of a 10% solution) or Calcium gluconate (0.6-1.2 mL/kg/h of a 10% solution) if necessary; serum ionized calcium assay every 2 hours; ECG monitoring

**IF NECESSARY (IN THE FOLLOWING ORDER)**

a) **Glucagon**: IV bolus 5 mg over 1 min (± 2nd and 3rd boluses every 10 min); if improvement → start infusion (2-15 mg/h); target MAP 60 mmHg; Antinausea treatment (Ondansetron)

b) **High-dose insulin / Glucose infusion**; 50 mL D50% if blood glucose < 8.25 mmol/L; Correct potassium

> **Bolus**: 1 unit/kg of regular insulin IV

> **Infusion**: 0.5 U/kg/h IV (titrate up to 2 U/kg/h according to response; increase by 0.5 U/kg/h every 20 min)

- **D5-10% infusion**: 0.5-1 g/kg/h of dextrose; additional bolus of D50% PRN (capillary blood glucose **every 15-30 min)**

- **Serum potassium** assay every 30 min (± $Mg^{2+}$); supplement as necessary

c) **IV vasopressor**: IV Norepinephrine

d) **IV fat emulsion (parenteral nutrition):** bolus 1-1.5 mL/kg x 1 min (20% solution); Infusion 0.25-0.5 mL/kg/min (30-60 min)

e) **Other measures**: Endovenous pacemaker (but does not improve contractility); IABP - Ventricular assist device

# DIGOXIN POISONING

**EXTRACARDIAC MANIFESTATIONS**: visual disorders; GI symptoms (nausea; vomiting); neurological symptoms (confusion; muscle weakness); hyperkalemia

**CARDIAC MANIFESTATIONS**: sinus bradycardia; sinus arrest; ectopic atrial tachycardia with AV block; "regularized" AF (junctional escape rhythm); junctional tachycardia; AV block; PVCs; ventricular bigeminy; VT; bidirectional VT; VF

> **Mechanisms**: A) ↗ **Delayed after-depolarizations** (due to ↗ intracellular $Ca^{2+}$); +
> B) ↗ **Automaticity**; C) ↗ Vagal tone; **D)** Associated hyperkalemia

> **Digoxin impregnation**: flattening / inversion of T waves; ↘ QT; "scooped" ST segment; ST depression (lateral leads); U waves

**ASSESSMENT**: Plasma digoxin (6 h post-ingestion if acute poisoning); electrolytes; K+; $Mg^{2+}$; Creatinine - BUN; ECG; Blood glucose

**MANAGEMENT:** ABC; Cardiac monitoring; Poison Center; Atropine 0.5 mg IV; Bolus NS; Activated charcoal if poisoning < 1-2 h

**CORRECT HYPOKALEMIA: as hypokalemia exacerbates the toxic effects**; correct hypomagnesemia associated with hypokalemia

> **Do not correct hyperkalemia,** which is corrected by Digibind

**ANTIDOTE:** Digibind (anti-Digoxin antibody)

> **Indications: A)** Threatening arrhythmia (symptomatic bradycardia; AV block; ventricular arrhythmia; asystole); **B)** Target organ damage (ARF; altered state of consciousness); **C)** Hyperkalemia (> 5 - 5.5 mmol/L)
> **1 vial of Digibind neutralizes 0.5 mg of Digoxin**

| EMPIRICAL TREATMENT (ACUTE POISONING WITH UNKNOWN DOSE) | ACUTE POISONING WITH KNOWN INGESTED DOSE | CHRONIC POISONING WITH KNOWN PLASMA DIGOXIN |
|---|---|---|
| **10 vials** (repeat in 30 min if insufficient) | Number of vials = [Ingested dose of Digoxin (mg) x 0.8] / 0.5 | Number of vials = [Serum concentration (ng/mL) x patient's weight (kg)] / 100 |

**MAINTAIN ON MONITOR > 72 H** if concomitant renal failure (delayed elimination)

**HEMODIALYSIS**: not indicated

# 9.14/ SWAN-GANZ CATHETER PLACEMENT

**INDICATIONS: A)** Cardiogenic shock; **B)** Mixed shock; **C)** Mechanical complication of myocardial infarction; **D)** PHT; **E)** Pretransplantation assessment

**1) VERIFICATIONS:** patency of ports; test balloon and pressure transducer

**2) CENTRAL VENOUS ACCESS**: insert the introducer (Cordis) under ultrasound guidance into the internal jugular vein (modified Seldinger technique)

**3) SWAN-GANZ CATHETER PLACEMENT**: insert the Swan-Ganz catheter by following the natural curvature towards the PA

> Inflate the balloon in the RA (RA hemodynamic curve); keep the balloon inflated while advancing the Swan-Ganz (deflate the balloon on withdrawal)
> Advance the Swan-Ganz while examining changes in the appearance of the hemodynamic curve displayed on the monitor (RA → RV → PA → Wedge)

| RA | RV | PA |
|---|---|---|
| **15-20 cm** | **30 cm** | **40 cm** |

> Withdraw the Swan-Ganz if **< 1 mL of NS** is necessary to inflate the balloon and obtain a Wedge pressure (the catheter tip is probably too distal)

**4) CXR**: catheter tip < 5 cm from the midline; West zone # 3 preferable

**CONSIDER FLUOROSCOPY** if chamber dilatation or significant TR

**AIR EMBOLISM**: left lateral decubitus position (to prevent RVOT obstruction); 100% $O_2$

### CARDIOPULMONARY ARREST

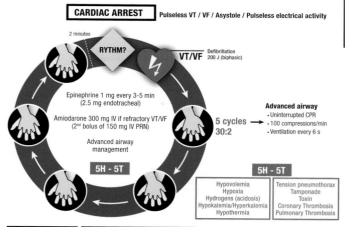

**CARDIAC ARREST** Pulseless VT / VF / Asystole / Pulseless electrical activity

2 minutes

RYTHM?

VT/VF — Defibrillation 200 J (biphasic)

Epinephrine 1 mg every 3-5 min
(2.5 mg endotracheal)

Amiodarone 300 mg IV if refractory VT/VF
(2nd bolus of 150 mg IV PRN)

Advanced airway
management

**5H - 5T**

5 cycles → **Advanced airway**
30:2 · Uninterrupted CPR
· 100 compressions/min
· Ventilation every 6 s

**5H - 5T**

| Hypovolemia | Tension pneumothorax |
| Hypoxia | Tamponade |
| Hydrogens (acidosis) | Toxin |
| Hypokalemia/Hyperkalemia | Coronary Thrombosis |
| Hypothermia | Pulmonary Thrombosis |

| **Improve CPR if:** | **Return of spontaneous circulation** |
|---|---|
| · $ETCO_2$ < 10 mmHg | · BP and Pulse |
| · DBP < 20 mmHg | · Abrupt ↑ of $ETCO_2$ ≥ 40 mmHg |
| · $SVO_2$ < 30 % | · Spontaneous waves on arterial recording |

**RECOGNIZE CARDIOPULMONARY ARREST**: unresponsive / breathing / pulse

> **Activate the survival chain:** 911 - Blue Code - Defibrillator / AED

**CARDIOPULMONARY RESUSCITATION**

> **Cycles: 30 compressions : 2 ventilations**
> **Compressions**: lower half of the sternum; 100-120 compressions / min; 5 cm deep (avoid > 6 cm); complete chest recoil between each compression; minimize interruptions
> **Ventilation**: Head tilt / Chin lift ("Jaw thrust" if cervical trauma); avoid excessive ventilation

**DEFIBRILLATION:** Pulseless VT or VF; perform as rapidly as possible

**AIRWAY MANAGEMENT**

> **Initial ventilation**: Ambu mask; 1 s; elevation of the rib cage; avoid excessive ventilation
> **Advanced airways support**: allows better ventilation and protects the airways; Endotracheal tube or Laryngeal mask or Combitube
> · **Confirmation of position: A)** Physical examination (expansion of rib cage; auscultation); **B)** Capnography / $CO_2$ detector; **C)** Esophageal detector (syringe); **D)** CXR (distal extremity of ETT > 3 cm from the carina)
> · **CPR cycles**: Continuous compressions at 100 bpm; Asynchronous ventilation every 6 sec

## BRADYCARDIA

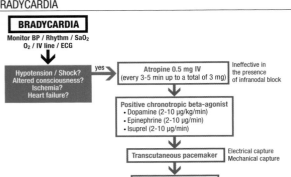

**BRADYCARDIA**

Monitor BP / Rhythm / SaO₂
O₂ / IV line / ECG

Hypotension / Shock?
Altered consciousness?
Ischemia?
Heart failure?

→ yes →

**Atropine 0.5 mg IV**
(every 3-5 min up to a total of 3 mg)

Ineffective in the presence of infranodal block

**Positive chronotropic beta-agonist**
• Dopamine (2-10 µg/kg/min)
• Epinephrine (2-10 µg/min)
• Isuprel (2-10 µg/min)

**Transcutaneous pacemaker** — Electrical capture / Mechanical capture

**Endovenous pacemaker**

## TACHYCARDIA

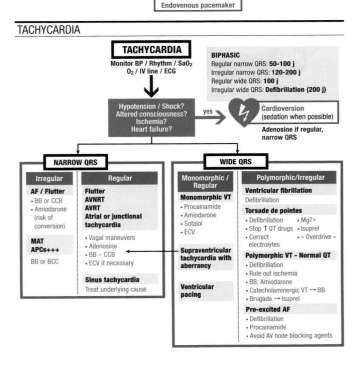

**TACHYCARDIA**

Monitor BP / Rhythm / SaO₂
O₂ / IV line / ECG

**BIPHASIC**
Regular narrow QRS: **50-100 j**
Irregular narrow QRS: **120-200 j**
Regular wide QRS: **100 j**
Irregular wide QRS: **Defibrillation (200 j)**

Hypotension / Shock?
Altered consciousness?
Ischemia?
Heart failure?

→ yes →

**Cardioversion**
(sedation when possible)

**Adenosine if regular, narrow QRS**

### NARROW QRS

| Irregular | Regular |
|---|---|

**Irregular**

**AF / Flutter**
• BB or CCB
• Amiodarone (risk of conversion)

**MAT**
**APCs+++**
BB or BCC

**Regular**

**Flutter**
**AVNRT**
**AVRT**
**Atrial or junctional tachycardia**
• Vagal maneuvers
• Adenosine
• BB – CCB
• ECV if necessary

**Sinus tachycardia**
Treat underlying cause

### WIDE QRS

**Monomorphic / Regular**

**Monomorphic VT**
• Procainamide
• Amiodarone
• Sotalol
• ECV

**Supraventricular tachycardia with aberrancy**

**Ventricular pacing**

**Polymorphic/Irregular**

**Ventricular fibrillation**
Defibrillation

**Torsade de pointes**
• Defibrillation   • Mg²⁺
• Stop ↑ QT drugs • Isuprel
• Correct        • « Overdrive »
  electrolytes

**Polymorphic VT - Normal QT**
• Defibrillation
• Rule out ischemia
• BB; Amiodarone
• Catecholaminergic VT → BB
• Brugada → Isuprel

**Pre-excited AF**
• Defibrillation
• Procainamide
• Avoid AV node blocking agents

| | | | |
|---|---|---|---|
| **Adenosine** | • 6 mg IV (push) then 20 mL NS<br>• 2nd bolus 12 mg IV PRN | • Supraventricular tachycardia | Bronchospasm; Hypotension; Flushing; Retrosternal chest pain; Can trigger AF |
| **Amiodarone** | • 150 mg IV x 10 min (repeat PRN)<br>• Infusion: 1 mg/min x 6 h then 0.5 mg/min (dilution: 450 mg / 250 mL D5%)<br>• Max: 2.2 g / 24 h | • Supraventricular tachycardia<br>• Stable monomorphic VT<br>• Polymorphic VT with normal QT | Bradycardia; ↗ QT; Long-term toxicity |
| **Beta-blockers** | • **Esmolol:** 0.5 mg/kg x 1 min then infusion of 0.05-0.3 mg/kg/min (dilution: 2500 mg / 250 mL)<br>• **Metoprolol:** 5 mg IV x 1 min (repeat every 5 min up to a total of 15 mg) | • Supraventricular tachycardia<br>• Polymorphic VT associated with ischemia or LQTS or catecholaminergic VT | Hypotension; Bradycardia; Negative inotrope; Bronchospasm |
| **Diltiazem** | • 15-20 mg IV x 2 min<br>• 2nd bolus (in 15 min): 20-25 mg IV<br>• Infusion: 5-15 mg/h IV<br>• Dilution: 125 mg/100 mL D5 % (= 1 mg/mL) | • Supraventricular tachycardia | Hypotension; Bradycardia; Negative inotrope |
| **Lidocaine** | • Bolus: 1-1.5 mg/kg IV<br>• Perfusion: 1-4 mg/min (30-50 µg/kg/min)<br>• Dilution: 2 g / 500 mL D5% | • Stable monomorphic VT | Altered state of consciousness; Seizures; Bradycardia |
| **Procainamide** | • 20-50 mg/min (until suppression of arrhythmia or hypotension or ↗ QRS > 50% or total dose 17 mg/kg)<br>• Dilution: 1000 mg / 250 mL NS | • Pre-excited AF<br>• Stable monomorphic VT | Bradycardia; Hypotension; ↗ QT; Torsade de pointes; Avoid in the presence of heart failure |
| **Sotalol** | • 1.5 mg/kg IV x 5 min | • Stable monomorphic VT | Bradycardia; Hypotension; ↗ QT; Torsade de pointes; Avoid in the presence of heart failure |
| **Magnesium sulfate** | • 1-2 g IV x 15 min | • Polymorphic VT with ↗ QT | Hypotension; Respiratory depression |
| **Epinephrine** | • **Dose:** 0.1-0.5 µg/kg/min<br>• **Dilution:** 5 mg / 250 mL D5% | | |

**09**

Miscellaneous

| Dobutamine | • **Dose**: 2-20 µg/kg/min<br>• **Dilution**: 250 mg / 100 mL D5% |
|---|---|
| Dopamine | • **Dose**: 1-20 µg/kg/min<br>• **Dilution**: 400 mg / 250 mL D5% |
| Isuprel | • **Dose**: 0.5-10 µg/min<br>• **Dilution:** 1 mg / 250 mL D5% |
| Milrinone | • **Bolus**: 50 µg/kg x 10 min<br>• **Dose**: 0.375 to 0.75 µg/kg/min<br>• **Dilution:** 10 mg / 100 mL D5%<br>(= 0.09 mg/mL) or 20 mg / 100 mL D5% (= 0.17 mg/mL) |
| Norepinephrine | • **Dose**: 0.1-0.5 µg/kg/min<br>• **Dilution:** 4 mg / 250 mL D5% (double PRN) |
| Phenylephrine | • **Dose**: 0.5-2 µg/kg/min<br>• **Dilution:** 10 mg / 250 mL NS |

## MANAGEMENT POST-CARDIAC ARREST

Look for and treat the cause of the cardiac arrest; Coronary angiography if necessary

**VENTILATION**: Tidal volume 6-8 mL/kg; $SaO_2 \geq 94\%$; $PaCO_2$ 40-45 mmHg

**TARGET ORGAN PERFUSION**: NaCl bolus; vasopressors (Epinephrine; Dopamine; Norepinephrine); treat any reversible causes; IABP - Ventricular assist device

> Stunned myocardium x 24-48 h and transient SIRS post-cardiac arrest
> **Targets:** SBP ≥ 90 mmHg; MAP ≥ 65 mmHg; $SVO_2 \geq 70 \%$

### TARGETED TEMPERATURE MANAGEMENT

> **Indications**: Comatose adult patients (no meaningful response to verbal commands) with return of spontaneous circulation after cardiac arrest
> **Benefits**: improvement of survival and neurological prognosis (★ Hypothermia after cardiac arrest study group)
> **Targets**: uncertain (between 32°C to 36°C for at least 24 h); intensive treatment of hyperthermia; ★ TTM → no demonstrated benefit of 33°C versus 36°C
> **Complications**: coagulopathy; arrhythmias; ↗ QT; bradycardias; hyperglycemia; infectious risk; hypokalemia / hypomagnesemia / hypophosphatemia

**NEUROLOGICAL ASSESSMENT:** neurological examination; EEG (rule out seizures in the presence of persistent coma); Brain CT / MRI

> **Factors of poor prognosis (valid after > 72 h)**: **A)** Bilaterally absent pupillary light reflex; bilaterally absent corneal reflexes; **B)** Status myoclonus (during the first 72 hours); **C)** EEG with persistent absence of reactivity to external stimuli or with persistent burst supression or with intractable status epilepticus; **D)** Somatosensory evoked potentials (bilateral absence of cortical response to median nerve stimulation); **E)** Imaging (extensive cortical / subcortical lesions; extensive brain edema)
> **Brain death**: consider organ donation

- Bonow RO, Mann DL, Zipes DP, Libby P. Braunwald's Heart Disease. *A textbook of cardiovascular medicine*. Saunders Elsevier. 2012. 1961 p.
- 2014 ACC/AHA Guideline on Perioperative Cardiovascular Evaluation and Management of Patients Undergoing Noncardiac Surgery. *JACC* 2014; *64;* 77-137
- 2014 ESC/ESA Guidelines on non-cardiac surgery: cardiovascular assessment and management. *EHJ* 2014; *35;* 2383-2431
- 2009 ACCF/AHA Focused Update on Perioperative Beta Blockade Incorporated Into the ACC/AHA 2007 Guidelines on Perioperative Cardiovascular Evaluation and Care for Noncardiac Surgery. *JACC* 2009; *54;* e13-e118.
- Canadian Cardiovascular Society/Canadian Anesthesiologists' Society/Canadian Heart Rhythm Society Joint Position Statement on the Perioperative Management of Patients With Implanted Pacemakers, Defibrillators, and Neurostimulating Devices. *CJC* 2012; *28;* 141-151
- Baron TH, Kamath PS, McBane RD. Management of antithrombotic therapy in patients undergoing invasive procedures. *NEJM* 2013; *368;* 2113-2124.
- Perioperative Management of Antithrombotic Therapy. Antithrombotic Therapy and Prevention of Thrombosis, 9th ed: American College of Chest Physicians Evidence-Based Clinical Practice Guidelines. *CHEST* 2012; *141;* e326S-e350S
- 2013 ACC/AHA guideline on the assessment of cardiovascular risk: a report of the American College of Cardiology/American Heart Association Task Force on Practice Guidelines. *Circulation* 2014; *129;* S49-73
- Core Components of Cardiac Rehabilitation / Secondary Prevention Programs: 2007 Update. *Circulation.* 2007; *115;* 2675-2682
- European Guidelines on cardiovascular disease prevention in clinical practice (version 2012). *EHJ* 2012; *33;* 1635-1701.
- AHA/ACCF Secondary Prevention and Risk Reduction Therapy for Patients With Coronary and Other Atherosclerotic Vascular Disease: 2011 Update. *Circulation* 2011; *124;* 2458-2473
- 2010 ACCF/AHA Guideline for Assessment of Cardiovascular Risk in Asymptomatic Adults. *JACC* 2010; *56;* e50-103
- The Use of Antiplatelet Therapy in the Outpatient Setting: Canadian Cardiovascular Society Guidelines. *CJC;* 2011; *27;* S1-S59
- Primary and Secondary Prevention of Cardiovascular Disease. Antithrombotic Therapy and Prevention of Thrombosis, 9th ed: American College of Chest Physicians Evidence-Based Clinical Practice Guidelines. *CHEST* 2012; *141;* e637S-e668S
- Smoking Cessation and the Cardiovascular Specialist: Canadian Cardiovascular Society Position Paper. *CJC;* 2011; *27;* 132-137
- Fiore MC, Baker TB. Treating Smokers in the Health Care Setting. *NEJM* 2011; *365;* 1222-31
- 2013 ACC/AHA guideline on the treatment of blood cholesterol to reduce atherosclerotic cardiovascular risk in adults: a report of the American College of Cardiology/American Heart Association Task Force on Practice Guidelines. *JACC* 2014; *63;* 2889-2934
- ESC/EAS Guidelines for the management of dyslipidaemias. *EHJ* 2011; *32;* 1769-1818.
- 2009 Canadian Cardiovascular Society/Canadian guidelines for the diagnosis and treatment of dyslipidemia and prevention of cardiovascular disease in the adult - 2009 recommendations. *CJC* 2009; *25;* 567-579.
- 2012 Update of the Canadian Cardiovascular Society Guidelines for the Diagnosis and Treatment of Dyslipidemia for the Prevention of Cardiovascular Disease in the Adult. *CJC* 2013; *29;* 151-167.
- Macini GB, Baker S, Bergeron J. Diagnosis, Prevention, and Management of Statin Adverse Effects and Intolerance: Proceedings of a Canadian Working Group Consensus Conference. *CJC* 2011; *27;* 635-662.

**09**

Miscellaneous

- 2014 evidence-based guideline for the management of high blood pressure in adults (JNC 8). *JAMA* 2014; *311;* 507-520.
- 2013 ESH/ESC Guidelines for the management of arterial hypertension. *EHJ* 2013; *34;* 2159-2219.
- The 2012 Canadian Hypertension Education Program Recommendations for the Management of Hypertension: Blood Pressure Measurement, Diagnosis, Assessment of Risk, and Therapy. *CJC* 2012; *28;* 270-287.
- Marik PE, Varon J. Hypertensive Crises, Challenges and Management. *Chest* 2007; *131;* 1949-1962.
- Resistant Hypertension: Diagnosis, Evaluation, and Treatment: A Scientific Statement From the American Heart Association Professional Education Committee of the Council for High Blood Pressure Research. *Hypertension* 2008; *51;* 1403-1419.
- ACCF/AHA 2011 Expert Consensus Document on Hypertension in the Elderly. *JACC* 2011; *57;* 2037-2114.
- ESC Guidelines on diabetes, pre-diabetes, and cardiovascular diseases developed in collaboration with the EASD. *EHJ* 2013; *34;* 3035-3087.
- Canadian Diabetes Association 2013 Clinical Practice Guidelines for the prevention and management of Diabetes in Canada. *Can J Diabetes* 2013; *37;* S1 - S212.
- Intensive Glycemic Control and the Prevention of Cardiovascular Events: Implications of the ACCORD, ADVANCE, and VA Diabetes Trials. *JACC* 2009; *53;* 298-304.
- Aspirin for Primary Prevention of Cardiovascular Events in People With Diabetes. *JACC* 2010; *55;* 2878-2886.
- Metkus TS, Baughman KL, Thompson PD. Exercise Prescription and Primary Prevention of Cardiovascular Disease. *Circulation* 2010; *121;* 2601-2604
- Physical Activity and Public Health Updated Recommendation for Adults From the American College of Sports Medicine and the American Heart Association. *Circulation.* 2007; 116: 1081-1093
- Thompson PD. Exercise Prescription and Proscription for Patients With Coronary Artery Disease. *Circulation.* 2005; 112: 2354-2363
- Exercise Standards for Testing and Training: A Statement for Healthcare Professionals. *Circulation.* 2001; *104:* 1694-1740
- 2013 AHA/ACC Guideline on Lifestyle Management to Reduce Cardiovascular Risk. *JACC* 2014; *63;* 2960-2984.
- Somers VK, White DP, Amin Raouf. Sleep Apnea and Cardiovascular Disease. *JACC* 2008; *52;* 686-717.
- CCS Consensus Conference 2003: Assessment of the cardiac patient for fitness to drive and fly. *CJC* 2004; *20;* 1313-1323.
- Canadian Cardiovascular Society Focused Position Statement Update on Assessment of the Cardiac Patient for Fitness to Drive: Fitness Following Left Ventricular Assist Device Implantation. *CJC* 2012; *28;* 137-140.
- 2015 American Heart Association Guidelines for Cardiopulmonary Resuscitation and Emergency Cardiovascular Care. *Circulation;* 2015; *132;* Section 1, 5, 6, 7, 8, 9 and 10. S315-S518.
- Haïat R, Leroy G. *Prescription guidelines in cardiology,* 5th edition. Éditions Frison-Roche. 2015. 350 p.
- UpToDate 2015

# Abbreviations

# A

**AAD**: Antiarrhythmic drug

**AAA**: Abdominal aortic aneurysm

**ABC**: Airway, Breathing, Circulation

**ABI**: Ankle-Brachial Index

**A/C**: Anticoagulant / Anticoagulation

**ACEi**: Angiotensin-converting enzyme inhibitor

**ACLS**: Advanced Cardiac Life Support

**ACS**: Acute coronary syndrome

**AF**: Atrial fibrillation

**AIVR**: Accelerated idioventricular rhythm

**ALT**: Alanine aminotransferase

**AML**: Anterior mitral leaflet

**ANA**: Antinuclear antibody

**Ao**: Aorta

**APC**: Atrial premature complex

**Apo**: Apoliprotein

**aPTT**: Activated partial thromboplastin time

**AR**: Aortic regurgitation

**ARB**: Angiotensin receptor blocker

**ARDS**: Adult respiratory distress syndrome

**ARF**: Acute renal failure

**ARVD**: Arrhythmogenic right ventricular dysplasia

**AS**: Aortic stenosis

**ASA**: Acetylsalicylic acid

**ASD**: Atrial septal defect

**AST**: Aspartate aminotransferase

**ATL**: Anterior tricuspid leaflet

**AV**: Atrioventricular

**AVM**: Arteriovenous malformation

**AVNRT**: Atrioventricular nodal reentrant tachycardia

**AVR**: Aortic valve replacement

**AVRT**: Atrioventricular reentry tachycardia

# B

**BB**: Beta-blockers

**BID**: Twice daily

**BMI**: Body mass index

**BMS**: Bare metal stent

**BNP**: Natriuretic peptide type B

**BOOP**: Bronchiolitis obliterans organizing pneumonia

**BP**: Blood pressure

**BSA**: Body surface area

**BUN**: Blood urea nitrogen

**BVR**: Balloon Valvuloplasty Registry

# C

**CABG**: Coronary artery bypass graft

**CAD**: Coronary artery disease

**CBC**: Complete blood count

**CCB**: Calcium channel blockers

**CCS**: Canadian Cardiology Society

**CCV**: Chemical cardioversion

**CK**: Creatinine kinase

**CM**: Cardiomyopathy

**CML**: Chronic myeloid leukemia

**CNS**: Central nervous system

**CO**: Cardiac output

**CoA**: Coarctation of the aorta

**CoNS**: Coagulase-negative Staphylococcus

**COPD**: Chronic obstructive pulmonary disease

**COX-1**: Cyclooxygenase-1

**CPB**: Cardiopulmonary bypass

**CRF**: Chronic renal failure

**CRP**: C-reactive protein

**CRT**: Cardiac resynchronization therapy

**CS**: Coronary sinus

**CSNRT**: Corrected Sinus Node Recovery Time

**CT**: Computed tomography

**cTn**: Cardiac troponin

**cTnT HS**: Highly sensitive cardiac troponin T

**cTnT**: Cardiac troponin T

**CTO**: Chronic total occlusion

**CVP**: Central venous pressure

**CXR**: Chest x-ray

# D

**DBP**: Diastolic blood pressure

**DCM**: Dilated cardiomyopathy

**DDx**: Differential diagnosis

**DES**: Drug-eluting stent

**DIC**: Disseminated intravascular coagulation

**DM**: Diabetes

dP/dt: Rate of LV pressure rise in early systole

**DTS**: Duke Treadmill score

**DVT**: Deep vein thrombosis

# E

**ECG**: Electrocardiogram

**ECMO**: Extracorporeal membrane oxygenation

**ECV**: Electrical cardioversion

**EEG**: Electroencephalogram

**EOA**: Effective orifice area

**EPO**: Erythropoietin

**EPS**: Electrophysiological study

**ESR**: Erythrocyte sedimentation rate

**EVAR**: Endovascular aortic repair

# F

**FAC**: Fractional Area Change

**FFP**: Fresh frozen plasma

**FFR**: Fractional flow reserve

**FMD**: Fibromuscular dysplasia

## G

**GERD**: Gastroesophageal reflux disease

**GFR**: Glomerular filtration rate

**GI**: Gastrointestinal

## H

**HbA1c**: Glycosylated hemoglobin

**HCM**: Hypertrophic cardiomyopathy

**HDCT**: High-definition computed tomography

**HDL**: High-density lipoprotein

**HELLP**: HELLP syndrome

**HIT**: Heparin-induced thrombocytopenia

**HR**: Heart rate

**HSM**: Hepatosplenomegaly

**HTN**: Hypertension

## I

**IABP**: Intra-aortic balloon pump

**IART**: Intraatrial reentry tachycardia

**ICD**: Implantable cardioverter-defibrillator

**IDU**: Intravenous drug user

**IMT**: Intima-media thickness

**INR**: International normalized ratio

**ISA**: Intrinsic sympathetic activity

**IUGR**: Intrauterine growth retardation

**IVC**: Inferior vena cava

**IVCT**: Isovolumic contraction time

**IVRT**: Isovolumic relaxation time

**IVS**: Interventricular septum

**IVUS**: Intravascular ultrasound

## J

**JVD**: Jugular vein distension

## L

**LA**: Left atrium

**LAA**: Left atrial appendage

**LAD**: Left anterior descending

**LAH**: Left atrial hypertrophy

**LAHB**: Left anterior hemiblock

**LAO**: Left anterior oblique

**LBBB**: Left bundle branch block

**LMCA**: Left main coronary artery

**LDH**: Lactate dehydrogenase

**LDL**: Low-density lipoprotein

**LFTs**: Liver function tests

**LGE**: Late gadolinium enhancement

**LIMA**: Left internal mammary artery

**LMWH**: Low molecular weight heparin

**LPHB**: left posterior hemiblock

**LPL**: Lipoprotein lipase

**LQTS**: Long QT syndrome

**LV**: Left ventricle

**LVAD**: Left ventricular assist device

**LVDD**: Left ventricular diastolic diameter

**LVEDP**: Left ventricular end-diastolic pressure

**LVEF**: Left ventricular ejection fraction

**LVH**: Left ventricular hypertrophy

**LVOT**: Left ventricular outflow tract

**LVSD**: Left ventricular systolic diameter

## M

**M**: Mitral

**MAC**: Mitral annular calcification

**MAO inhibitor**: Monoamine oxidase inhibitor

**MAP**: Mean arterial pressure

**MCP**: Metacarpophalangeal

**MET**: Metabolic Equivalent of Task

**MIBIP**: MIBI-Dipyridamole

**MPA**: Main pulmonary artery

**MR**: Mitral regurgitation

**MS**: Mitral stenosis

**MSK**: Musculoskeletal

**MTX**: Methotrexate

**MVP**: Mitral valve prolapse

**MVR**: Mitral valve replacement

## N

**NGT**: Nasogastric tube

**NIHSS**: NIH Stroke Scale

**NNT**: Number needed to treat

**NPO**: Nil per os

**NPV**: Negative predictive value

**NSAID**: Non-steroidal anti-inflammatory drug

**NSVT**: Non-Sustained Ventricular Tachycardia

**NYHA:** New York Heart Association

## O

**OH**: Orthostatic hypotension

**OR**: Operating room

**OSAHS**: Obstructive sleep apnea / hypopnea syndrome

**OTP**: Orthopnea

## P

**PA**: Pulmonary artery

**PAD**: Peripheral artery disease

**PAH**: Pulmonary arterial hypertension

**PAN**: Polyarteritis nodosa

**PAP**: Pulmonary artery pressure

**PAT**: Paroxysmal atrial tachycardia

**PCI**: Percutaneous coronary intervention

**PCR**: Polymerase chain reaction

**PDE-5**: Phosphodiesterase-5

**PET**: Positron emission tomography

**PET-FDG**: Fluorodeoxy-glucose positron emission tomography

**PFO**: Patent foramen ovale

**PFTs**: Pulmonary function tests

**PHT**: Pressure half time

**PHT**: Pulmonary hypertension

**PISA**: Proximal isovolumic surface area

**PDA**: Posterior interventricular artery

**PJRT**: Paroxysmal junctional reentry tachycardia

**PLAX**: Parasternal long axis

**PML**: Posterior mitral leaflet

**PMR**: Polymyalgia rheumatica

**PMT**: Pacemaker-mediated tachycardia

**PNC**: Penicillin

**PND**: Paroxysmal nocturnal dyspnea

**PO**: Per os

**POTS**: Postural orthostatic tachycardia syndrome

**PPD**: Purified Protein Derivative (Mantoux test)

**PPI**: Proton pump inhibitor

**PPM**: Permanent pacemaker

**PPV**: Positive predictive value

**PR**: Pulmonary regurgitation

**PRN**: As needed

**PS**: Pulmonary stenosis

**PSAX**: Parasternal short axis

**PSVT**: Paroxysmal lsupraventricular tachycardia

**PT**: Prothrombin time

**PTCA**: Percutaneous coronary angioplasty

**PTL**: Posterior tricuspid leaflet

**PTU**: Propylthiouracil

**PV**: Pulmonary vein

**PVAB**: Post-ventricular atrial blanking

**PVARP**: Post-ventricular atrial refractory period

**PVE**: Prosthetic valve endocarditis

**PVR**: Pulmonary valve replacement

**PVR**: Pulmonary vascular resistance

## Q

**QD**: Once daily

**QID**: Four times a day

## R

**RA**: Rheumatoid arthritis

**RA**: Right atrium

**RAA**: Right atrial appendage

**RAH**: Right atrial hypertrophy

**RAO**: Right anterior oblique

**RBBB**: Right bundle branch block

**RCA**: Right coronary artery

**RCM**: Restrictive cardiomyopathy

**RCT**: Randomized controlled trial

**RF**: Radiofrequency

**RF**: Rheumatoid factor

**RF**: Risk factor

**RPA**: Right pulmonary artery

**RUQ**: Right upper quadrant

**RV**: Right ventricle

**RVAD**: Right ventricular assist device

**RVG**: Radionuclide ventriculography

**RVH**: Right ventricular hypertrophy

**RVOT**: Right ventricular outflow tract

**RVSP**: Right ventricular systolic pressure

**RWMA**: Regional wall motion abnormality

**RWT**: Relative wall thickness

## S

**SA**: Sinoatrial

**SAECG**: Signal-averaged ECG

**SAH**: Subarachnoid hemorrhage

**SAM**: Systolic anterior movement of mitral leaflet

**SaO₂**: Oxygen saturation

**SBP**: Systolic blood pressure

**SIRS**: Systemic inflammatory response syndrome

**SLE**: Systemic lupus erythematosus

**SPEP**: Serum protein electrophoresis

**SQTS**: Short QT syndrome

**SR**: Sinus rhythm

**SSRI**: Selective serotonin reuptake inhibitor

**SSS**: Sick sinus syndrome

**STS**: Society of Thoracic Surgeons

**STEMI**: ST segment elevation myocardial infarction

**STL**: Septal tricuspid leaflet

**SVC**: Superior vena cava

**SVO$_2$**: Venous oxygen saturation

**SVR**: Systemic vascular resistance

## T

**T**: Tricuspid

**TARP**: Total atrial refractory period

**TAVI**: Transcatheter aortic valve implantation

**TB**: Tuberculosis

**TEE**: Transesophageal echocardiography

**TG**: Triglycerides

**TGV**: Transposition of the great arteries

**TIA**: Transient ischemic attack

**TID**: Three times a day

**TNK**: Tenecteplase

**TNT**: Nitroglycerin

**TOF**: Tetralogy of Fallot

**TR**: Tricuspid regurgitation

**TTE**: Transthoracic echocardiography

**TTR**: Transthyretin

**TVR**: Tricuspid valve replacement

**TXA**-2: Thromboxane-2

## U

**ULN**: Upper limit of normal

**URI**: Upper rate interval

**URTI**: Upper respiratory tract infection

**US**: Ultrasound

## V

**VAC**: Vacuum assisted closure

**VF**: Ventricular fibrillation

**VLDL**: Very low density lipoprotein

**VO$_2$**: Oxygen consumption

**VPC**: Ventricular premature complex

**VSD**: Ventricular septal defect

**VT**: Ventricular tachycardia

**VTI**: Velocity-time integral

**vW**: von Willebrand

## W

**WMSI**: Wall motion score index

**WPW**: Wolff-Parkinson-White

**Abbreviations**

★ Clinical
Trials cited

**4D** (statins in dialysis)..... 322
**4S** (statins) ..................... 322
**AATAC-AF** (PVI in congestive HF)........ 122; 215
**ACAS** (carotid revascularization)........... 294
**ACCEPT-D** (ASA in DM)... 332
**ACCOMPLISH** (HTN)....... 326
**ACCORD** (fibrates) .......... 321
**ACCORD** (glycemic control) .............................. 330
**ACCORD-BP** (BP control in DM) ............................. 332
**ACST** (carotid revascularization) ........... 294
**ACT** (N-acetyl-L-cysteine)... 48
**ACT** (Vernakalant) ........... 213
**ACTION** (Nifedipine) ........ 77
**ACTIVE-A** (Clopidogrel)... 216
**ACUITY** (Bivalirudin) .... 87
**ADVANCE** (glycemic control) .............................. 330
**ADVANCE** (Perindopril and DM) ........................... 332
**AFASAK 1 and 2** (Warfarin).......................... 216
**AFCAPS / TexCAPS** (statins) .......................... 322
**AF-CHF** (AF) ............122, 211
**AFFIRM** (AF)................... 211
**A-HEFT** (Hydralazine - Nitrate) ........................... 121
**AIM-HIGH** (Niacin) ..321, 322
**AIRE** (ACE Inhibitors - Ramipril) ...................96, 118
**ALLHAT** (HTN) ............... 326
**ALLIANCE** (statins) ........ 322
**AMPLIFY** (Apixaban in venous thromboembolism).......... 299
**ANDROMEDA** (Dronedarone)...121, 212, 231
**Antithrombotic Trialists'** (ASA)..........76, 86, 96, 287, 314, 315
**APAF** (AF)....................... 211
**ARISTOTLE** (Apixaban in AF) ............................... 217
**ARMYDA** (statins) .......... 106
**ARMYDA-2** (Clopidogrel)..106
**ARTS** (CABG / PCI)........... 79

**ASCEND** (ASA in DM)...... 331
**ASCEND-HF** (Nesiritide) . 128
**ASCOT-BP** (HTN) ........... 326
**ASCOT** (statins) ............. 322
**ASPIRE** (ASA in venous thromboembolism).......... 299
**ASSERT** (AF detected by pacemaker) ................ 219
**ASSET** (thrombolysis) ...... 93
**ASSOCIATE** (Ivabradine) ... 77
**ATHENA** (Dronedarone).........212, 231
**ATLAS** (Lisinopril) .......... 118
**ATLAS ACS** (Rivaroxaban in ACS)........................... 87
**A-to-Z** (statins) ............... 322
**AURORA** (statins in dialysis)......................... 322
**AVERROES** (Apixaban in AF) ............................... 217
**AVID** (ICD) ..................... 241
**AVRO** (Vernakalant) ........ 213
**BAATAF** (Warfarin).......... 216
**BARI** (CABG / PCI) ........... 79
**BASIL** (critical limb ischemia)........................ 288
**B-CONVINCED** (BB) ........ 118
**BEAT** (beta-blockers) ..... 118
**BEST** (CABG / PCI) ........... 79
**BLOCK-HF** (CRT) ............ 211
**BRIDGE** (AF / surgery) ..... 313
**CAFA** (Warfarin) ............. 216
**CAMELOT** (Amlodipine) ... 77
**CANPAP** (OSAHS) ........... 123
**CAPRICORN** (Carvedilol) ................96, 118
**CAPRIE** (Clopidogrel) ......76, 287, 315
**CARDS** (statins in DM) .... 332
**CARE** (statins) ............... 322
**CARE-HF** (CRT) ..............122, 239, 240
**CARESS-HF** (ultrafiltration)................. 120
**CARESS-in-AMI** (pharmaco-invasive strategy)............. 95
**CARISA** (Ranolazine) ........ 77
**CARP** (preop revascularization)............ 312
**CASH** (ICD) ..................... 241
**CASS** (CABG) ................... 79

**CAST** (post-myocardial infarction PVCs).......102, 121, 212, 230
**CHARISMA** (Clopidogrel) ............287, 315
**CHARM** (ARB - Candesartan) .............96, 120
**CHARM-PRESERVED** (ARB - Candesartan) ....... 124
**CHEST** (Riociguat in thromboembolic PHT) ........................305, 306
**Cholesterol Treatment Trialists'** (statins)............ 322
**CIBIS** (Bisoprolol)............ 118
**CIDS** (ICD) ..................... 241
**CLARITY** (Clopidogrel) ...... 95
**CLOSURE-1** (patent foramen ovale) ............... 250
**CLOT** (venous thromboembolism).......... 299
**COMET** (beta-blockers)... 118
**COMMIT** (beta-blockers) .. 95
**COMMIT** (Clopidogrel)....... 95
**COMPANION** (resynchronization) .........122, 239, 240
**CONFIRM HF** (iron therapy) .................. 123
**CONSENSUS** (ACE inhibitors - Enalapril)....... 118
**COPE** (Colchicine)........... 174
**COPERNICUS** (Carvedilol) ...................... 118
**COPPS-POAF** (Colchicine)...................... 107
**CORAL** (renovascular disease)........................ 289
**CORONA** (statins in heart failure) .................. 322
**CORONARY** (beating heart surgery) ............... 107
**CORP** (Colchicine) .......... 174
**COURAGE** (CABG / PCI) .... 79
**CREST** (stent in carotid stenosis) ...................... 294
**CRYSTAL-AF** (Subclinical AF) .............................. 291
**CTAF** (antiarrhythmics in AF) .......................... 212
**CTOPP** (pacing) ............. 233

**CTSN** (functional mitral regurgitation) .................. 123

**CTSN AF** (Maze during mitral surgery) .........151, 215

**CURE** (Clopidogrel) ......86, 96

**CURRENT-OASIS** (ASA / Clopidogrel) ........ 86

**Dal-OUTCOMES** (Dalcetrapib) .................... 322

**DANISH** (pacing) ............. 233

**DANPACE** (pacing) ......... 233

**DAPT** (dual antiplatelet therapy) .......................... 106

**DAVID** (pacing) ......233, 240

**DCCT** (glycemic control) . 330

**DECREASE-V** (preop revascularization)............. 312

**DEFINITE** (ICD) .............. 241

**DIAMOND** (Dofetilide) ..... 231

**DIG** (Digoxin) ................. 120

**DIGAMI** (glycemic control) 97

**DINAMIT** (ICD) ............... 241

**DOSE** (diuretics) ............ 129

**DREAM** (abdo Ao aneurysm treatment)...................... 283

**DREAM** (thiazolidinediones) ......... 330

**EAFT** (Warfarin in stroke) 294

**EARLY-ACS** (GPIIb/IIIa inhibitors) ......................... 87

**EAST** (CABG / PCI) ........... 79

**ECASS-3** (thrombolysis in stroke) ............................ 292

**ECSS** (CABG) .................. 79

**ECST** (carotid revascularization) ............. 294

**Eikelboom** (Heparin) ........ 87

**EINSTEIN** (Rivaroxaban in VTE) ........................... 299

**EMBRACE** (Subclinical AF) ............... 291

**EMERAS** (thrombolysis).... 94

**EMPA-REG** (Empagliflozin) ................ 332

**EMPHASIS-HF** (Eplerenone) .................... 118

**EPHESUS** (Eplerenone) ...............96, 118

**ERICA** (Ranolazine).......... 77

**ESCAPE** (Stroke - Revascularization)............. 293

**ESPRIT** (antiplatelet therapy in stroke)............. 294

**ESPS-2** (antiplatelet therapy in stroke)............. 294

**EUROPA** (ACE inhibitors - Perindopril) ..........76, 96, 332

**EVAR** (abdo Ao aneurysm treatment)...................... 283

**EVEREST** (Mitraclip) ...... 154

**EVEREST** (Tolvaptan)...... 119

**EXAMINE** (DDP-4 inhibitor) ......................... 331

**EXTRACT-TIMI 25** (Enoxaparin) ...................... 95

**FAIR-HF** (anemia) .......... 123

**FAME** (FFR).............52, 104

**FAME-2** (FFR)................. 52

**FREEDOM** (CABG / PCI)................79, 333

**Freemantle** (BB) ............. 96

**FRISC-II** (early invasive strategy) ............................ 86

**GISSI** (thrombolysis) ........ 93

**GISSI-HF** (omega-3 or statins in HF) .......121, 322

**GOPCABE** (beating heart surgery) .......................... 107

**Haïssaguerre** (AF)......... 214

**HEARMATE II** (LVAD) ...... 135

**HEAT-PPCI** (Bivalirudin)... 94

**HF-ACTION** (exercise)..................121, 334

**HOPE** (ACE inhibitors - Ramipril) ......76, 96, 287, 332

**HORIZONS-AMI** (Bivalirudin) ...................... 94

**HPS** (statins) ...........322, 332

**HPS2-THRIVE** (Niacin) .............321, 322

**Hypothermia after cardiac arrest** ............. 350

**HYVET** (HTN in the elderly) ............................ 327

**IABP-SHOCK** (IABP) ........ 99

**ICAP** (Colchicine)............ 174

**ICTUS** (ischemia-guided strategy) ............................ 86

**IDEAL** (statins)................ 322

**INITIATIVE** (Ivabradine)..... 77

**IONA** (Nicorandil) ............. 77

**I-PRESERVE** (ARB - Irbesartan) ...................... 124

**IRIS** (ICD) ...................... 241

**ISAR-SAFE** (double antiplatelet therapy)........ 106

**ISCHEMIA** (revascularization)............ 123

**ISIS-1** (beta-blockers) ...... 95

**ISIS-2** (thrombolysis) ..93, 95

**ISSUE-3** (PPM in vasovagal syncope) .......... 228

**JUPITER** (statins) ...318, 322

**LATE** (thrombolysis).......... 94

**LIPID** (statins) ................ 322

**Lyon Diet Heart Study** (Mediterranean diet) ........ 338

**MADIT-I** (ICD) ........241, 242

**MADIT-II** (ICD).121, 241, 242

**MADIT-CRT** (CRT) ......122, 239, 240

**MADIT-RIT** (ICD - programming) .................... 242

**MATCH** (antiplatelet therapy in stroke) ............ 294

**MATRIX** (Bivalirudin)....87, 94

**MERIT-HF** (Metoprolol) ... 118

**MELODY-1** (Macitentan) . 306

**MERLIN-TIMI 36** (Ranolazine) ....................... 77

**MIAMI** (beta-blockers) ...... 95

**MOST** (pacing) ............... 233

**MR CLEAN** (Stroke - Revascularization)............ 293

**MUSTT** (ICD) ..........241, 242

**NAPLES II** (statins) ......... 106

**NASCET** (carotid stenosis) .......................... 294

**NORDIC-BALTIC** (bifurcation) ...................... 105

**NICE-SUGAR** (glycemic control) ............................. 97

**NINDS rtPA Stroke Study** (thrombolysis in stroke).... 292

**NEAT-HFpEF** (Nitrates in HFpEF) .......... 124

**OASIS 5 and 6** (Fondaparinux).............87, 95

**ODYSSEY long term** (Alirocumab) .................... 322

**ONTARGET** (Telmisartan)................... 332

**OPTIC** (Amiodarone) ....... 221
**OPTIME-HF** (Milrinone)... 128
**OSLER** (Evolocumab)...... 322
**PABA-CHF**
(AF).................122, 211, 215
**PAIN FREE RX II** (ATP) ... 242
**PALLAS**
(Dronedarone)..........212, 231
**PARADIGM-HF** (Neprilysin
inhibition).......................... 121
**PARTNER** (TAVI) ........... 144
**PATENT** (Riociguat
in PAH) .............................. 305
**PC** (patent foramen
ovale) ................................. 250
**PEGASUS** (Ticagrelor
post MI) ........................86, 96
**PEITHO** (pulmonary
embolism).......................... 298
**PEP-CHF** (ACE inhibitors -
Perindopril) ...................... 124
**PLATO**
(Ticagrelor) ...........86, 94, 96
**POISE** (periop
beta-blockers) ................. 312
**Primary Pulmonary
Hypertension Study**
(Epoprostenol)................. 305
**PREDIMED** (Mediterranean
diet).................................... 338
**PROFESS** (antiplatelet
therapy in stroke) .......... 294
**PROMISE** (CCTA vs.
Functionnal testing
in CAD) ............................... 65
**PROTECT AF** (LAA
occlusion)................218, 294
**PROVE IT** (statins) .....96, 322
**RACE-II** (AF).................. 211
**RAFT** (CRT)......122, 239, 240
**RALES** (Spironolactone).. 118
**REACT** (rescue PCI) ....... 95
**RED-HF** (anemia in heart
failure).............................. 123
**RELY** (Dabigatran in AF).. 217
**REMATCH** (LVAD)......... 135
**REMEDY** (Dabigatran
in VTE) ............................... 299
**RESONATE** (Dabigatran
in VTE) ............................... 299
**RESPECT** (patent
foramen ovale)................. 250

**RE-VERSE**
(Idarucizumab)................. 217
**RITA-3** (early invasive
strategy) ............................. 86
**ROCKET-AF** (Rivaroxaban
in AF) .................................. 217
**ROMICAT-II** (coronary CT
angiography)........................ 66
**ROOBY** (beating heart
surgery) ............................. 107
**ROSE AHF** (Nesiritide).. 128
**SAPPHIRE**
(revascularization in
carotid stenosis) ............ 294
**SAVE** (ACE inhibitors -
Captopril)....................96, 118
**SAVOR** (DPP-4 inhibitor) . 331
**SCD-HEFT**
(ICD) ..............121, 241, 242
**SEARCH** (statins).......... 322
**SENIORS** (Nebivolol)...... 118
**SERVE-HF** (servo-ventilation
in HF)................................. 123
**SHARP** (Statin and
Ezetimibe in CRF)........... 318
**SHIFT** (Ivabradine) ....... 120
**SHOCK** (cardiogenic
shock) ..........................98, 99
**SIGNIFY** (Ivabradine) ...... 77
**Sil-HF** (PDE-5 inhibitors
in heart failure)............... 306
**SOAP-II** (Dopamine) ...... 128
**SOLVD** (Enalapril)......... 118
**SOS** (CABG / PCI) .......... 79
**SPAF 1, 2 and 3**
(Warfarin)......................... 216
**SPARCL** (statins and
stroke).......................294, 322
**SPINAF** (Warfarin) ........ 216
**SPRINT** (HTN target)...... 326
**STAR-AF** (persistent AF)...214
**STICH** (revascularization)...123
**STREAM**
(thrombolysis) .............92, 93
**SURVIVE**
(Levosimendan) ............... 128
**SWORD** (post-myocardial
infarction PVCs) ......102, 231
**Symplicity-HTN-3** (renal
denervation) ..................... 329
**SYNERGY** (LMWH) ......... 87
**SYNTAX** (CABG / PCI)........ 79

**TACTICS** (early invasive
strategy) ............................. 86
**TASTE** (thrombectomy)... 104
**TECOS** (Sitagliptin) ........ 331
**TNT** (statins) ................. 322
**TOPCAT** (Spironolactone) 124
**TOTAL** (Manual
thrombectomy) ................ 104
**TRACE** (ACE inhibitors -
Trandolapril)..............96, 118
**TRANSCEND**
(Telmisartan)..................... 332
**TRANSFER-AMI** (pharmaco-
invasive strategy)............. 95
**TRENDS** (AF detected
by pacemaker) ................. 219
**TRIMPOL II**
(Trimetazidine) .................. 77
**TRITON-TIMI 38**
(Prasugrel)...................94, 96
**TRYTON** (bifurcation) ...... 105
**TTM** (hypothermia after
cardiac arrest) ................. 350
**UKPDS** (glycemic
control)......................330, 331
**UNLOAD** (ultrafiltration) ... 120
**VA Cooperative** (CABG) .... 79
**VACS** (carotid stenosis)... 294
**VADT** (glycemic control)... 329
**VALIANT** (ARB -
Valsartan)...................96, 120
**V-HEFT** (Hydralazine -
Nitrate) .............................. 121
**VPS-II** (neurocardiogenic
syncope)....................228, 235
**WARCEF** (Warfarin)........ 123
**WARFASA** (ASA in venous
thromboembolism).......... 299
**WOSCOPS** (statins) ........ 321
**WOEST** (dual antiplatelet
therapy)............................. 218
**Yusuf** (CABG) .................. 79

# Index

AAI .................................................. 235
ABCD2 score ................................... 291
Abciximab
    STEMI ......................................... 94
Abdominal aortic aneurysm ................ 282
    EVAR ......................................... 283
    Management ............................... 283
    Surgery ..................................... 283
Aberrant conduction ..................... 12, 220
Abnormal automaticity ...................... 200
ABPM .............................................. 323
Accelerated idioventricular rhythm ...... 221
    Accessory pathway ..................... 208
    Electrocardiogram ...................... 208
    Localization ................................. 15
Acetylsalicylic acid
    Acute coronary syndrome ............. 96
    CAD ............................................ 76
    Diabetes ................................... 332
    Peripheral vascular disease ........ 287
    Primary prevention ..................... 314
    Secondary prevention ................. 315
    STEMI ......................................... 94
    Stroke ....................................... 293
    Unstable angina and NSTEMI ....... 86
Acromegaly ...................................... 342
Action potential ................................ 200
Acute aortic syndrome ....................... 279
Acute coronary syndrome
    Anticoagulation ........................... 87
    Antiplatelet therapy ..................... 86
    Arrhythmias and blocks .............. 102
    Early invasive strategy .......... 86, 88
    Management ........................... 85, 88
    Risk ........................................... 84
    STEMI ......................................... 88
    Unstable angina and NSTEMI ....... 83
Acute ischemia of lower limbs ............. 288
Adenosine ........................................ 232
    Cardiopulmonary resuscitation .... 349
    Vasoreactivity test ..................... 303
Adrenaline
    Cardiopulmonary
    resuscitation ....................... 347, 349
    Heart failure ............................. 129
Afterdepolarization
    Early ........................................ 200
    Delayed .................................... 200
Agatston score ............................ 65, 75
AH interval ...................................... 203
Air travel ......................................... 341
ALCAPA syndrome ............................ 268
Alcoholic cardiomyopathy ................... 184
Aldosterone antagonists
    Heart failure ................ 117, 118, 119

Alpha-blocking agents
    Hypertension ............................. 327
Alpha-glucosidase inhibitors
    Diabetes ................................... 331
Ambrisentan
    Pulmonary hypertension ............. 305
Ambulant blood pressure monitor ........ 323
Amiodarone ..................................... 231
    Adverse effects .......................... 232
    Atrial fibrillation ......................... 212
    Cardiopulmonary
    resuscitation ....................... 347, 349
    Drug interactions ....................... 233
    Follow-up .................................. 233
    Gastrointestinal toxicity .............. 232
    Pulmonary toxicity ..................... 232
    Thyroid toxicity ......................... 232
Amlodipine
    CAD ........................................... 77
    Hypertension ............................. 326
    Pulmonary hypertension ............. 305
Anaphylaxis ....................................... 53
Anemia
    Heart failure ............................. 123
    Post-myocardial infarction ............ 97
Anginal equivalent ............................... 72
Angiosarcoma .................................. 195
Angiotensin receptor antagonists
    Acute coronary syndrome ............. 96
    Diabetes ................................... 332
    Heart failure ....................... 117, 120
    Hypertension ............................. 326
Angiotensin-converting enzyme inhibitors
    Acute coronary syndrome ............. 96
    Coronary artery disease ............... 76
    Diabetes ................................... 332
    Heart failure ....................... 117, 118
    Hypertension ............................. 326
Ankle-brachial index ......................... 286
Ankylosing spondylitis ....................... 285
Anomalous pulmonary venous
connection ....................................... 268
Anthracycline cardiotoxicity ............... 196
Antianginal agents .............................. 76
Antiarrhythmics ................................ 229
Anticoagulation ..................................
    Bleeding risk ............................. 216
    Heart failure ............................. 123
    Noncardiac surgery ................... 313
    Post-myocardial infarction ............ 96
    Pregnancy ................................ 272
    Prosthetic valve ......................... 159
    Pulmonary embolism ................. 298
    STEMI ......................................... 94
    Stroke ....................................... 294
    Unstable angina and NSTEMI ....... 87
Antiphospholipid syndrome ................. 342

**Antiplatelet therapy.** See Acetylsalicylic acid

STEMI .................................................. 94
Unstable angina and NSTEMI......... 86

**Antitachycardia pacing** ........................... 242

**Aortic arch aneurysm** ............................. 277
Management .................................... 278

**Aortic atherosclerotic plaque**................ 283
Complex plaque ............................... 283
Embolism ......................................... 283

**Aortic dissection** .................................... 279
Chest x-ray ...................................... 281
Classification ................................... 279
Clinical features .............................. 280
Complications .................................. 280
Echocardiography............................ 280
False lumen ..................................... 280
Follow-up.......................................... 282
Management..................................... 281
Presentation .................................... 280
Risk factors...................................... 280

**Aortic regurgitation** ............................... 145
Acute aortic regurgitation .............. 148
Angiographic assessment .............. 59
Auscultation.................................... 146
Echocardiography............................. 37
Etiologies ........................................ 145
Hemodynamic consequences........ 145
Management..................................... 148
Peripheral signs .............................. 147
Pregnancy........................................ 272
Prognosis......................................... 147
Severity............................................ 146
Signs and symptoms...................... 146
Surgical indication.......................... 148

**Aortic root** ............................................. 276

**Aortic sclerosis** ..................................... 140

**Aortic stenosis** ...................................... 140
Aortic pseudostenosis .................... 143
Auscultation.................................... 141
Bicuspid aortic valve ...................... 140
Cardiac catheterization .................... 59
Degenerative................................... 140
Echocardiography............................. 35
Hemodynamic consequences........ 140
Investigations.................................. 142
Low flow, low gradient ................... 143
Management..................................... 143
Noncardiac surgery ........................ 312
Percutaneous balloon
valvuloplasty ................................... 143
Pregnancy........................................ 271
Prognosis......................................... 142
Severity............................................ 141
Signs and symptoms...................... 141
Subvalvular ..................................... 254
Supravalvular .................................. 253
Surgical indications........................ 143
TAVI.................................................. 144

**Apex, physical examination** ...................... 4

**Apical impulse** ........................................... 4

**Apixaban**
Atrial fibrillation.............................. 217
Pulmonary embolism....................... 299

**Apnea-hypopnea index** ........................... 339

**ApoA1** ..................................................... 316

**ApoB** ....................................................... 316

**Arcus senilis** .......................................... 317

**Arrhythmia, mechanisms** ....................... 200

**Arrhythmogenic right ventricular dysplasia** ................................................. 188
Biopsy.............................................. 189
Cardiac MRI .................................... 189
Diagnosis......................................... 189
Differential diagnosis..................... 190
Echocardiography............................ 189
Electrocardiogram ........................... 189
Genetic testing ............................... 226
Management..................................... 190

**Arterial switch** ....................................... 260
Complications .................................. 260
Indications for surgery.................... 260

**ARVD.** See Arrhythmogenic right ventricular dysplasia

**Ascending aortic aneurysm** ................... 276
Familial ............................................ 284
Indications for surgery.................... 277
Management..................................... 277
Risk factors ..................................... 276
Surveillance .................................... 277

**Ashman phenomenon**.............................. 13

**Asystole**
Cardiopulmonary resuscitation ..... 347

**Atheroembolism** ............................... 53, 283

**Atherosclerosis of the arms** .................. 288

**Atherosclerotic coronary disease.** See Stable angina

**Atherosclerotic renovascular disease** .... 289
Management..................................... 289

**Athlete's heart** ....................................... 181

**Atrial appendages** .................................. 248

**Atrial fibrillation**.................................... 210
CCS SAF scale................................ 210
CHA2DS2-VASc .............................. 216
CHADS2 ........................................... 215
Chemical cardioversion .................. 213
Classification................................... 210
Rate control........................... 211, 212
Rhythm control..................... 211, 212
Coronary disease............................. 218
Digoxin............................................. 212
Electrical cardioversion ................. 213
Electrocardiogram ........................... 210
HAS-BLED ....................................... 216
Heart failure.................................... 122
Management..................................... 211
Noncardiac surgery ........................ 313

Occlusion of left atrial
appendage ......................................218
Paroxysmal ........................................214
Persistent ..........................................214
Post-cardiac surgery ........................107
Pre-excited ..............................219, 348
Pregnancy .........................................273
Pulmonary vein isolation...................214
Reversible cause ...............................211
Stroke ...............................................294
Subclinical .........................................219
Surgical ablation ...............................215
Thromboembolic prevention...............215
**Atrial flutter**...........................................206
Atypical .............................................206
Electrocardiogram .............................206
Management ......................................206
Typical ...............................................206
**Atrial premature complex** ....................204
Blocked..............................................204
Noncompensatory pause....................204
**Atrial septal aneurysm** ........................250
**Atrial septal defect** ..............................248
Chest x-ray .......................................249
Clinical features ................................249
Complications ....................................249
Coronary sinus ASD ..........................248
Echocardiography...............................249
Electrocardiogram .............................249
Indications for closure .......................249
Percutaneous closure ........................250
Pregnancy .........................................250
Primum ASD.......................................248
Secundum ASD...................................248
Sinus venosus ASD............................248
**Atrial septostomy**
Severe pulmonary hypertension ...306
**Atrial situs**............................................248
**Atrial switch**..........................................259
**Atrial waves**
A wave .................................................56
C wave .................................................56
V wave .................................................56
X descent .............................................56
Y descent .............................................56
**Atrioventricular canal defect** ..............251
Complete............................................251
Complications ....................................252
Electrocardiogram .............................251
Indications for repair .........................252
Partial ................................................251
**Atrioventricular nodal reentrant**
**tachycardia** ...........................................207
Atypical .............................................207
Electrocardiogram .............................207
Management ......................................208
Typical ...............................................207
**Atrioventricular reentrant**
**tachycardia** ...........................................208

Antidromic.........................................209
Electrocardiogram .............................209
Management ......................................209
Orthodromic ......................................209
**Atropine**................................................232
Cardiopulmonary resuscitation ...348
**Auscultation** .........................................
Heart sounds .........................................4
Murmurs ................................................6
Dynamic auscultation ...........................8
**Austin-Flint murmur** ......................7, 146
**AV block** ...............................................202
2:1 .....................................................202
Complete............................................203
First degree .......................................202
High-grade .........................................202
Mobitz I .............................................202
Mobitz II ............................................202
Pacemaker .........................................234
Post-myocardial infarction..................102
Variable conduction ............................11
**AV conduction** ...........................11, 203
**AV dissociation** ......................................11
**AV fistula**
Post-coronary angiography ........53
**AV node disease** .................................202
Pacemaker .........................................234
**AVNRT. See Atrioventricular nodal**
**reentrant tachycardia**
**AVRT. See Atrioventricular reentrant**
**tachycardia**
**Axis deviation** .......................................12
**Azathioprine**
Heart transplantation...................132

## B

**Bachmann's bundle** ...............................11
**Balloon mitral valvuloplasty**...............150
**Bariatric surgery**.................................337
**Bayes' theorem** .....................................73
**Bazett's equation** .................................18
**Beck's triad** .........................................174
**Becker muscular dystrophy** ................342
**Behçet's disease** .................................285
**Bentall procedure** ...............................263
**Beta-blockers** ......................................230
Acute coronary syndrome ........95, 96
Adverse effects ...................................78
Antianginal .................................76, 78
Cardiopulmonary resuscitation .....349
Heart failure .....................................117
Hypertension .....................................327
Intrinsic sympathetic activity .........77
Perioperative ....................................312
Poisoning ..........................................344
Types ...................................................77
**Bezold-Jarish reflex** ...........................102

**Bicuspid aortic valve** .................................. 140
**Bidirectional Glenn** ................................... 265
**Bifascicular block** ........................... 14, 202
     Pacemaker .................................... 234
**Bile acid absorption inhibitors** .............. 321
**Biomarkers** ................................................ 80
**Bioprosthesis** ........................................ 158
**Bivalirudin**
     STEMI ............................................. 94
     Unstable angina and NSTEMI ........ 87
**Biventricular hypertrophy** ........................ 17
**Blalock-Taussig shunt** ............................ 267
**Blood pressure** ......................................... 2
     Measurement ................................ 324
**Blue toe** ................................................ 283
**BMI** ....................................................... 336
**BNP** ....................................................... 114
**Body surface area** ...................................... 3
**Borg scale** .............................. 66, 336
**Bosentan**
     Pulmonary hypertension ............... 305
**Bradyarrhythmias** .................................. 201
**Bradycardia**
     Cardiopulmonary resuscitation ..... 348
**Brockenbrough-Braunwald-Morrow**
**sign** ....................................................... 182
**Bruce protocol** .......................................... 23
**Brugada pattern** ..................................... 225
**Brugada syndrome** ................................. 225
     Electrocardiogram ........................ 225
     Genetic testing ............................. 226
**B-type natriuretic peptide** ...................... 114
**Bundle branch block. See Left (or Right)**
**bundle branch block**
**Bundle branch reentry tachycardia** ........ 221
**Bupropion**
     Smoking cessation ........................ 315
**Burn** ....................................................... 343
**Burst** ..................................................... 242
**BVR score** .............................. 35, 150

## C

**Cabrera's sign** ............................................ 13
**Calcineurin inhibitors**
     Heart transplantation .................... 132
**Calcium channel blockers** ...................... 231
     Adverse effects .............................. 78
     Antianginal .................................... 77
     Dihydropyridines ............. 77, 78, 326
     Hypertension ............................... 326
     Nondihydropyridine ......... 77, 78, 326
     Poisoning .................................... 345
     Pulmonary hypertension ............... 305
**Cancer, cardiac complications** ............... 196
**Capture failure** ...................................... 238
**Car. See Driving**
**Carabello's sign** ........................................ 59

**Carcinoid syndrome** ............................... 186
**Cardiac amyloidosis** ............................... 187
     Cardiac MRI ................................. 187
     Clinical features .......................... 187
     Diagnosis .................................... 187
     Echocardiography ......................... 187
     Electrocardiogram ........................ 187
     Familial amyloidosis ..................... 188
     Management ................................ 188
     Primary amyloidosis ..................... 187
     Senile amyloidosis ....................... 188
**Cardiac catheterization.**
**See Hemodynamic assessment**
**Cardiac computed tomography,**
**Cardiac CT** ................................................ 65
**Cardiac index** ..................................... 54, 66
**Cardiac lymphoma** ................................. 196
**Cardiac mass**
     Echocardiography ........................... 39
**Cardiac metastasis** ................................ 194
**Cardiac MRI** ............................. 63, 64, 65
     Arrhythmogenic right ventricular
     dysplasia .................................... 189
     Cardiac amyloidosis ..................... 187
     Hypertrophic cardiomyopathy. ...... 182
     Indications .................................... 65
     Late gadolinium enhancement ....... 64
     Myocarditis .................................. 192
     Precautions .................................... 63
     Sarcoidosis ................................. 186
**Cardiac output**
     Angiographic .................................. 55
     Echocardiographic .......................... 29
     Fick ............................................... 55
     Normal values ............................... 54
     Thermodilution .............................. 55
**Cardiac resynchronization therapy** ........ 239
     Electrocardiogram ........................ 241
     Evidence ..................................... 239
     Heart failure ................................ 122
     Indications .................................. 240
     Programming ............................... 240
**Cardiac surgery. See Coronary artery**
**bypass graft**
**Cardiac tumor** ........................................ 194
     Malignant .................................... 195
     Metastasis ................................... 194
     Primary ....................................... 194
**Cardioembolism** ..................................... 291
**Cardiogenic shock** ........................... 98, 125
     Management .................................. 99
**Cardiomyopathies, classification** ........... 179
**Cardioprotection** ...................................... 76
**Cardiopulmonary arrest** ......................... 347
**Cardiopulmonary resuscitation** ............. 347
     Neurological assessment ............. 350
     Post-cardiac arrest management. 350
     Therapeutic hypothermia ............. 350
**Cardiopulmonary exercise testing** ......... 66

Cardiorenal syndrome ............................ 130
Cardiothoracic index .............................. 47
Cardiovascular implantable electronic
device infection ...................................... 167
Cardiovascular syndrome X .................. 108
Cardioversion
    Atrial fibrillation ............................ 213
    Tachycardia ................................... 348
Carey-Coombs murmur ...................... 7, 168
Carney complex ...................................... 194
Carotid angioplasty ............................... 294
Carotid artery stenosis,
revascularization ................................... 294
Carotid endarterectomy ........................ 294
Carotid pulse ..................................... 3, 58
Carotid revascularization ..................... 294
Carotid sinus hypersensitivity ............. 229
    Pacemaker .................................... 235
Carotid sinus massage .................... 3, 229
Carotids
    Physical examination ................. 3, 58
    Revascularization ......................... 294
Carpenter classification ....................... 152
CARPREG score ..................................... 270
Catecholaminergic polymorphic
ventricular tachycardia ......................... 225
    Genetic testing ............................. 226
Cavotricuspid isthmus .......................... 206
Central alpha-adrenergic agonists
    Hypertension ................................ 327
Central sleep apnea syndrome
    Heart failure ................................. 123
Central venous pressure ........................... 3
Cerebrovascular disease ...................... 290
    Etiologies ..................................... 290
    Intracranial hemorrhage .............. 295
    Ischemic stroke ........................... 291
    Transient ischemic attack ............ 290
CHA2DS2-VASc score ............................ 216
CHADS2 score ....................................... 215
Chagas disease ...................................... 184
Chagas cardiomyopathy ........................ 184
Channelopathies .................................... 224
    Genetic testing ............................. 226
Chapman's sign ........................................ 13
Chemical cardioversion ........................ 213
Chemotherapy, cardiotoxicity ............... 196
Chest pain. See Retrosternal chest pain
Chest x-ray .............................................. 45
    Aortic dissection .......................... 281
    Cardiothoracic index ...................... 47
    Dilatation of heart chambers ......... 47
    Heart failure ................................. 114
    Pulmonary vascularization ............. 47
Cheyne-Stokes respiration .................... 123
Cholesterol absorption inhibitor .......... 320
Cholesterol crystals .............................. 283

Chronic obstructive pulmonary disease
    Electrocardiogram .......................... 20
Chronic renal failure ..................... 333, 343
Chronic total occlusion ........................ 104
Chronotropic incompetence .......... 26, 201
    Pacemaker .................................... 233
Churg and Strauss syndrome ................ 342
Chylomicrons .......................................... 316
Cilostazol
    Peripheral vascular disease .......... 287
CK-MB ........................................................ 81
Clopidogrel
    Acute coronary syndrome .............. 96
    Atrial fibrillation ............................ 216
    STEMI ............................................. 94
    Unstable Angina and NSTEMI ........ 86
Coarctation of the aorta ....................... 254
    Chest x-ray ................................... 254
    Clinical features ........................... 254
    Complications ............................... 255
    Diagnosis ..................................... 254
    Echocardiography ......................... 254
    Indications for repair .................... 255
    Management ................................. 255
    Percutaneous repair ..................... 255
    Pregnancy .................................... 255
    Surgical repair ............................. 255
Cocaine .................................................. 344
    Myocardial infarction ................... 344
Commotio cordis .................................... 343
Compensatory pause .............................. 204
Concertina effect ..................................... 14
Concordance, precordial ........................ 220
Conduction tissue
    Blood supply ................................ 103
    Electrophysiological study ............ 203
Congenital coronary artery anomalies ... 268
Congenitally corrected transposition
of the great arteries .............................. 261
    Complications ............................... 261
    Indications for surgery ................. 261
Connective tissue diseases ................... 342
Constrictive pericarditis ....................... 177
    Cardiac catheterization ................. 178
    Clinical features ........................... 177
    Echocardiography ......................... 177
    Etiologies ..................................... 177
    Management ................................. 178
    Pathophysiology ........................... 178
    Versus restrictive cardiomyopathy 185
    Versus tamponade ....................... 175
Contraception ........................................ 273
Contrast nephropathy .............................. 53
Cor triatriatum ...................................... 270
Cornell protocol ...................................... 23
Cornell voltage ........................................ 16
Coronary anatomy ............................ 49, 50
    Dominance ..................................... 49

Ectopic origin of coronary artery.... 268
**Coronary aneurysm** ........................ 341, 342
**Coronary angiography** ......................... 48
    Angiographic views ................ 49, 50
    Atheroembolism ......................... 53
    Cardiac allograft vasculopathy...... 133
    Complications ............................ 52
    Contrast nephropathy .................. 53
    Coronary anatomy ................. 49, 50
    Coronary artery stenosis .............. 51
    FFR ......................................... 52
    IVUS ........................................ 52
    Preparation ............................... 48
    Pretest probability ...................... 73
    Vascular access ........................ 48
    Vein graft ................................. 49
**Coronary arteriovenous fistula** .......... 269
**Coronary arteritis** .............................. 82
**Coronary artery bypass graft** ............ 106
    Arterial graft ............................ 107
    Beating heart ........................... 107
    Benefits .................................... 79
    Complications .......................... 107
    EuroSCORE............................. 106
    Minimally invasive surgery .......... 107
    Perioperative risk ..................... 106
    STS score................................ 106
    SYNTAX score .......................... 79
    Vein graft ................................ 107
**Coronary artery stenosis** .................... 51
    Bifurcation .............................. 105
    Characteristics .......................... 51
    Chronic total occlusion .............. 104
    Coronary reserve ....................... 62
    FFR .................................. 52, 104
    Ischemic cascade ...................... 73
    IVUS ................................. 52, 104
    Noninvasive stratification ............ 73
    Pretest probability ...................... 73
    Prognosis ................................. 79
    Revascularization ......... 79, 103, 106
    Severity .............................. 51, 103
    TIMI flow ................................. 51
**Coronary atherosclerosis. See Coronary
artery stenosis**
**Coronary balloon angioplasty** ............. 103
**Coronary blood flow** ........................... 52
**Coronary dominance** .......................... 49
**Coronary embolism** ............................ 82
**Coronary perfusion** ............................ 61
**Coronary reserve** ............................... 62
**Coronary revascularization**
    Acute coronary syndrome ............ 86
    Bypass graft........................ 79, 106
    Diabetes.................................. 333
    Indications ............................... 78
    Left main coronary artery ............. 79
    Objectives ................................ 78

    Percutaneous coronary
    intervention......................... 79, 103
    Preoperative ............................ 312
    Primary PCI .............................. 94
    SYNTAX score .......................... 79
**Coronary thromboaspiration** ............... 104
**Coronary thrombosis**........................... 83
**Coronary vasospasm** ......................... 108
**Corrigan's pulse** ........................ 58, 147
**Corticosteroids**
    Heart transplantation................. 132
**Cox-Maze procedure** ......................... 215
**Critical leg ischemia** ......................... 288
**Crosstalk** ........................................ 238
**CT coronary angiography** ..................... 65
    Prognosis ................................. 75
**Cushing syndrome** ..................... 325, 342
**Cyanotic heart disease** ...................... 267
    Pregnancy ............................... 272
**Cyclosporine**
    Heart transplantation................. 132

## D

**Dabigatran**
    Atrial fibrillation....................... 217
    Pulmonary embolism................... 299
**Dallas criteria** ................................. 191
**David procedure** .............................. 263
**Davies disease** ................................ 186
**DDD** ............................................. 235
**D-Dimers** ....................................... 295
**DeBakey classification** ...................... 279
**Decompensated heart failure**............... 125
    Hemodynamic targets ................ 129
    Management............................ 126
    Precipitating factors .................. 126
    Scenarios................................ 125
**Deep vein thrombosis**........................ 296
    Anticoagulation ........................ 299
    Local catheter thrombolysis......... 299
    Noncardiac surgery ................... 313
    Post-thrombotic syndrome .......... 299
    Thromboprophylaxis................... 299
    Upper limb .............................. 299
**Defibrillation** ................................... 347
**Defibrillator shock** ............................ 243
**Delta wave** ................................ 14, 208
**Descending thoracic aorta aneurysm**.... 278
**Dextrocardia** ................................... 248
    Electrocardiogram ...................... 20
**Dextro-transposition of the great
vessels. See Transposition of
the great arteries**
**Diabetes** ........................................ 329
    Abnormal fasting blood glucose.... 330
    Antiplatelet therapy ................... 332
    Cardiovascular risk..................... 332

Diabetic nephropathy .................. 333
Diagnosis ............................. 330
Drug treatment ....................... 330
Glucose intolerance .................. 330
Glycemic control ..................... 330
Hypoglycemia ........................ 333
Insulin therapy ...................... 330
Macrovascular complications ........ 330
Microalbuminuria .................... 333
Microvascular complications ........ 330
Nondrug treatment ................... 330
Post-myocardial infarction
glycemic control ..................... 97
Revascularization ................... 333
Screening ............................ 330
Statins .............................. 332
Targets .............................. 330
**Diabetic nephropathy** ................... 333
**Diastolic function** ................... 32, 124
**Diastolic heart failure** ................. 123
Management .......................... 124
**Dicrotic pulse** ......................... 58
**Dicrotic wave** ......................... 57
**Diet** .................................. 337
Targets .............................. 338
**Differential cyanosis** .................. 252
**Differential pressure** ............... 2, 57
**DiGeorge syndrome** .................... 258
**Digibind** .............................. 346
**Digoxin** .............................. 232
Antidote ............................. 346
Heart failure .................... 117, 120
Poisoning ............................ 345
**Digoxin glycoside impregnation** ....... 21, 345
**Digoxin toxicity** ....................... 345
Electrocardiogram ..................... 21
**Dilated cardiomyopathy** ................ 184
Cardiac MRI .......................... 64
Complications ....................... 184
Echocardiography..................... 184
Electrocardiogram ................... 184
Genetic testing ...................... 226
Pregnancy ........................... 272
**Diltiazem** ............................. 231
Adverse effects ...................... 78
Antianginal .......................... 78
Atrial fibrillation ................... 212
Cardiopulmonary resuscitation ..... 349
Hypertension ........................ 326
Pulmonary hypertension .............. 305
**Direct oral anticoagulants** ............ 217
Bleeding ............................ 217
Pulmonary embolism.................. 299
Switch ............................... 218
Surgery .............................. 218
**Direct renin inhibitor** ................. 326
**Disopyramide** ......................... 229

**Diuretics**
Decompensated heart failure........ 129
Heart failure .................... 118, 119
Hypertension ........................ 327
Resistance ........................... 120
**Dobutamine**
Cardiopulmonary resuscitation ..... 350
Heart failure ........................ 128
**Dobutamine echocardiography. See
Stress echocardiography**
**Dofetilide** ............................ 231
Atrial fibrillation ................... 212
**Dopamine**
Cardiopulmonary resuscitation ..... 350
Heart failure ........................ 128
**Double chamber right ventricle** ....... 256
**Double product** ........................ 26
**Down syndrome** ........................ 251
**Doxorubicin cardiotoxicity** ............ 196
**DPP-4 inhibitors** ...................... 331
**Dressler syndrome** ................ 101, 173
**Driving** ............................... 339
**Dronedarone** .......................... 231
Atrial fibrillation ................... 212
**Duchenne dystrophy** ................... 342
**Ductus arteriosus** ..................... 248
**Ductus venosus** ....................... 248
**Duke criteria** ......................... 162
**Duke treadmill score** ................... 26
**Duroziez sign** ......................... 147
**Dysautonomia** ........................ 228
**Dyslipidemia** ......................... 316
Genetic disorders .................... 317
Management .......................... 318

Nondrug treatment ................... 321
Screening ............................ 317
Secondary causes .................... 317

**E**

**Early repolarization** ................. 17, 89
**Ebstein anomaly** ...................... 262
Clinical features .................... 262
Complications ....................... 262
Indications for repair .............. 262
Pregnancy ........................... 263
Repair ............................... 263
**ECMO** ................................. 130
**Ectopic origin of coronary artery** ..... 268
**Ehlers-Danlos syndrome** ............... 284
**Eisenmenger syndrome** ................. 266
Clinical features .................... 266
Complications ....................... 266
Heart transplantation ............... 267
Management........................... 267
Pulmonary hypertension.............. 306

**Ejection click**
Valvular ...................................................5
Vascular ..................................................5
**Electrical alternans** ..................................16
**Electrical storm** .......................................223
**Electrocardiogram** .......................................8
Chamber hypertrophy.....................16
Clinical entities............................20
Frontal axis..................................12
Intraventricular conduction...........12
Ischemia .............................19, 84
Lead inversion.............................10
Myocardial
infarction..............19, 84, 88, 90, 91
Normal values ...............................9
P wave.........................................11
Pericarditis.................................173
Precordial transition .....................15
Q wave........................................19
Repolarization .............................17
**Electrocution**...........................................343
**Electromagnetic interference**................238
**Electrophysiological study** ...................203
Programmed ventricular
stimulation .................................228
Syncope...........................227, 228
**Elephant trunk procedure** ......................278
**Emery-Dreifuss dystrophy** .....................343
**Endoleak** ................................................278
**Endomyocardial biopsy**
Complications .............................193
Indications .................................193
**Endomyocardial fibrosis**.........................186
**Endothelial dysfunction** .........................108
**Endothelin receptor antagonists**
Pulmonary hypertension...............305
**Enoxaparin**
Thrombolysis ................................95
Unstable angina and NSTEMI .........87
**Eplerenone**
Heart failure ...............................117
Post-myocardial infarction..............96
**Epoprostenol**
Pulmonary hypertension...............305
Vasoreactivity test .......................303
**Epsilon wave**.........................................189
**Eptifibatide**
Unstable angina and NSTEMI .........87
**Ergonovine provocation test** .................108
**Erythrocytosis, secondary**.....................267
**Esmolol**
Atrial fibrillation...........................212
Cardiopulmonary resuscitation .....349
Hypertensive crisis.......................329
**EuroSCORE** ............................................106
**EVAR** .....................................................283
**Everolimus**
Heart transplantation...................132

**External counterpulsation**
Stable angina ...............................77
**Exudative enteropathy**...........................265
**Ezetimibe** ..............................................321

# F

**Fabry disease**.........................................186
**Fallot, tetralogy of. See Tetralogy
of Fallot**
**False lumen**............................................280
**Familial aortic syndromes**......................284
**Familial combined hyperlipidemia**..........318
**Familial dysbetalipoproteinemia**........2, 317
**Familial hypercholesterolemia**..........2, 317
**Far-field**.................................................238
**Fetal circulation**.....................................248
**FFR** ..........................................51, 52, 104
**Fibrates** .................................................321
**Fibroelastoma**.........................................194
**Fibroma** ..................................................195
**Fibromuscular dysplasia** ........................289
**Fick equation** .....................................55, 66
**Filling pressure** .....................................124
Echocardiography...........................33
**Flash pulmonary edema**
Heart failure ...............................125
Renovascular atherosclerotic disease289
**Flecainide**..............................................230
Atrial fibrillation....................212, 213
**Focal atrial tachycardia** .........................206
Electrocardiogram .......................207
Management ...............................207
**Fondaparinux**
Pulmonary embolism....................298
Unstable angina and NSTEMI .........87
**Fontaine classification**...........................286
**Fontan procedure**...................................265
Clinical features ..........................265
Complications .............................265
Protein-losing enteropathy ...........265
Management ...............................266
Pregnancy ..................................266
Reoperation ................................266
**Foramen ovale** .......................................250
**Framingham score**.........................314, 318
**Free wall rupture** ...................................100
**Friedreich's ataxia** .................................343
**Functional capacity**
According to age ...........................25
**Functional class**
CCS ............................................72
NYHA.........................................112
**Fundoscopy**...............................................2

## G

Gadolinium ................................................. 63
    Late enhancement ................................. 64
Gallavardin phenomenon .......................... 141
Gestational hypertension .......................... 273
Ghent criteria ............................................ 264
Giant-cell myocarditis ............................... 192
Giant-cell arteritis .................................... 285
Glagov phenomenon .................................... 52
GLP-1 analog ............................................ 330
Glucose
    Post-myocardial infarction .................... 97
Gorlin formula ............................................. 59
GpIIb/IIIa inhibitors
    STEMI ................................................. 94
    Unstable angina and NSTEMI ............... 86
GRACE score .............................................. 84
Graham-Steell murmur ......................... 7, 302
Guillain-Barré syndrome .......................... 343

## H

Haïssaguerre pattern ................................ 223
Hakki formula .............................................. 59
Hampton hump ......................................... 296
Handgrip ........................................................ 8
HAS-BLED score ....................................... 216
HDL ........................................... 316, 317, 321
Heart disease in pregnant women.
See Pregnancy
Heart failure ............................................. 112
    Assessment ........................................ 114
    Definition ........................................... 112
    Etiologies .......................................... 113
    Palliative care .................................... 136
    Pathophysiology ................................. 113
    Signs and symptoms ........................... 112
Heart sounds ................................................ 4
Heart transplantation ............................... 130
    Allocation system .............................. 131
    Assessment ........................................ 131
    Cardiac allograft vasculopathy ............ 133
    Complications ..................................... 132
    Contraindications ............................... 131
    Corticosteroids .................................. 132
    Immunosuppression ............................. 132
    Indications ......................................... 130
    Induction ........................................... 132
    Opportunistic infection ....................... 133
    Prophylactic antibiotics ...................... 165
    Pulmonary vascular resistance ............ 131
    Rejection ........................................... 132
Hemangioma ............................................. 195
Hemochromatosis ...................................... 186
Hemodynamic assessment ........................... 53
    Arterial recording ................................ 57
    Atrial recording .................................. 56

    Curves ................................................ 55
    Hemodynamic data .............................. 54
    Indications ........................................... 53
    Intracardiac shunt ............................... 60
    Qp/Qs ................................................ 60
    Valvular regurgitation .......................... 59
    Valvular stenosis ................................. 59
    Ventricular recording ........................... 56
Hemodynamic curves ................................... 55
    Arterial curve ...................................... 57
    Atrial curve ........................................ 56
    Ventricular curve ................................. 56
Hemopericardium ...................................... 172
Heparin
    Antidote ............................................. 53
    Noncardiac surgery ............................ 313
    Pulmonary embolism .......................... 298
    STEMI ................................................. 94
    Thromboprophylaxis ........................... 299
    Unstable angina and NSTEMI ............... 87
Heparin-induced thrombocytopenia ........... 300
    4T score ............................................ 300
    Management ....................................... 301
    Pathophysiology ................................. 300
Hepatojugular reflux ..................................... 3
Hill sign .................................................... 147
HIV .......................................................... 341
HMG-CoA reductase inhibitors .................. 321
Holt-Oram syndrome ................................. 249
Hollenhorst plaques ............................... 2, 283
HV interval ............................................... 203
Hydralazine
    Heart failure ................................ 117, 121
    Hypertension ...................................... 328
Hyperaldosteronism, primary .................... 324
Hypercalcemia
    Electrocardiogram ................................ 21
Hypercholesterolemia, familial ............. 2, 317
Hypereosinophilic syndrome ...................... 186
Hyperkalemia
    Electrocardiogram ........................... 21, 90
Hyperparathyroidism ................................ 341
Hypertension ............................................ 323
    ABPM ................................................ 323
    Assessment ........................................ 323
    Cushing syndrome .............................. 325
    Elderly ............................................... 328
    Hypertensive crisis ............................. 329
    Management ....................................... 325
    Masked HT .......................................... 324
    Nondrug treatment ............................. 326
    Percutaneous renal denervation ... 329
    Pheochromocytoma ............................ 325
    Pregnancy .......................................... 273
    Primary hyperaldosteronism ............... 324
    Pseudohypertension ........................... 328
    Target organ damage .......................... 324
    Treatment-resistant ........................... 328
    Underlying causes .............................. 324

White coat syndrome................... 324
**Hypertensive crisis** ............................ 329
**Hypertensive retinopathy** ...................... 2
**Hyperthyroidism** ................................ 342
**Hypertriglyceridemia** ........... 2, 316, 317, 321
**Hypertrophic cardiomyopathy**............. 181
    Alcohol septal ablation ............... 183
    Cardiac catheterization............... 182
    Cardiac MRI ...................... 64, 182
    Clinical features ......................... 181
    Differential diagnosis.................. 181
    Echocardiography....................... 182
    Electrocardiogram ................. 20, 181
    Genetic testing .......................... 226
    Management............................... 183
    Myomectomy .............................. 183
    Obstructive................................. 181
    Pathophysiology ......................... 181
    Pregnancy.................................. 273
    Presentation............................... 181
    Stress test.................................. 182
    Sudden death.............................. 183
    Versus athlete's heart.................. 181
**Hyperviscosity syndrome** ..................... 267
**Hypocalcemia**
    Electrocardiogram ......................... 21
**Hypoglycemia** ................................... 332
**Hypothermia**
    Electrocardiogram ......................... 22
    Therapeutic ............................... 350
**Hypothyroidism**................................ 342
    Electrocardiogram ......................... 22
**Hysteresis** ...................................... 237


# I

**IART**............................................. 206
**Ibutilide** ........................................ 231
    Atrial fibrillation............................ 213
**If current inhibitor**
    Antianginal ................................. 77
    Heart failure ....................... 117, 120
**Iloprost**
    Pulmonary hypertension............... 305
**Immunosuppression**
    Heart transplantation................... 132
**Impella** ......................................... 130
**Implantable cardiac monitor**................. 227
**Implantable cardioverter-defibrillator** .... 241
    Antitachycardia pacing ................ 242
    Discriminators............................. 242
    Evidence .................................... 241
    Heart failure .............................. 121
    Inappropriate shock...................... 243
    Indications ................................. 242
    Ineffective shock ......................... 243
    Magnet ..................................... 312
    Perioperative.............................. 312

    Postshock management.............. 243
    Primary prevention...................... 241
    Programming .............................. 242
    Secondary prevention................... 241
**Inappropriate sinus tachycardia
syndrome** ........................................ 205
**Incretins** ....................................... 331
**Infectious aortitis** ............................. 285
**Infective endocarditis** ......................... 160
    Antibiotics.................................. 164
    Complications ............................. 163
    Duke criteria .............................. 162
    Echocardiography........................ 163
    Embolism................................... 163
    Management............................... 164
    Prophylactic antibiotics................ 165
    Prosthetic valve................... 161, 166
    Renal failure............................... 163
    Risk factors ............................... 161
    Signs and symptoms.................... 162
    Signs................................. 2, 162
    Stroke ...................................... 163
    Surgical indications ..................... 166
    Vegetation ................................. 163
**Inferior vena cava filter** ....................... 299
**Inotropes, positive**
    Cardiopulmonary resuscitation ..... 350
    Heart failure ....................... 128, 129
**Insulin therapy**................................. 330
**Insulins** ........................................ 332
**INTERMACS classification** ................... 134
**Intermittent claudication**...................... 286
**Intermittent pneumatic compression** ..... 299
**Intraaortic balloon pump**........................ 99
    Acute heart failure...................... 130
**Intraatrial conduction disorder** ............... 11
**Intracardiac shunt**
    Cardiac catheterization ................. 60
    Contrast echocardiography............. 39
**Intracerebral hemorrhage** ........ 95, 290, 295
**Intracranial hypertension**...................... 295
**Intramural hematoma, spontaneous**....... 282
**Intraventricular gradient** ...................... 182
**Intrinsic automaticity** .......................... 200
**Intrinsic sympathetic activity**
    Beta-blockers............................... 76
**Ischemic cascade** ............................... 73
**Isuprel**
    Cardiopulmonary resuscitation ..... 350
    Heart failure .............................. 129
**Ivabradine**
    Antianginal ................................. 77
    Heart failure ....................... 117, 120
**IVUS** ............................... 51, 52, 104


# J

**Janeway lesion** .................................. 162

**Jatene procedure** ............................... 260
**Jervell and Lange-Nielsen syndrome** ..... 224
**Jones criteria** ..................................... 168
**Jugular veins** ......................................... 3
**Jugular waves** ....................................... 3
**Junctional tachycardia** ....................... 210
    Focal paroxysmal ......................... 210
    Nonparoxysmal ........................... 210

## K

**Kawasaki disease** ............................... 341
**Kent bundle** ....................................... 208
**Killip classification** ............................. 93
**Konno procedure** ............................... 254
**Kussmaul sign** ............................. 3, 177
    Differential diagnosis .................. 177

## L

**Labetalol**
    Hypertensive crisis ..................... 329
    Stroke ....................................... 293
**Lactescent serum** ............................... 317
**Lake Louise criteria** ........................... 192
**Lambl's excrescence** ............................ 39
**Laser myocardial revascularization** ........ 77
**LDL** ................................................... 316
    Calculation ................................. 316
**Lecompte maneuver** ........................... 260
**Left anterior hemiblock** ........................ 13
**Left atrial appendage**
    Echocardiography .......................... 40
    Occlusion ........................... 218, 294
    Thrombus ..................................... 40
**Left bundle branch block** ...................... 13
    Acute myocardial infarction ...... 13, 89
    Electrocardiogram ......................... 13
**Left posterior hemiblock** ...................... 13
**Left ventricular aneurysm** ................... 100
    Electrocardiogram ................... 20, 89
**Left ventricular end-diastolic
pressure** ....................................... 54, 56
**Left ventricular hypertrophy** ................. 16
**Left ventricular noncompaction** ............ 190
    Echocardiography ........................ 190
    Management ............................... 190
**Left ventricular outflow tract
obstruction** ........................................ 253
**Leiomyosarcoma** ................................ 196
**LEOPARD syndrome** ........................... 257
**Levocardia** ........................................ 248
**Levosimedan**
    Heart failure .............................. 128
**Levo-transposition of the great vessels.
See Congenitally corrected transposition
the great arteries**

**Libman-Sacks endocarditis** ................. 342
**Lidocaine** ........................................... 230
    Cardiopulmonary resuscitation ..... 349
**Limb-girdle muscular dystrophy** .......... 343
**Lipemia retinalis** ............................... 317
**Lipoma** .............................................. 194
**Lipomatous hypertrophy of atrial
septum** ............................................... 195
**Lipoproteins** ...................................... 316
**Loeys-Dietz syndrome** ........................ 284
**Löffler endocarditis** ............................ 186
**Long QT**
    Acquired .................................... 223
    Causes ...................................... 223
    Genetic testing ........................... 226
    Syndrome .................................. 224
**Loop diuretics**
    Decompensated heart failure ........ 129
    Heart failure ...................... 117, 119
    Hypertension .............................. 327
    Resistance ................................. 120
**Loss of consciousness**
    Differential diagnosis .................. 227
**Low molecular weight heparin**
    Noncardiac surgery ..................... 313
    Pulmonary embolism ................... 298
    Thrombolysis ............................... 95
    Thromboprophylaxis .................... 299
    Unstable angina and NSTEMI ....... 87
**Low voltage, ECG** ................................ 15
**Lp(a)** ................................................ 316
**LPL, familial deficiency** ...................... 317
**Lutembacher syndrome** ................. 7, 249
**Lymphangioma** ................................... 195
**Lymphoma, cardiac** ............................ 196

## M

**Macroalbuminuria** ............................... 333
**Magnesium sulfate** .................................
    Cardiopulmonary resuscitation ..... 349
**Magnet**
    Pacemaker ................................. 312
**Magnetic resonance imaging.
See Cardiac RMI**
**Mahaim's bundle** ................................ 209
**Mahan's formula** ................................ 303
**Marfan syndrome** ............................... 263
    Aortic disease ............................ 284
    Ghent criteria ............................. 264
    Indications for surgery ................. 263
    Management ............................... 263
    Pregnancy .................................. 263
    Surgery ..................................... 263
**Mass, cardiac**
    Echocardiography .......................... 39
**McConnell's sign** ................................ 296

**Mechanical support**
Assessment...................................134
Complications................................136
ECMO.........................................130
Impella........................................130
Indications...................................133
Long-term....................................133
LVAD..........................................135
Medium-term...............................130
Percutaneous...............................130
Scenarios....................................134
Short-term...................................130
TandemHeart...............................130
**Mediastinitis**...........................................107
**Medina classification**...............................51
**Meglitinide**...............................................331
**Mesocardia**...............................................248
**Metabolic syndrome**...............................338
**Metastasis, cardiac**.................................194
**Metformin**.................................................331
**Metoprolol**
Acute coronary syndrome.............96
Atrial fibrillation...........................212
Cardiopulmonary resuscitation.....349
Heart failure................................118
**Mexiletine**.......................................221, 230
**MIBI-Dipyridamole**.....................................61
Prognosis.....................................75
Sensitivity and specificity.............74
**MIBI-Persantin. See MIBI-Dipyridamole**
**Microalbuminuria**....................................333
**Microvascular disease**............................108
**Midsystolic click (MVP)**...............................5
**Milrinone**
Cardiopulmonary resuscitation.....350
Heart failure................................128
**Mitochondrial diseases**...........................343
**Mitraclip**....................................................154
Heart failure................................123
**Mitral regurgitation**
Acute mitral regurgitation............155
Angiographic assessment..............59
Carpentier classification..............152
Echocardiography...................36, 42
Etiology.......................................151
Functional...................................151
Heart failure................................123
Hemodynamic consequences.......153
Involved segment..........................42
Ischemic.....................................151
Management................................154
Mitraclip......................................154
Mitral valve prolapse...................155
Pregnancy...................................272
Severity.......................................152
Signs and symptoms...................153
Surgical indications.....................154
**Mitral stenosis**
Auscultation................................149

Balloon valvuloplasty...................150
Cardiac catheterization.................59
Echocardiography..........................35
Etiology.......................................148
Hemodynamic consequences.......149
Management................................150
Open commissurotomy.................151
Pregnancy...................................271
Prognosis....................................150
Severity.......................................149
Signs and symptoms...................149
**Mitral valve prolapse**..............................155
Dynamic auscultation..................155
**Mitral valve, morphological criteria**......248
**Mobitz I, AV block**...................................202
**Mobitz II, AV block**..................................202
**Mode switch**............................................237
**m-TOR inhibitors**
Heart transplantation...................132
**Mueller's maneuver**................................156
**Müller's sign**............................................147
**Multifocal atrial tachycardia**..................207
Electrocardiogram.......................207
**Murmur**
Benign.............................................6
Continuous......................................7
Diastolic..........................................7
Mammary murmur of pregnancy.....7
Systolic...........................................6
**Muscular dystrophies**.............................342
**Musset's sign**...........................................147
**Mustard procedure**.................................259
Clinical features..........................259
Complications..............................260
Echocardiography........................259
Indications for surgery.................260
Pregnancy...................................260
**MVO$_2$**.......................................................333
**Myasthenia gravis**...................................343
**Mycophenolate mofetil**
Heart transplantation...................132
**Myocardial bridge**...................................269
**Myocardial contusion**.............................343
**Myocardial hibernation**.............................63
**Myocardial infarction**
Absence of atherosclerosis............82
Arrhythmias and blocks...............102
Classification................................82
Cocaine.......................................344
Complications................................98
Coronary embolism.......................82
Definition......................................81
Electrocardiogram...................90, 91
NSTEMI. see NSTEMI....................83
Reinfarction..................................81
Right ventricle.......................91, 100
Secondary.....................................82
STEMI. see STEMI.........................88

**Myocardial performance index**
Left ventricle .................................. 29
Right ventricle ................................. 31
**Myocardial perfusion** ................................ 34
**Myocarditis** ................................................ 191
Cardiac MRI ......................... 64, 192
Diagnosis ..................................... 192
Etiologies ...................................... 191
Fulminant ...................................... 192
Giant-cell ...................................... 192
Management ................................. 193
Pathophysiology ........................... 192
Presentation ................................. 192
**Myomectomy, septal** ................................. 183
**Myopathy, statin-induced** ....................... 322
**Myotonic dystrophies** ............................. 343
**Myxoma** ..................................................... 194

# N

**Narrow QRS tachycardia** ................. 204, 348
**Naughton protocol** ..................................... 23
**Neck venous hum** ......................................... 7
**Nesiritide**
Heart failure ................................. 128
**Neuromodulation** ........................................ 77
**Niacin** ......................................................... 322
**Nicardipine**
Hypertensive crisis ....................... 329
**Nicorandil**
Antianginal .................................... 77
**Nicotine replacement therapy** ................ 315
**Nicotinic acid** ............................................ 322
**Nifedipine**
Hypertension ................................ 326
Pulmonary hypertension ............... 305
Stable angina ................................. 78
**Nitroglycerin**
Acute coronary syndrome ............. 95
Adverse effects ............................. 78
Antianginal ............................... 77, 78
Heart failure ................................. 128
Hypertensive crisis ....................... 329
**Nitroprusside**
Heart failure ................................. 128
Hypertensive crisis ....................... 329
**NO**
Vasoreactivity test ........................ 303
**Noncardiac surgery, preoperative
assessment** ................................................ 310
Anticoagulation ............................ 313
Atrial fibrillation ........................... 313
Functional capacity ...................... 311
Noninvasive stratification ............. 312
Prosthetic valve ............................ 313
Risk assessment ........................... 311
Thromboembolic disease .............. 313

**Noncompensatory pause** ........................ 204
**Non-HDL cholesterol** .............................. 316
**Noninvasive stratification** ........................ 74
Prognosis ....................................... 75
**Nonspecific intraventricular conduction
disorder** ..................................................... 14
**Non-steroidal anti-inflammatory drugs** .... 97
**Nonsustained ventricular tachycardia** ... 219
**Noonan syndrome** .................................... 257
**No-reflow phenomenon** ............................ 105
**Norepinephrine** ........................................ 129
Heart failure ................................. 129
Cardiopulmonary resuscitation ..... 350
**NSTEMI** ........................................................ 83
Anticoagulation .............................. 87
Antiplatelet therapy ....................... 86
Arrhythmias and blocks ............... 102
Assessment .................................... 83
Complications ................................. 98
Early invasive strategy .............. 86, 88
Management ............................... 85, 88
TIMI score ...................................... 93
**NT-proBNP** ................................................ 114
**Nuclear medicine** ....................................... 60
Myocardial perfusion imaging ........ 60
Positron emission tomography ........ 62
Radionuclide ventriculography ....... 62

# O

**Obesity** See Weight
**Obesity cardiomyopathy** .......................... 184
**Obstructive sleep apnea syndrome** ........ 338
Apnea-hypopnea index .................. 339
Diagnosis ...................................... 339
Heart failure ................................. 123
**Omega-3**
Heart failure ................................. 121
**Opening snap** ..................................... 6, 150
**Orthostatic hypotension** ................... 2, 228
Dysautonomia ............................... 228
**Ortner syndrome** ...................................... 149
**Osborn wave** .............................................. 22
**Osler maneuver** ........................................ 328
**Osler nodes** .............................................. 162
**Output failure, pacemaker** ...................... 238
**Oversensing** ............................................. 238

# P

**P wave** ......................................................... 11
**Pacemaker lead** ........................................ 237
Maturation ................................... 238
**Pacemaker syndrome** ............................... 239
**Pacemaker-mediated tachycardia** .......... 239
**Paget-Schroetter syndrome** ................... 299

**Palliative care** .......................................... 136
**Palliative shunts** ...................................... 267
**Pancarditis, rheumatic fever** .............. 168
**Pancreatic lipase inhibitor** ................. 337
**Pannus** ........................................................ 38
**Papillary fibroelastoma** ......................... 194
**Papillary muscle rupture** ...................... 101
**Parasternal heave** ....................................... 4
**Patent ductus arteriosus** ...................... 252
    Complications ..................................... 253
    Echocardiography ............................... 253
    Indications for repair ....................... 253
    Percutaneous closure ....................... 253
    Pregnancy ........................................... 253
    Severity ................................................ 252
**Patent foramen ovale** ............................. 250
    Cryptogenic stroke ........................... 250
**PCSK9 inhibitors** ..................................... 322
**PDE-5 inhibitors** ......................................
    Pulmonary hypertension ................. 305
**Penetrating atherosclerotic ulcer** ....... 282
**Percutaneous coronary intervention** ...... 103
    Adjuvant therapy ............................... 106
    Benefits ................................................. 79
    Bifurcation .......................................... 105
    Chronic total occlusion .................... 104
    Left main coronary artery ...... 79, 105
    Complications ..................................... 105
    Early chest pain post-PCI ................ 106
    Risk ........................................................ 51
    Rotational atherectomy .................... 104
    STEMI .................................................... 93
    Stent thrombosis ............................... 106
    SYNTAX score ...................................... 79
    Thromboaspiration ............................ 104
    Vein graft ............................................ 104
**Pericardial cyst** ........................................ 179
**Pericardial disease**
    Etiologies ............................................ 172
**Pericardial effusion**
    Chronic ................................................ 173
    Metastatic ........................................... 173
**Pericardial friction rub** ...................... 6, 173
**Pericardial knock** ................................ 6, 177
**Pericardial window** ................................. 176
**Pericardiectomy** ...................................... 178
**Pericardiocentesis** .................................. 176
**Pericarditis**
    Acute ................................................... 173
    Bacterial .............................................. 173
    Complications ..................................... 174
    Diagnosis ............................................ 174
    Dressler syndrome ................... 101, 173
    Electrocardiogram ............ 20, 89, 173
    Incessant ............................................ 174
    Management ....................................... 174
    Post-myocardial infarction.... 101, 173
    Post-radiotherapy ............................. 173
    Recurrent ............................................ 174

**Pericardium, congenital absence** ........... 179
**Peripartum cardiomyopathy** ................. 272
**Peripheral artery disease** ...................... 285
    Acute ischemia of lower limbs ...... 288
    Ankle-brachial index ......................... 286
    Atherosclerosis of upper limbs ...... 288
    Clinical features ................................. 286
    Critical ischemia of lower limbs ..... 288
    Differential diagnosis ....................... 286
    Management ....................................... 287
    Revascularization .............................. 287
**Peripheral pulmonary artery stenosis** .... 256
**Periprosthetic regurgitation** ................. 159
    Echocardiography ......................... 38, 42
**Permanent pacemaker** ........................... 233
    Capture failure ................................... 238
    Classification ...................................... 235
    Diaphragmatic stimulation ............. 239
    Dysfunction ........................................ 238
    Follow-up ............................................ 237
    Indications .......................................... 233
    Indications, post-myocardial
    infarction ............................................ 102
    Infection .............................................. 167
    Intervals .............................................. 236
    Magnet ................................................ 312
    Output failure .................................... 238
    Oversensing ....................................... 238
    Pacemaker- mediated
    tachycardia ........................................ 239
    Pacemaker syndrome ....................... 239
    Perioperative ..................................... 312
    Sensitivity ........................................... 237
    Stimulation ......................................... 237
    Undersensing ..................................... 238
**Persistent juvenile pattern** ............. 18, 89
**Phenylephrine**
    Cardiopulmonary resuscitation ..... 350
    Heart failure ....................................... 129
**Pheochromocytoma** ......................... 325, 342
**Physical examination** ................................. 2
**Physical activity** ...................................... 333
    Benefits .............................................. 334
    Heart failure ....................................... 121
    Intensity ............................................. 334
    Isometric ............................................ 336
    Physiology .......................................... 333
    Prescription ........................................ 336
    Pretraining assessment ................... 334
    Risks .................................................... 333
    Targets ................................................. 336
**Pill in the pocket** ..................................... 212
**PJRT** ............................................................ 209
**Plane. See Air travel**
**Poisoning** ....................................................
    Beta-blockers .................................... 344
    Calcium channel blockers ............... 345
    Cocaine ............................................... 344
    Digoxin ................................................ 345

Polyarteritis nodosa..................................342
Polymyositis.............................................342
Positron emission tomography................62
    Viability ...........................................63
Postural orthostatic tachycardia
syndrome..................................................206
Potassium channel blocking agents......231
POTS syndrome.......................................206
Potts shunt...............................................267
PR interval..................................................11
Prasugrel
    Acute coronary syndrome ..............96
    STEMI ..............................................94
Precordial transition.................................15
Precordium, physical examination ..........4
Pre-eclampsia..........................................273
Pregnancy
    Anticoagulation ...........................272
    Aortic regurgitation......................272
    Aortic stenosis.............................271
    Atrial fibrillation...........................273
    Contraindications..........................271
    Cyanotic heart disease .................272
    Dilated cardiomyopathy.................272
    Gestational hypertension...............273
    Hemodynamic changes .................270
    Hypertension.................................273
    Hypertrophic cardiomyopathy.......273
    Mitral regurgitation......................272
    Mitral stenosis.............................271
    Peripartum cardiomyopathy..........272
    Physical examination.....................270
    Preeclampsia.................................273
    Prosthetic valve............................272
    Pulmonary hypertension................272
    Risk of cardiac events ...................270
    Supraventricular tachycardia.........273
    WHO classification........................271
Preoperative assessment. See
Noncardiac surgery
Primary hyperaldosteronism....................324
Primary prevention of cardiovascular
disease.....................................................314
Prinzmetal angina....................................108
Procainamide............................................229
    Atrial fibrillation...........................213
    Cardiopulmonary resuscitation......349
Programmed ventricular stimulation
    Electrophysiological study ............228
Propafenone.............................................230
    Atrial fibrillation....................212, 213
Prophylactic antibiotics, endocarditis....165
Prostacyclins
    Pulmonary hypertension................305
Prostanoids
    Pulmonary hypertension................305
Prosthetic thrombosis.............................159
Prosthetic valve.......................................158

Antithrombotic.........................................159
Bioprostheses..........................................158
Complications..........................................159
Dysfunction...............................................38
Echocardiography.......................................38
Follow-up.................................................160
Mechanical prostheses............................158
Noncardiac surgery..................................313
Pannus.......................................................38
Patient-prosthesis mismatch.....................38
Pregnancy.................................................272
Prophylactic antibiotics...........................165
Prosthetic thrombosis..............................159
Regurgitation..............................38, 42, 159
Thrombus...................................................38
Protamine...................................................53
Protein-losing enteropathy.....................265
Proton pump inhibitors.............................97
Pseudoaneurysm
    Aorta .............................................276
    Femoral artery ...............................53
    Left ventricle ................................100
Pseudohypertension.................................328
Pseudoinfarction........................................20
Pulmonary artery pressure.............54, 303
Pulmonary capillary wedge
pressure ...........................................54, 56
Pulmonary congestion ..............................47
Pulmonary embolism...............................295
    Anticoagulation ....................298, 299
    Assessment...................................297
    Chest x-ray....................................296
    Clinical features ...........................295
    Consequences...............................296
    Deep vein thrombosis....................296
    Echocardiography..........................296
    Electrocardiogram .........20, 90, 296
    Embolectomy .......................298, 299
    Inferior vena cava filter.................299
    Intravenous thrombolysis......298, 299
    Management..................................298
    Noncardiac surgery .......................313
    Thrombophilia...............................295
    Wells criteria ................................297
Pulmonary hypertension.........................301
    Assessment...................................302
    Atrial septostomy..........................306
    Cardiac MRI..................................303
    Catheterization..............................303
    Clinical features ...........................302
    Congenital heart disease ..............306
    Disproportionate...........................306
    Drug treatment.............................305
    Echocardiography..................302, 303
    Etiologies .............................301, 302
    Lung transplantation ....................306
    Management..................................304
    Post-capillary ...............................301
    Pregnancy.....................................272

Transpulmonary gradient..............306
Vasoreactivity test ......................303
**Pulmonary regurgitation** .........................157
**Pulmonary stenosis** .......................157, 256
Auscultation ...........................256
Clinical features ......................256
Complications .........................257
Indications for repair ................257
Pregnancy...............................257
Subvalvular .............................256
Supravalvular ..........................256
**Pulmonary vascular resistance** ....... 55, 303
Heart transplantation..................131
**Pulmonary vein isolation**......................214
**Pulmonary veins**
Anomalous connection .................268
Echocardiography ......................41
**Pulse**
Alternans................................58
Bisferiens......................58, 146, 181
Bounding................................58
Dicrotic................................58
Paradoxus...............................58
Parvus et tardus ...............58, 141
**Pulseless electrical activity**
Cardiopulmonary resuscitation .....347
**Pulsus bisferiens** ................58, 146, 181
**Pulsus paradoxus** .......................2, 58, 175
Differential diagnosis..................175
**Pulsus parvus et tardus** ..............58, 141
**Purine synthesis inhibitors**
Heart transplantation..................132
**PVAB**.....................................................236
**PVARP**...................................................236

**Q**

**Qp/Qs**.....................................................60
**QRS**
Chamber hypertrophy..................16
Frontal axis ...........................12
Intraventricular conduction ............12
Low voltage.............................15
Precordial transition ..................15
**QT interval**.............................................18
Long QT syndrome ......................224
Short QT syndrome .....................224
**Quincke's sign** .......................................147
**Quinidine** ...............................................229

**R**

**Radiation exposure** ..................................67
**Radionuclide ventriculography** ...............62
**Radiotherapy**
Cardiac complications .................197
Pericarditis ...........................173

**RAMP protocol** ..........................................24
**Ramp, ICD** ..............................................242
**Ranolazine**
Antianginal.............................77
**Rastelli procedure** .................................260
**Rate drop response** .................................237
**Recovery pressure phenomenon** ...............38
**Reentry** .................................................200
**Reinfarction** ............................................81
**Renal denervation** ..................................329
**Repolarization** ........................................200
**Reserve, heart rate** .................................336
**Resins** ...................................................321
**Resting potential**....................................200
**Restrictive cardiomyopathy** ....................184
Clinical features ......................184
Echocardiography......................185
Electrocardiogram .....................185
Management............................185
Versus constrictive pericarditis.....185
**Retroperitoneal hematoma** ........................53
**Retrosternal chest pain** .............................72
Differential diagnosis .................72
Noncoronary ...........................72
**Rhabdomyolysis**
Statin .................................322
**Rhabdomyoma** .........................................195
**Rhabdomyosarcoma** .................................196
**Rheumatic fever** ......................................168
Jones criteria .........................168
Pancarditis ............................168
Secondary prevention..................168
**Rheumatoid arthritis** ...............................342
**Right bundle branch block**.........................14
**Right heart failure**...........................125, 136
Assessment.............................136
Etiologies .............................136
Management............................136
Signs and symptoms...................136
**Right ventricular hypertrophy** ....................17
**Right ventricular outflow tract**
**obstruction**...........................................256
**Right ventricular stroke work index** ..........134
**Rivaroxaban**
Acute coronary syndrome ..............87
Atrial fibrillation.....................217
Pulmonary embolism...................299
**Romano-Ward syndrome**..............................224
**Romhilt-Estes score** ..................................16
**Ross procedure** .......................................254
**Rotational atherectomy** ............................104
**Roth spot** ...............................................162
**Rupture of papillary muscle**......................101
**Rytand's murmur** ........................................7

**S**

**S1** ..........................................................4

S2 ...................................................... 5
    Paradoxical splitting ......................... 5
    Physiological splitting ....................... 5
**S3** ...................................................... 6
**S4** ...................................................... 6
**Sarcoidosis** ..................................... 186
**Schwartz score** ............................... 224
**Scimitar syndrome** .......................... 268
**Scleroderma** ................................... 342
    Restrictive cardiomyopathy ..........185
**SCORE model** ......................... 314, 319
**Seattle Heart Failure Model** ............ 115
**Secondary prevention of cardiovascular disease** ...........................................314
**Segmental contractility** ..................... 34
**Selective serotonin agonist**
    Obesity ........................................ 337
**Senning procedure** .......................... 259
**Septal curvature** ............................... 30
**Sgarbossa criteria** ...................... 13, 89
**Shone complex** ............................... 254
**Shunt, intracardiac**
    Cardiac catheterization ................ 60
    Contrast echocardiography ............ 39
    Pulmonary arterial hypertension ... 306
**Sildenafil**
    Pulmonary hypertension .............. 305
**Simpson's method** ............................. 29
**Sinoatrial block** ............................... 201
    Pacemaker ................................. 233
**Sinoatrial nodal reentrant tachycardia** ... 206
**Sinoatrial node disease** .................. 201
    Pacemaker ................................. 233
**Sinotubular junction** ....................... 276
**Sinus arrest** .................................... 201
**Sinus arrhythmia** .............................. 10
**Sinus bradycardia** ........................... 201
    Pacemaker ................................. 233
**Sinus node recovery time** ................ 203
**Sinus of Valsalva** ............................ 276
    Aneurysm .................................... 269
**Sinus pause** .................................... 201
    Pacemaker ................................. 233
**Sinus rhythm** .................................... 10
**Sinus tachycardia** ........................... 205
**Sirolimus**
    Heart transplantation ................... 132
**Sitaxsentan**
    Pulmonary hypertension .............. 305
**Sleep-disordered breathing** ...... 123, 338
**Smoking** .......................................... 315
    Drug therapy ............................... 315
**Sodium channel blocking agents** ....... 229
**Sokolow-Lyon criteria** ....................... 16
**Sotalol** ........................................... 231
    Atrial fibrillation .......................... 212
    Cardiopulmonary resuscitation ..... 349
**Splinter hemorrhages** ...................... 162
**Spondyloarthropathies** .................... 342

**Square root sign** ............................. 178
**Squatting** ........................................... 8
**ST segment**
    Depression ............................ 18, 84
    Elevation ............................... 17, 88
    Male pattern ................................. 88
**Stable angina** ................................... 72
    Assessment ................................. 73
    Functional class ........................... 72
    Ischemic cascade ......................... 73
    Management ................................. 76
    Noninvasive stratification .............. 73
    Prognosis .................................... 75
**Stanford classification** ..................... 279
**Statins** ..................................... 321, 322
    Acute coronary syndrome ............. 96
    Coronary artery disease .............. 76
    Diabetes .................................... 332
    Follow-up ................................... 322
    Myalgia ...................................... 322
    Primary prevention ...................... 322
    Rhabdomyolysis .......................... 322
    Secondary prevention .................. 322
    Toxicity ...................................... 322
**STEMI** ............................................. 88
    Arrhythmias and blocks ............... 102
    Complications ............................... 98
    Electrocardiogram ......................... 91
    Killip classification ........................ 93
    Management ................................. 92
    Pharmacoinvasive strategy ............ 95
    Primary PCI ................................. 93
    Rescue PCI ................................. 95
    Thrombolysis ................................ 93
    TIMI score .................................. 93
**Stent thrombosis** ............................ 106
**Stent** .............................................. 103
    Drug-eluting ................................ 103
    Metallic ...................................... 104
    Noncardiac surgery ..................... 313
    Restenosis ................................. 104
    Thrombosis ................................. 106
**Stress echocardiography** .................. 43
    Ischemia ...................................... 44
    Prognosis .................................... 75
    Sensitivity and Specificity ............. 74
**Stress test** ...................................... 22
    Contraindications ......................... 22
    Electrocardiographic evaluation ...... 24
    Exaggerated hypertensive response ... 26
    Factors of poor prognosis .............. 26
    Indications to terminate the test ..... 25
    Post-myocardial infarction ....... 24, 97
    Prognosis .................................... 75
    Protocols .................................... 23
    Sensitivity and Specificity ............. 74
    Submaximal ............................ 24, 97
**Stroke** ............................................ 290
    Atrial fibrillation .......................... 294

Blood pressure control ................. 293
Cardioembolic source ................. 291
Carotid revascularization ............. 294
Differential diagnosis ................. 292
Intraarterial thrombolysis ........... 293
Intracranial hemorrhage ............. 295
Intravenous thrombolysis ..... 292, 293
Lacunar ................................ 290
Management ........................... 292
Mechanical thrombolysis ........... 293
Mechanisms ........................... 290
NIH scale ............................... 291
Patent foramen ovale ............... 250
Secondary prevention ............... 294
Thrombophilia ......................... 294
**STS score** ................................. 106
**Subarachnoid hemorrhage** ............... 290
**Subclavian steal syndrome** ............. 288
**Subendocardial ischemia** .................... 19
**Sulfonylurea** ............................... 331
**Summation gallop** ............................ 6
**Supraventricular tachycardia** ............. 204
Cardiopulmonary resuscitation ... 348
Pregnancy ............................. 273
**Swan-Ganz catheter** ...................... 346
Heart failure .......................... 129
**Sydenham's chorea** ....................... 168
**Syncope** .................................... 227
Assessment ............................ 227
Cardiogenic ........................... 227
Differential diagnosis ............... 227
Electrocardiogram .................... 227
Neurocardiogenic ..................... 228
Orthostatic hypotension ............. 228
Pacemaker ................... 233, 234, 235
**SYNTAX score** .............................. 79
**Systemic lupus erythematosus** ............. 342
Coronary arteritis .................... 82
Drug-induced Lupus ................. 342
**Systemic vascular resistance** .............. 55
**Systolic function**
Echocardiography ...................... 29
**Systolic heart failure**
Management ........................... 115

**T wave**
Inversion ......................... 18, 84
Juvenile pattern ..................... 89
Peaked ................................ 18
Symmetrical ........................... 18
**Tachy-bradycardia syndrome** ............. 201
Pacemaker ............................ 233
**Tachycardia**
Cardiopulmonary resuscitation ..... 348
**Tachycardiomyopathy** ......................... 184

**Tacrolimus**
Heart transplantation ................. 132
**Tadalafil**
Pulmonary hypertension ............... 305
**Takayasu disease** ......................... 285
**Takotsubo cardiomyopathy** ............... 191
Differential diagnosis ................. 191
Management ............................. 191
**Tamponade** ................................ 174
Clinical features ...................... 174
Echocardiography ..................... 175
Electrocardiogram ..................... 175
Pathophysiology ....................... 175
Versus constriction ................... 175
**TARP** ..................................... 236
**TAVI** ..................................... 144
**Temporal arteritis** ...................... 285
**Tetralogy of Fallot** ..................... 257
Clinical features ...................... 258
Complications ......................... 258
Echocardiography ..................... 258
Electrocardiogram ..................... 258
Indications for surgery ............... 258
Pregnancy ............................. 259
Surgery ............................... 258
Ventricular arrhythmia ............... 259
**TEVAR** ................................... 278
**Thermodilution** ............................ 55
**Thiazide diuretics**
Heart failure .................... 117, 119
Hypertension .......................... 327
**Thiazolidinedione** ....................... 331
**Thienopyridines**
STEMI ................................. 94
Unstable angina and NSTEMI ......... 86
**Thoracic aorta** .......................... 276
Aneurysm .............................. 276
Aortic dissection ..................... 279
Atherosclerotic plaque ............... 283
Echocardiography ...................... 42
Normal dimensions .................... 276
**Thorax, physical examination** .............. 4
**Thrombolysis**
Adjuvant therapy ...................... 95
Contraindications ..................... 94
Intracranial hemorrhage .............. 95
Prosthetic valve thrombosis ......... 159
Pulmonary embolism ................... 299
STEMI ................................. 93
Stroke ................................ 292
**Thrombophilia, hereditary** ......... 290, 295
**Thrombus**
Echocardiography ...................... 39
Intraventricular ...................... 101
Prosthetic valve ...................... 38
**Ticagrelor**
Acute coronary syndrome .............. 96
STEMI ................................. 94
Unstable Angina and NSTEMI ......... 86

**Tilt table** .................................................. 228
**TIMI flow** ..................................................... 51
**TIMI score**
    STEMI ........................................................ 93
    Unstable angina and NSTEMI ....... 84
**Tirofiban**
    Unstable angina and NSTEMI ........ 87
**Tolvaptan**
    Heart failure .......................................... 117
**Torsade de pointes** ....................... 222, 348
**Transesophageal echocardiography** ....... 39
    Endocarditis ......................................... 163
    Indications .............................................. 39
    Periprosthetic regurgitation ........... 42
    Standard views ..................................... 40
**Transient ischemic attack** ................... 290
**Transmural ischemia** ................................ 19
**Transposition of the great arteries** ... 259
    Arterial Switch .................................... 260
    Complications ..................................... 260
    Indications for surgery ................... 260
    Mustard procedure ........................... 259
    Rastelli procedure ........................... 260
**Transpulmonary gradient** ..................... 306
**Transthoracic echocardiography** .......... 27
    Atria ........................................................ 31
    Contrast ................................................. 39
    Diastolic function ................................ 32
    Endocarditis ......................................... 163
    Left ventricle ......................................... 28
    Mass ........................................................ 39
    Prosthetic valve ................................... 38
    Pulmonary arterial pressure .... 31, 303
    Right ventricle ...................................... 29
    Segmental contractility ................... 34
    Septal curvature ................................. 30
    Speckle tracking .................................. 39
    Standard views ..................................... 27
    Strain ....................................................... 39
    Thrombus ................................................ 39
    Tissue Doppler .................................... 39
    Valvular heart disease ...................... 35
**Traube's sign** .......................................... 147
**Trauma**
    Aortic rupture ..................................... 285
    Cardiovascular complications .... 343
    Management ........................................ 344
**Traumatic aortic rupture** ..................... 285
**Treprostinil**
    Pulmonary hypertension ............... 305
**Tricuspid regurgitation** ....................... 156
**Tricuspid stenosis** ................................. 156
**Tricuspid valve, morphological criteria** .. 248
**Triggered activity** .................................. 200
**Triglycerides** ........................................... 316
**Trimetazidine**
    Antianginal ............................................ 77
**Troponin** ....................................................... 80
    Differential diagnosis of elevation .... 80

    High sensitivity ................................... 81
**Trypanosoma cruzi** ................................ 184
**Tumor, cardiac** ......................................... 194
**Tumor plop** ................................................... 6
**Turner's syndrome** .................................. 254
    Aortic involvement ............................ 284

## U

**U wave** ........................................................... 18
**Undersensing** ........................................... 238
**Unstable angina** ......................................... 83
    Anticoagulation .................................... 87
    Antiplatelet therapy .......................... 86
    Assessment ............................................ 83
    Management ........................................... 85
**Use-dependent effect** ........................... 230

## V

**Valsalva** .................................................... 2, 8
**Valvular heart disease** ........................... 139
    Multivalvular disease ...................... 158
**Valvular prosthesis. See Prosthetic valve**
**Varenicline**
    Smoking cessation ............................ 316
**Vascular ring** ........................................... 269
**Vascular territories** ................................. 34
**Vasculitis** .................................................. 341
    Aortic involvement ............................ 285
**Vasodilators**
    Heart failure ........................................ 128
    Hypertension ........................................ 328
**Vasopressin antagonist**
    Heart failure ............................... 117, 119
**Vasopressors**
    Cardiopulmonary resuscitation ..... 350
    Heart failure ........................................ 129
**Vasoreactivity test**
    Pulmonary hypertension ............... 303
**Vasospastic angina** ................................ 108
**Vaughan Williams classification** .......... 229
**VDD** ............................................................. 236
**Vegetation** ................................................ 163
**Ventilation**
    Cardiopulmonary resuscitation .... 347
**Ventilatory anaerobic threshold** .............. 66
**Ventricle, morphological criteria** ......... 248
**Ventricular fibrillation** ................. 223, 347
    Cardiopulmonary resuscitation .... 347
**Ventricular pre-excitation** ........... 14, 208
**Ventricular premature complex** ........... 219
**Ventricular safety pacing** ..................... 237
**Ventricular septal defect** ..................... 250
    AV canal defect ................................. 251
    Clinical features ................................. 251
    Complications ..................................... 251

Indications for closure ................ 251
Membranous .............................. 250
Muscular ................................... 250
Percutaneous closure ................. 251
Pregnancy ................................. 251
Severity ..................................... 251
Subarterial ................................ 250
**Ventricular septal rupture** ..................... 101
**Ventricular tachycardia** ........................ 221
Bundle branch reentry ................ 221
Cardiopulmonary resuscitation ..... 347
Electrocardiogram ...................... 221
Fascicular .................................. 222
Idiopathic .................................. 222
Management ............................... 221
Monomorphic ..................... 221, 348
Outflow tract ............................. 222
Polymorphic ....................... 221, 348
Torsade de pointes ..................... 222
**Ventriculography** .............................. 54
**Verapamil** ..................................... 231
Adverse effects .......................... 78
Antianginal ................................ 78
Atrial fibrillation ......................... 212
Hypertension ............................. 326
**Vernakalant**
Atrial fibrillation ......................... 213
**Viability** ...................................... 63
**Vital signs** ................................... 2
**VLDL** .......................................... 316
**VO2 max** ..................................... 66
**VOO** ........................................... 235
**VVI** ............................................ 235

**Waist** ........................................... 337, 338
**Wall motion score index** ........................... 34
**Warfarin**
Acute coronary syndrome ............. 96
Antidote ...................................... 216
Atrial fibrillation ........................... 216
Bleeding risk ............................... 216
Noncardiac surgery ....................... 313
Pulmonary embolism .................... 298
Stroke ......................................... 295
**Watchman system** ......................... 218, 294
**Waterston shunt** .................................... 267
**Wedge** ........................................... 54, 56
**Weight** .................................. 336, 337, 338
Bariatric surgery .......................... 337
Benefit of control ......................... 337
Drug treatment ............................ 337
Nondrug treatment ....................... 337
**Wellens waves** ........................................ 18
**Wells criteria** ................................. 296, 297
**Wenckebach** .......................................... 202
**Westermark's sign** ................................. 296
**White coat syndrome** ............................... 324
**Wide QRS tachycardia** ..................... 220, 348
**Williams' syndrome** ................................ 253
**Wolff-Parkinson-White syndrome** ........... 208

**Xanthelasmas** ........................................ 317
**Xanthomas** .............................................. 2
Eruptive ...................................... 317
Palmar ........................................ 317
Tendon ........................................ 317
Tuberous ..................................... 317

**Index**

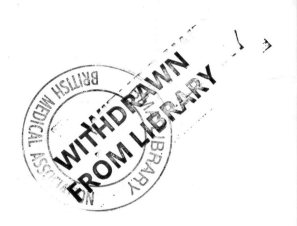

Printed in EU in february 2016